CATECHOLAMINES AND BEHAVIOR · 1

Basic Neurobiology

Volume 1: Basic Neurobiology

Volume 2: Neuropsychopharmacology

CATECHOLAMINES AND BEHAVIOR · 1

Basic Neurobiology

Edited by
Arnold J. Friedhoff

*Millhauser Laboratories of
the Department of Psychiatry*
New York University School of Medicine
New York, New York

PLENUM PRESS • NEW YORK AND LONDON

Library of Congress Cataloging in Publication Data

Main entry under title:

Catecholamines and behavior.

  Includes bibliographies and indexes.
  CONTENTS: v. 1. Basic neurobiology. — v. 2. Neuropsychopharmacology.
  1. Catecholamines. 2. Psychopharmacology. I. Friedhoff, Arnold J. [DNLM: 1.
Behavior — Drug effects. 2. Catecholamines — Physiology. QV129 C357]
QP981.C25C37   599'.01'88   75-11697
ISBN 0-306-38411-6 (v. 1)

© 1975 Plenum Press, New York
A Division of Plenum Publishing Corporation
227 West 17th Street, New York, N.Y. 10011

United Kingdom edition published by Plenum Press, London
A Division of Plenum Publishing Company, Ltd.
Davis House (4th Floor), 8 Scrubs Lane, Harlesden, London, NW10 6SE, England

Printed in the United States of America

Foreword

The editor of these volumes has asked me to contribute a brief foreword. When I accepted this honor I suddenly became aware of the enormous progress that has taken place in this field in the 50 years since I began as a medical student, in a humble way, to take interest in the catecholamine system.

At about that time some evidence was forthcoming to the effect that catecholamines were an important factor in eliciting emotional reactions, thus secondarily influencing behavior. The great physiologist Walter B. Cannon showed in his classic experiments that when a cat was exposed to a dog it responded not only with overt signs of aversion and dislike, but also with an increased flow of adrenaline from its adrenals. The relationships between catecholamines and behavior have since then become the subject of intense research by physiologists, pharmacologists, and psychologists. Infusion of adrenaline in man was shown to provoke a typical pattern of emotional and behavioral changes.

The development of more convenient methods for the measurement of catecholamines in blood and urine led to important new findings. A close association between emotional stress and catecholamine release could be established. This was further extended to psychiatric disorders in which characteristic disturbances in catecholamine release patterns were described.

Still an important link was missing. To what extent did the release of catecholamines from the adrenal medulla and the sympathetic nerve endings reflect the central mechanisms responsible for the behavioral manifestations? Catecholamine analyses from our own and other laboratories had shown the presence of such compounds—noradrenaline as well as dopamine and some adrenaline—in the CNS, but it was still uncertain to which kind of nervous structures they were bound, and their distribution. The final breakthrough came with the application of the Falck–Hillarp histochemical fluorescence technique to the CNS. Today various systems of catecholaminergic neurons have been described including lately even adrenaline-producing neurons. It is not my intention to make even a brief survey of the remarkable results that have been achieved during the last ten years but only to point out that the dopaminergic system controlling motility has become just one element in a total system of high complexity. We now have good reason to believe that catecholamine-producing neurons in the CNS control or modulate a large number of autonomic functions, including circulation, respiration, and motility. The same is true for the CNS mental activity. In this realm, it may be assumed that disturbances in the controlling or modulating mechanisms cause behavioral alterations of manifold types, some of a serious character.

The reader of these volumes is presented with a broad view of a variety of dysfunctions in which the associations to catecholamine production, release, turnover, and inactivation are gaining a clearer contour each day. The combined efforts of research workers in many areas offer good hope for a better understanding of the role of catecholamines in behavioral patterns and consequently new opportunities for successful treatment of a variety of disorders.

Dr. Friedhoff is to be congratulated on successfully editing this valuable survey presented by distinguished experts in the field.

Stockholm   U. S. von Euler

Preface

This volume is intended to provide students and investigators of brain–behavior relationships with an understanding of the current concepts of the role of catecholamines in the regulation of behavior. Catecholamines are now believed to be modulators or transmitters in systems regulating a number of important aspects of behavioral function. The present intense interest in catecholamines is reflected by the large number of scientific reports dealing with these compounds. Even those reports which are relevant to behavior are staggering in number. The contributors to this book have drawn on the salient literature, as well as on their own work, with a view toward clarifying relationships between the basic neurobiology of catecholaminergic neural systems and normal and abnormal behavioral function. Current work in this field is heavily dependent on the use of psychotropic drugs to produce model behavioral states, or as biological probes. As a result psychopharmacological studies are generously represented. In the last chapter of Volume 2 the editor has attempted to further relate and develop the material in the two volumes from the conceptual and theoretical standpoint.

New York   AJF

Contributors

Murray Alpert, *Department of Psychiatry, New York University School of Medicine, New York, New York.*

I. H. Ayhan, *Department E, Hans Hospital, Roskilde, Denmark*

N. P. Bechtereva, *Institute of Experimental Medicine, Leningrad, USSR*

E. Costa, *Laboratory of Preclinical Pharmacology, National Institute of Mental Health, Saint Elizabeths Hospital, Washington, D. C.*

R. Fog, *Department E, Hans Hospital, Roskilde, Denmark*

Arnold J. Friedhoff, *Millhauser Laboratories of the Department of Psychiatry, New York University School of Medicine, New York, New York*

Christo Goridis, *Centre de Neurochimie du CNRS, and Institut de Chimie Biologique, Faculte de Medecine, Strasbourg, France*

O. Hornykiewicz, *Department of Psychopharmacology, Clarke Institute of Psychiatry, Toronto, Ontario, Canada*

A. K. Kambarova, *Institute of Experimental Medicine, Leningrad, USSR*

George M. Krauthamer, *College of Medicine and Dentistry of New Jersey, Rutgers Medical School, New Brunswick, New Jersey*

K. G. Lloyd, *Department of Pharmacology, University of Toronto, Toronto, Canada*

Gérard Mack, *Centre de Neurochimie du CNRS, and Institute de Chimie Biologique, Faculte de Medecine, Strasbourg, France*

Paul Mandel, *Centre de Neurochimie du CNRS and Institut de Chimie Biologique, Faculte de Medecine, Strasbourg, France*

I. Munkvad, *Department E, Hans Hospital, Roskilde, Denmark*

V. K. Pozdeev, *Institute of Experimental Medicine, Leningrad, USSR*

A. Randup, *Department E, Hans Hospital, Roskilde, Denmark*

Jack W. Schweitzer, *Millhauser Laboratories of the Department of Psychiatry, New York University School of Medicine, New York, New York*

M. Trabucchi, *Laboratory of Preclinical Pharmacology, National Institute of Mental Health, Saint Elizabeths Hospital, Washington, D. C.*

Contents

Chapter 2

Catecholamines in Regulation of Motor Function

K. G. Lloyd and O. Hornykiewicz

Chapter 3

**Catecholamines in Behavior and Sensorimotor Integration: The
Neostriatal System**

George M. Krauthamer

Chapter 7

Mammalian Biosynthesis of Potential Psychotogens Derived from Dopamine

Arnold J. Friedhoff and Jack W. Schweitzer

Chapter 8

Regulation of Brain Dopamine Turnover Rate: Pharmacological Implications

E. Costa and M. Trabucchi

Chapter 1

Function of the Central Catecholaminergic Neuron: Synthesis, Release, and Inactivation of Transmitter

Paul Mandel, Gérard Mack, and Christo Goridis

Centre de Neurochimie du CNRS, and Institut de Chimie Biologique
Faculté de Médecine
Strasbourg, France

1. INTRODUCTION

The term "catecholamine" refers to a series of organic compounds which have a benzene nucleus with two adjacent hydroxyl groups (the catechol nucleus) and amine group. Thus dopamine (dihydroxyphenylethylamine), noradrenaline (β-hydroxy dihydroxyphenylethylamine), and adrenaline (N-methyl-β-hydroxy dihydroxyphenylethylamine) and certain of their metabolites are catecholamines.

2. ANALYTICAL METHODS

2.1. Biological Methods

The biological assays for noradrenaline and adrenaline are extremely sensitive and have been used to estimate the catecholamines of biological fluids or tissue extracts. For this purpose, they have advantages since they do not require the often laborious preparations necessary for chemical assay. Nevertheless, chemical assays, which are more specific and easier to standardize have now generally replaced the bioassays.

2.2. Histochemical Methods: Mapping of Catecholaminergic Pathways

The histofluorescence method for detecting catecholamines was developed by Falck and Hillarp (1959), Falck and Torp (1961), Falck, (1962), Falck *et al.* (1962), Carlsson *et al.* (1962a, 1962b), Falck and Owman (1965). It is based upon the formation of fluorescent products from hydroxylated phenylethylamines, indolylamines, and their respective amino acids, when tissue sections which contain these compounds, are exposed to dry formaldehyde vapors. The fluorescence is due to the formation of a new cycle by reaction of the formaldehyde with the amino group. The derivatives obtained differ by their excitation and emission spectra, and thus various phenylethylamine, indolylamine, and histamine derivatives can be distinguished.

These fluorescent techniques have been used to map catecholaminergic pathways, particularly when coupled with pharmacological agents such as monoamine oxidase inhibitors or precursors which increase the normal fluorescence. These techniques have also been coupled with anterograde or retrograde degeneration after mechanical or chemical lesions. Unfortunately, it is difficult to distinguish between adrenaline, noradrenaline, and dopamine in tissue slices, although refined techniques do allow this.

Recently glyoxylic acid has been used instead of formaldehyde since it forms more intensely fluorescent products than formaldehyde (Lindvall *et al.*, 1973). This has enabled fine catecholaminergic axons to be followed without using the pharmacological tools which cannot be used on human tissues.

Little is known about the localization of the biogenic amines in adult human brain in view of the rapid decrease of fluorescence after death. This is surprising in view of the fact that the actual levels of the catecholamines decrease very little (Bertler and Rosengren, 1959a; Joyce, 1962; McGeer and McGeer, 1962). However, the catecholaminergic pathways have been mapped in human fetal brains (Nobin and Björklund, 1973). Groups of catecholaminergic neurons have been detected in the medulla oblongata, in the pons, in particular in the locus coeruleus and the subcoeruleus zone, and in the central and median mesencephalon, above all in the substantia nigra and the ventromedian tegmentum. Catecholaminergic neurons have also been detected in the hypothalamus and the diencephalon. The catecholaminergic pathways have been identified, and pathways corresponding to the ascending and descending pathways in the rat have been detected. In general, the organization of the pathways in man and the rat are very similar.

On the basis of a vast literature related to the anatomy of the monoamine pathways in the brain, it is possible to outline a descending and an ascending catecholamine neuron system in the rat brain (Dahlström and Fuxe, 1965; Ungerstedt, 1971a). The descending pathway represents a system of fibers from the most caudal norepinephrine neuron system to the anterior funiculus, and the ventral and dorsal part of the lateral funiculus. The ascending catecholaminergic pathways can be divided into the major neuron systems: (i) the ventral noradrenaline bundle which includes the intermediate bundles coming from the cell bodies in the pons and the medulla and ending in the mesencephalon, the hypothalamus, and the preoptic region; (ii) the dorsal noradrenaline bundle which starts in the locus coeruleus and finishes in the cerebellar cortex, the reticular formation as well as in several subcortical regions, the hippocampus, the thalamus, and hypothalamus; (iii) the dopaminergic nigrostriatal system which starts in the zona compacta of the substantia nigra and ends in the striatum (nucleus caudatus and putamen) and the dopaminergic mesolimbic system which starts in the dorsal and lateral cells of the interpenduncular nucleus and ends in the nucleus accumbens and the olfactory tubercle.

Well-localized lesions have been used to define these pathways, and to relate them to certain behaviors. The specificity of these techniques has been considerably increased by stereotaxic injection of 6-hydroxydopamine (Ungerstedt, 1968, 1971a). This technique has been combined with the use of drugs and lesions by Ungerstedt and Ljungberg (1973) to study the effects of hypo- and hyperactivity of certain catecholaminergic neuron systems. Ungerstedt's suggestion (1971a,b,c,d) that the vast majority of the noradrenergic nerve endings in the telencephalon are derived from the locus coeruleus has been recently confirmed by Moore (1973).

2.3. Electron Microscopy

Cytochemical techniques have been used at the electron microscope levels to localize catecholaminergic synaptic vesicles (see Bloom, 1972). The enzymes involved in catecholamine metabolism have been localized immunochemically by electron microscopy. Thus the antigenic zone of dopamine-β-hydroxylase is on the outer surface of the synaptic vesicle membrane (Thomas et al., 1973). Freeze-etching has been used to study the chromaffin granule taken as a model of the adrenergic synaptic vesicle. Small granular vesicles appear to parallel in distribution catecholamine histofluorescence, while the large vesicles contain dopamine-β-hydroxylase and ATP. It seems likely that the granular vesicles of adrenergic neurons are formed somewhere in the Golgi apparatus and transported to the nerve endings by axonal flow (Hökfelt, 1973). Two populations of vesicles (large and small granular vesicles) are seen in adrenergic nerve endings, whereas in the axons, only the large dense-core vesicles are seen. In addition, recent work has demonstrated a third tubular reticulum compartment which exists in the axon and probably in the neuronal cell body (Tranzer, 1973). These three storage compartments are probably formed in the cell body and transported to the nerve endings by axoplasmic flow (see section 4, Storage).

Immunohistochemical evidence has been presented to demonstrate the depletion of dopamine-β-hydroxylase in parallel with exocytosis (Geffen and Rush, 1973).

2.4. Chemical Methods

2.4.1 Fluorometric Techniques

After conversion of the catecholamines into fluorescent derivatives, condensation either with ethylene diamine (Weil-Malherbe and Bone, 1952; Weil-Malherbe, 1961) or with trihydroxyindol (Lund, 1949; Udenfriend, 1962) is used. The former method is less specific and gives similar fluorescent products with the different catecholamines, and thus it generally requires preliminary separation. The trihydroxyindol method is more specific since it requires the catechol nucleus, an α-substituted alkylamine and a β-hydroxyl group. These methods are extremely sensitive, although they are not adequate for all problems.

2.4.2. Dansylation

This method can be used to determine the levels of catecholamines either by measuring the fluorescence of the dansyl derivatives, or by the use of labeled dansyl reagents (Seiler and Wiechmann, 1967; Diliberto and Di-Stefano, 1969). These methods require that the catecholamines be separated by thin-layer chromatography. The method using radioactive dansyl chloride is the most reliable since the fluorescence of dansyl derivatives is relatively labile. Moreover, labeled dansyl facilitates metabolic studies since the ratio of the dansyl and the precursor labels gives the specific activity, while the absolute level of dansyl label gives the quantity of the compound.

2.4.3. Gas-Liquid Chromatography

Very low amounts of the catecholamines can be separated, characterized, and quantified by gas-liquid chromatography, most commonly as their trifluoroacetate derivatives. Coupling this technique with mass spectrometry increases its sensitivity and at the same time the compound measured can be unequivocally identified (Cattabeni *et al.*, 1972; Koslow *et al.*, 1972).

2.4.4. Enzymatic Radiochemical Methods

This method is based on the transformation of noradrenaline or adrenaline into their *O*-methyl derivatives with *S*-adenosyl-L-methionine-$^{14}CH_3$ and partially purified catechol *O*-methyl transferase (COMT) or acetylation with acetyl nitrate (Saelens *et al.*, 1967; Nikodijevik *et al.*, 1969; Cuello *et al.*, 1973). This method is extremely sensitive, and for metabolic studies it has the same advantages as dansylation.

3. THE DISTRIBUTION OF THE CATECHOLAMINES

The first observations of the Euler school demonstrated noradrenaline in sympathetic ganglia, and in nonmyelinated fibers (von Euler, 1956). The discovery of noradrenaline in the spleen and the splenic nerve revealed a system which has often been used as a model for noradrenaline metabolism, storage, and liberation. Noradrenaline exists in all tissues, and its level can be correlated with the degree of sympathetic innervation and the number of blood vessels. The vas deferens, the heart and the arteries, and the spleen are particularly rich in noradrenaline. The high content of noradrenaline in the spleen is due to the richness in noradrenaline of the splenic nerve and the vessels which irrigate it.

The demonstration of noradrenaline in the brain (von Euler, 1946; Holtz, 1960) and the observation of marked regional variation in its concentration (Vogt, 1954) suggested that it might have a role in the central nervous system other than that correlated with the blood vessels. The highest concentrations of noradrenaline have been found in the hypothalamus and the medulla oblongata. In general, gray matter is richer in noradrenaline than is white matter. The cerebellum contains very little.

Dopamine was demonstrated in the central nervous system by Bertler and Rosengren (1959*a,b*) and represents more than 50% of the total catecholamine content in the brain and spinal cord of many species (Carlsson *et al.*, 1958; Montagu, 1957, 1963). It was shown to be concentrated in some regions, particularly in the basal ganglia where there is very little noradrenaline (Sano *et al.*, 1959; Ehringer and Hornykiewicz, 1960; Bertler, 1961). In the striatum, dopamine is contained exclusively in nerve terminals, whereas in the substantia nigra this amine is found in neuronal pericarya only. Ehringer and Hornykiewicz (1960) showed that cerebral dopamine levels were markedly reduced in Parkinson's disease. The severity of the main symptoms also correlates significantly with the degree of striatal dopamine deficiency. The treatment of the disease with L-dopa was developed by Birkmayer and Hornykiewicz (1961) and by Barbeau (1961).

There is very little adrenaline in the central nervous system, but certain regions such as the olfactory bulb and tubercule are relatively rich in phenylethanolamine *N*-methyl transferase and can thus synthesize this catecholamine (Pohorecky *et al.*, 1969). Therefore it seems unlikely that the adrenaline detected in these regions is due to errors in methodology, and it might have a role as a transmitter in the olfactory system.

4. STORAGE

Electron microscopic and subcellular fractionation techniques have been used to localize the catecholamines in nerve endings in association with synaptic vesicles (Chrusciel, 1960; Gray and Whittaker, 1962; Laverty *et al.*, 1963; Potter and Axelrod, 1963). The observation that a significant part of the noradrenaline is localized in the granules or synaptic vesicles of chromaffin cells or nerve endings (Palade and Palay, 1954; Sjöstrand, 1954; De Robertis and Bennett, 1954; De Robertis and Pellegrino de Iraldi, 1961*a,b* Lever and Esterhuizen, 1961; Richardson, 1962, Wolfe *et al.*, 1962; Tranzer *et al.*, 1969; Hökfelt, 1968, 1973) has been essential for understanding the mode of action of the catecholamines in synaptic transmission. In the granules, the catecholamines are associated with ATP in a molecular ratio of around 4:1, and with protein. In this manner high concentration of ATP and catecholamines can be maintained in the granules without the significant hypertonicity which would have been associated with the free compounds. In addition to noradrenaline and ATP, the chromaffin granules of the adrenal gland, and the synaptic vesicles of the splenic nerve contain dopamine-β-hydroxylase and a soluble protein: chromogranin (Whittaker, 1966; Tranzer and Thoenen, 1967, 1968; Lapetina *et al.*, 1968; Thuoreson-Klein *et al.*, 1970; Woods, 1970; Fillenz, 1971; Bisby *et al.*, 1973; Hökfelt, 1968, 1969, 1973). These vesicles store the catecholamines, and at the same time protect them from the action of monoamine oxidase. Moreover the vesicles would seem to be the site of formation of noradrenaline from dopamine. The mode of formation of the synaptic vesicles is still unknown, but given the inability of nerve endings to synthesize proteins, it is highly likely that the vesicles are formed in the cell body from where they are transported to the nerve endings by axoplasmic flow (Dahlström, 1965, 1971; Dahlström *et al.*, 1965; Kappeler and Major, 1967; Smith *et al.*, 1970). In fact, the constriction of an axon provokes an accumulation of vesicles containing noradrenaline proximal to the constriction (Dahlström, 1965, 1971; Kapeller and Major, 1967). Recent studies suggest that only large granular vesicles are formed in the cell body, transported to the axon terminals, and after release of the amines and vesicular proteins by exocytosis are transformed into small granular vesicles (Geffen and Ostberg, 1969; Smith, 1971). Evidence in favor of such a process has also been obtained by De Potter *et al.* (1973) in the splenic nerve. According to this hypothesis large granular vesicles are "young" granules, whereas the small granular vesicles represent a more mature state (Hökfelt, 1973).

5. BIOSYNTHESIS OF CATECHOLAMINES

The catecholamines are synthesized in adrenergic neurons of the central nervous system, in the cells of sympathetic ganglia, and in the adrenal chromaffin cells from the amino acids phenylalanine and tyrosine. Tyrosine is normally present in blood at a concentration of $5-8 \times 10^{-5}$M and is concentrated in the central nervous system and the sympathetic nervous system by active transport.

The conversion of tyrosine into noradrenaline and adrenaline was first demonstrated in the adrenal gland, by using labeled tyrosine (Demis *et al.*, 1955; Hagen, 1956; Kirshner and Goodall, 1956; Masuoka *et al.*, 1956; Udenfriend and Wyngaarden, 1956; Pellerin and D'Iorio, 1957); this has been confirmed in the nervous system and in sympathetically innervated tissues (heart, arteries, and veins) (Masuoka *et al.*, 1961, 1963). Tyrosine can also be produced in mammals from phenylalanine (Ikeda *et al.*, 1965): both are present in the central nervous system at concentrations around 5×10^{-5} M. Only a small fraction of the tyrosine is converted to catecholamines.

The major pathway for catecholamine synthesis is that proposed by Blaschko in 1939 from tyrosine → dopa → dopamine → noradrenaline → adrenaline using the enzymes: tyrosine hydroxylase; dopa decarboxylase; dopamine-β-hydroxylase; and phenylethanolamine N-methyl transferase (see Figure 1).

In parallel to this major pathway, there is a minor pathway since in liver there is a NADPH- and oxygen-dependent enzyme which can convert the monophenolic phenylethylamines into the corresponding catecholamines (Axelrod, 1962*a*, 1963; Molinoff and Axelrod, 1971). There is also, in rat brain, a "ring dehydroxylase" which converts the diphenolic to the

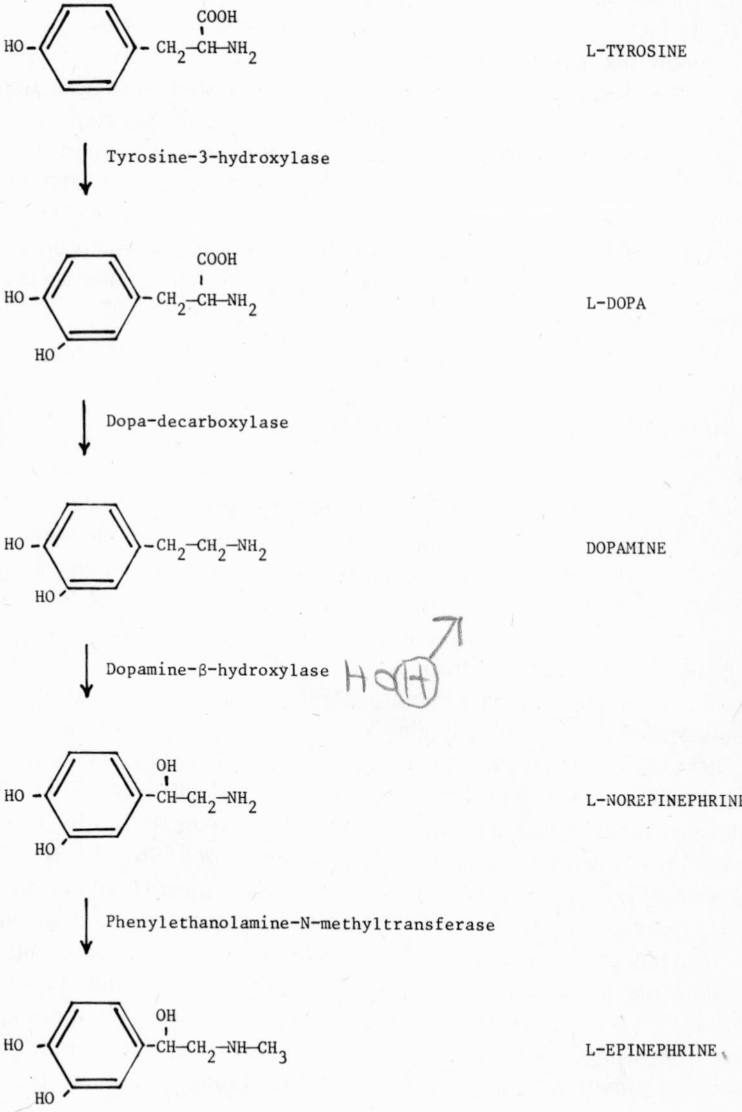

Figure 1. Biosynthesis of catecholamines.

monophenolic amines (Brandau and Axelrod, 1973). Recently the central dogma of the major biosynthetic pathway for the catecholamines has been questioned by Laduron (1973), but his data need to be confirmed.

5.1. The Enzymes of Catecholamine Biosynthesis

5.1.1. Tyrosine Hydroxylase

The first enzyme involved in the synthesis of noradrenaline, dopamine, and adrenaline from tyrosine is tyrosine hydroxylase, which was demonstrated by Nagatsu et al. (1964), Bagchi and McGeer (1964), and Udenfriend (1966). This enzyme is found in the central nervous system, in sympathetic ganglia, and in the adrenal glands. After denervation of sympathetically innervated tissues, the enzyme activity disappears.

Brain tyrosine hydroxylase is at present regarded as a soluble enzyme which has a marked tendency to aggregate, and to stick to membranes in high ionic strength media. A quantity equal to 60% of the brain enzyme is found in the synaptosomal fraction (Coyle, 1972), but of this 82% is liberated by lysis of the synaptosomes. The intrinsic properties of the enzyme vary from one tissue to another, and from one animal to another (Petrack et al., 1973). The beef adrenal enzyme has been the most extensively studied kinetically and ultrastructurally. It is a soluble enzyme with a molecular weight of 150,000 and a sedimentation coefficient of 9.2 S (Musacchio and Craviso, 1973). Nevertheless, the tendency of the enzyme to aggregate, which contrasts with the guinea pig adrenal enzyme, can be decreased by mild trypsinization, which gives a slightly more active product with mol. wt. of 34,000 and a sedimentation coefficient of 3.4 S. This product is easier to study kinetically. The K_m of the native enzyme is 4.76×10^{-5} M for tyrosine, 12.33% for oxygen, and 5.65×10^{-5} M for 6,7-dimethyltetrahydropterin, whereas for the trypsinized enzyme the corresponding figures are 2.38×10^{-5} M, 4.20%, and 6.24×10^{-5}, respectively.

The enzyme is stereospecific for L-tyrosine, and is inactive with D-tyrosine, D,L-m-tyrosine, and tyramine. It requires as cofactors tetrahydropteridine, oxygen, and iron (Ikeda et al., 1966). The enzyme is quite different from tyrosinase in reaction mechanism. Moreover, phenylalanine hydroxylase is not inhibited by inhibitors of tyrosine hydroxylase. While it is almost certain that the adrenal enzyme, requires tetrahydropteridine as a cofactor, the concentration of this biopterine in brain seems too low (1×10^{-6} M) to be the sole cofactor since the K_m for the cofactor is 2.5×10^{-4} M. Other tetrahydropterines are generally used in vitro such as 6-methyltetrahydropterin, 7-methyltetrahydropterin, and above all 6,7-dimethyltetrahydropterin (DMPH$_4$) (Kaufman, 1973; Musacchio and Craviso, 1973).

The effectors of the enzyme compete either with the substrates, the cofactor, or the Fe^{++}. Thus α-methyl-β-tyrosine, which is used to block catecholamine biosynthesis in turnover studies, is competitive for the substrate and noncompetitive for DMPH$_4$. The catecholamines and dopa inhibit by competing with the cofactor, in particular dopamine (K_i 2.1 $\times$ 10^{-5}) which is more inhibitory than norepinephrine (K_i 4.6 $\times$ 10^{-5}). Although dopamine is less concentrated in noradrenergic neurons than is noradrenaline, the fact that it is localized in the cytoplasm makes it an important factor in the feedback regulation of tyrosine hydroxylase, and hence of catecholamine biosynthesis (Musacchio and Craviso, 1973).

5.1.2. Dopa Decarboxylase

Dopa decarboxylase was the first enzyme involved in catecholamine biosynthesis to be discovered (Holtz *et al.*, 1938). The enzyme was renamed L-aromatic amino acid decarboxylase by Lovenberg *et al.* (1962) in view of its lack of specificity. The enzyme decarboxylates dopa, tyrosine, 5-hydroxytryptophan, histidine, α-methyldopa, *m*-tyrosine, and tryptophan. However, it is not certain that all these activities are associated with one enzyme, although antibodies to the purified pig kidney enzyme inhibit all these activities in brain and adrenal gland. Sims and Bloom (1973) and Sims *et al.* (1973) have suggested that there may be two enzymes, a dopa decarboxylase and a 5-hydroxytryptophan decarboxylase. This hypothesis is supported by differences in reaction kinetics, sensitivity to pyridoxal phosphate, subcellular distribution, and sensitivity to 6-hydroxydopamine (which destroys the dopa decarboxylase activity while leaving the 5-hydroxytryptophan decarboxylase activity). However, Bender and Coulson (1972) have suggested that the enzyme could have two different binding sites, with a common catalytic site.

The enzyme is not exclusive to adrenergic tissues and has been isolated and purified from pig kidney and beef adrenal. Soluble enzymes ranging from 112,000 to 90,000 mol. wt. (Christenson *et al.*, 1970; Lancaster and Sourkes, 1972; Dairman *et al.*, 1973) have thus been obtained. The enzyme is cytoplasmic, and is not associated with the vesicles as is shown by the slower rates of axonal flow of the enzyme and dopamine-β-hydroxylase. Pig kidney dopa decarboxylase has a K_m for dopa of 5 $\times$ 10^{-4} M and a pH optimum of 7.2. The high affinity for dopa explains why it is difficult to detect this compound which is rapidly converted to dopamine.

During vitamin B deficiency, the dopa decarboxylase activity decreases, but in deficiencies which are not lethal, the reduction of catecholamine synthesis is not particularly menacing.

The best known pharmacological effector is α-methyldopa. It is a competitive inhibitor, of which the product is α-methyl dopamine, a false transmitter with a hypotensive effect (Sourkes, 1954; Hess *et al.*, 1961; Sjoerdsma, 1961). There are many pharmacological inhibitors: the hydrazines, benzyloxyamines, *N*-diethylmaleimide, and borohydride (Molinoff and Axelrod, 1971). In contrast to tyrosine hydroxylase, the dopa decarboxylase is not regulated transsynaptically. In rat liver the activity drops by 50% after chronic administration of L-dopa, pyridoxal phosphate deficiency being excluded (Dairman *et al.*, 1972).

5.1.3. Dopamine-β-Hydroxylase (EC 1.14.17.1)

The β-hydroxylation of dopamine to noradrenaline was demonstrated *in vivo* by Leeper and Udenfriend (1956), then *in vitro* by Neri *et al.* (1956). The enzyme catalyzing the reaction is a "mixed function oxidase" specific to adrenergic tissues. It is found in adrenal medullary cells, and in adrenergic neurons of the peripheral system. The enzyme disappears after chronic denervation of the sympathetic system. The enzyme has been localized by immunochemical techniques in the cell bodies, axons, and nerve endings of noradrenergic structures using optic and electron microscopy (Goldstein *et al.*, 1973; Thomas *et al.*, 1973). Subcellular fractionation has confirmed that it is localized in the synaptic vesicles from which it is released in parallel with the catecholamines. The enzyme is essentially particulate, but can be solubilized with certain detergents. Although the enzyme has been purified from pheochromocytoma and human serum (Levin and Kaufman, 1961; Goldstein, 1972; Miras-Portugal *et al.*, 1975a), the bovine adrenal enzyme has been the most studied (Levin and Kaufman, 1961; Aunis *et al.*, 1973a, 1974). However, it must be noted that there are marked species differences since antibodies to the human and bovine enzymes do not cross-react.

The bovine enzyme is a cuproprotein of mol. wt. 280,000–300,000 which has four identical subunits of 77,000 mol. wt. (Aunis *et al.*, 1974), and the subunit has been demonstrated to be similar to the chromogranin A (Aunis *et al.*, 1975), a constituent of chromaffin granules. Each subunit consists of two polypeptide chains. The copper has an essential role in the enzymatic mechanism which is ping-pong. The first substrate, the cofactor, ascorbic acid, is oxidized to dehydroascorbate while the Cu^{++} is reduced to Cu^{+}. Then the second substrate, dopamine or oxygen, becomes involved. Fumarate, phosphate, and antiperoxide agents such as catalase stimulate the activity of dopamine-β-hydroxylase *in vitro*. The K_m is 5×10^{-3} mM, and the enzyme is not markedly specific since all the phenylethylamines, and phenylethanolamines, such as tyramine (forming octopamine) and methyldopa (forming methylnoradrenaline), can be β-hydroxylated. The derivatives thus formed may be false transmitters.

Natural inhibitors of dopamine-β-hydroxylase have been described in the heart (Chubb *et al.*, 1969). Thiol reagents (mercaptoethanol, cysteine, dithiothreitol, and glutathion) are known to be reversible inhibitors of the enzyme. The inhibition is due to copper chelation and is reversible with *N*-ethylmaleimide.

Some endogenous and exogenous inhibitors active *in vivo* and *in vitro* react with the Cu^{++}. This is the case of disulphuram and FLA-63 after reduction (Molinoff and Axelrod, 1971). Other inhibitors of bacterial origin, such as fusaric acid, dopastin, and aquayamycin, are extremely active (over 50% inhibition at 10^{-9}–10^{-6}) (Hidaka, 1973; Nagatsu *et al.*, 1973). The inhibition is uncompetitive for the substrate and competitive for ascorbic acid. Finally, 6-hydroxydopamine inhibits the enzyme *in vitro* by forming peroxides, as is shown by the protective effect of catalase (Aunis *et al.*, 1973*b*). Ascorbic acid deficiency leads to a 40% reduction of the dopamine-β-hydroxylase activity in guinea pig adrenals (Goldstein *et al.*, 1973).

Dopamine-β-hydroxylase is present in plasma where it shows marked individual differences in activity. The plasma activities change in a number of pathological conditions (Miras-Portugal *et al.*, 1975*b*; for review see Geffen, 1974).

Stimulation of peripheral adrenergic nerves provokes a parallel liberation of dopamine-β-hydroxylase and the transmitter (Smith, 1968). This is also found for the adrenal gland. This release of dopamine-β-hydroxylase may explain the serum enzymatic activities which seem to correlate with the sympathetic tonus of the subject. Acute stress increases the serum dopamine-β-hydroxylase activity, whereas this enzymatic activity decreases in the adrenal gland or in a sympathetically innervated tissue such as the mesenteric artery. By contrast, chronic stress increases the synthesis of the enzyme, as do injections of ACTH in hypophysectomized animals (Fuxe *et al.*, 1972; Goldstein, 1972; Goldstein *et al.*, 1973; Roffman *et al.*, 1973).

5.1.4. Phenylethanolamine N-methyltransferase (PNMT, EC 2.2.1)

The last step in catecholamine biosynthesis is the conversion of noradrenaline to adrenaline by PNMT which uses the cofactor *S*-adenosylmethionine as methyl donor (Kirshner and Goodall, 1957). The enzyme methylates noradrenaline, normetanephrine, octopamine, synephrine, and metanephrine, the last two being thus dimethylated. There are, however, dif-

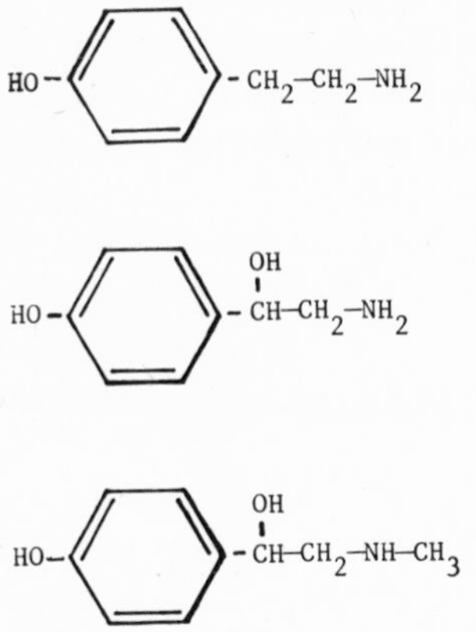

Figure 2

ferences in specificity depending upon the species from which the enzyme is isolated. Thus the monkey, rabbit, rat, and human enzymes methylate β-hydroxylated phenylethylamines only, whereas the dog and beef enzymes methylate all the phenylethylamines (Ciaranello, 1973). Species differences are also observed in the biochemical, kinetic, and immunological characteristics of the enzymes (Axelrod, 1962b; Axelrod and Vessel, 1970; Fuller et al., 1970).

The PNMT is found in specific populations of adrenal medullary cells suggesting that there may be two types of cells: adrenergic and noradrenergic (Eränko, 1952; Hillarp and Hökfelt, 1953). There is also a low activity in sympathetic ganglia (Ciaranello et al., 1973), heart, and in some brain regions such as the olfactory bulbs (Pohorecky et al., 1969) or the perifornical region of the hypothalamus (Goldstein et al., 1973). The beef adrenal enzyme is the most studied and has been shown to be a soluble enzyme with a molecular weight of 37,000 to 41,000. In view of the difference in electrophoretic mobility and chromatographic behavior, the existence of several enzymes has been suggested (Joh and Goldstein, 1973). Recently PNMT from ox brain tissue has been isolated and purified by Eagles and Iqbal (1974). The enzyme is strongly inhibited in vitro by the substrate noradrenaline, and by the reaction product adrenaline (Fuller and Hunt, 1967). Thiol reagents stimulate the enzyme activity, whereas heavy metals (Cd^{++}, Hg^{++}, and Cu^{++}) inhibit (Kitabchi and Williams, 1969). It should be stressed that in view of the cytoplasmic localization of the soluble enzyme, noradrenaline synthesized in the chromaffin granules would seem to need to leave the granules to be methylated before being restocked (Axelrod and Weinshilboum, 1972). However, in view of the localization of dopamine-β-hydroxylase activity on the exterior of adrenergic vesicles, an

14

Paul Mandel *et al.*

alternate hypothesis of a more efficient process can be suggested. Dopamine can be hydroxylated on the exterior of the vesicles, the noradrenaline formed will be methylated and then taken up for storage into vesicles.

Pharmacological inhibitors include tranylcypromine (a competitive inhibitor), 2-cyclohexylcyclopropaneamine, and 8-amino-1,2-methanoindane chloride (Krakoff and Axelrod, 1967).

6. REGULATION OF THE BIOSYNTHESIS

6.1. Tyrosine Hydroxylase

The rate of catecholamine biosynthesis is adjusted to the physiological needs of the organism by at least two different mechanisms: feedback inhibition and induction of tyrosine hydroxylase.

The feedback inhibition of tyrosine hydroxylase by catecholamines has been repeatedly demonstrated *in vitro* and *in vivo* (Udenfriend *et al.*, 1965; Costa and Neff, 1966; Alousi and Weiner, 1966; Spector, *et al.*, 1967; Musacchio and Craviso, 1973). The increased tyrosine hydroxylase activity by induction results from increased enzyme protein synthesis (Mueller *et al.*, 1969*a,b*). However, there are still some aspects of these mechanisms which are not entirely clear.

It is obvious that the catecholamine pool which controls the activity of tyrosine hydroxylase has to be in contact with the enzyme. The localization in brain of tyrosine hydroxylase in a soluble fraction of synaptosomes (Coyle, 1972; Kuczenski and Mandell, 1972) is consistent with the pharmacological data which suggest that there is a small, cytoplasmic pool of catecholamines which is an important regulatory factor in the biosynthesis of catecholamines (Alousi and Weiner, 1965; Weiner and Selvaratnam, 1968; Kopin *et al.*, 1969; Goldstein *et al.*, 1970*a*).

Native tyrosine hydroxylase is inhibited by catecholamines and dopa. This inhibition is competitive with the $DMPH_4$ and with tetrahydrobiopterin (Udenfriend *et al.*, 1965; Ikeda *et al.*, 1966; Musacchio *et al.*, 1971*a, b;* Nagatsu *et al.*, 1972). The relative effectiveness of dopamine, noradrenaline, and adrenaline in inhibiting native tyrosine hydroxylase shows that dopamine is twice as effective as noradrenaline and adrenaline as a feedback inhibitor of tyrosine hydroxylase (Musacchio *et al.*, 1973). Since dopamine is found in the cytosol, it is possible that dopamine may be the amine which controls the activity of tyrosine hydroxylase. This is consistent with the high amount of dopamine in the heart and the rapid transformation of dopamine to norepinephrine when it is taken up in the storage vesicles (Costa *et al.*,

1972). The atmospheric concentration of oxygen inhibits tyrosine hydroxy-lase and the inhibition is more pronounced at low levels of tetrahydrobiop-terin. Native bovine adrenal tyrosine hydroxylase can also be inhibited by high concentrations of oxygen. This inhibition is more marked at low levels of $DMPH_4$. Two important regulatory properties of tyrosine hydroxylase are lost or attenuated when tetrahydrobiopterin is substituted by $DMPH_4$ (Shiman and Kaufman, 1970; Shiman et al., 1971): inhibition by excess tyrosine and inhibition by dopa. Taking into account the K_m values and the concentration of the cofactor, it would appear that the activity of adrenal tyrosine hydroxylase may be limited by the availability of the cofactor. Moreover, there is some uncertainty about whether biopterin is the cofactor for tyrosine hydroxylase in the brain (Kaufman, 1973).

6.2. Dopa Decarboxylase

Dopa decarboxylase is a soluble enzyme according to axoplasmic transport studies and cannot be contained within or bound to dopamine-β-hydroxylase and norepinephrine-containing vesicles (Dairman et al., 1973). In response to acute changes in sympathetic nerve activity which modifies catecholamine synthesis, dopa decarboxylase activity does not change. Simi-larly, during the induction of tyrosine hydroxylase and dopamine-β-hydroxylase in sympathetic tissues, dopa decarboxylase activity remains un-changed (Thoenen et al., 1971). In Parkinsonian patients and in animals submitted to a chronic administration of L-dopa, a decrease in the activity of liver dopa decarboxylase was observed (Yahr et al., 1969; Whitsett et al., 1970; Cotzias et al., 1971; Dairman et al., 1971). This may be of great im-portance in the therapeutic treatment of Parkinsonian patients with L-dopa. Using monospecific antigens to dopa decarboxylase, it has been demonstrated in L-dopa-treated animals that the reduced activity of liver dopa decarboxylase is due to a net reduction in enzyme protein (Dairman et al., 1971). The ability of the substrate to decrease the enzyme activity is rather unique. The aromatic amino acids themselves do not seem to be directly responsible for the decreased dopa decarboxylase activity. The amines formed via the decarboxylation or the nondeaminated amine me-tabolites are probably responsible for this effect (Dairman et al., 1972).

6.3. Dopamine-β-Hydroxylase

Several findings are consistent with the idea that chronic stress induces de novo dopamine-β-hydroxylase synthesis. In rats, the acute and chronic stress leads to an increase of dopamine-β-hydroxylase activity in the serum. The chronic stress also increases the enzyme activity in the cervical ganglion and in adrenal glands (Roffman *et al.*, 1973).

Dopamine-β-hydroxylase activity is increased in rat serum and different tissues after hypophysectomy. ACTH but not dexamethasone administration decreases the activity (Fuxe *et al.*, 1971, 1972). In contrast, in the cervical ganglion and in the mesenteric artery of rats the dopamine-β-hydroxylase activity is markedly reduced after pituitary ablation. The activity is partially restored by treatment with ACTH (Fuxe *et al.*, 1971; 1972).

Ascorbic acid deficiency reduces adrenal dopamine-β-hydroxylase (Goldstein *et al.*, 1973). Similarly, a reduction of tyrosine hydroxylase in adrenals was reported in scorbutic guinea pigs (Nakashima *et al.*, 1972). Evidence has been presented that agents which stimulate or block dopamine receptors, affect the rate of dopamine synthesis in the striatum (Goldstein *et al.*, 1970b; Kehr *et al.*, 1972).

6.4. The Effects of Cyclic AMP on Catecholamine Biosynthesis

Dibutyryl cyclic AMP increases the formation of labeled dopamine from ^{14}C-tyrosine in striatal slices, and stimulates the synthesis of dopamine from tyrosine (Goldstein *et al.*, 1973). This stimulation may occur prior to, or at the tyrosine hydroxylase step. It is conceivable that the dibutyryl cyclic AMP reduces the end-product inhibition of catecholamine synthesis. It is assumed that the activation of tyrosine hydroxylase activity due to increased nerve impulses is associated with catecholamine release followed by a reduction in end-point inhibition. It is also conceivable that cyclic AMP may contribute to the activation of tyrosine hydroxylase and the increased rate of catecholamine synthesis.

Depolarizing agents like potassium or ouabain stimulate the synthesis of dopamine in striatal slices (Goldstein *et al.*, 1970a; Harris and Roth, 1971) and stimulate cAMP formation (Shimizu and Daly, 1972). The effects of cyclic AMP and potassium on dopamine synthesis are synergic. The stimulation of dopamine synthesis is less marked in a calcium-free medium. It seems probable that calcium inhibits striatal adenylate cyclase and that the stimulation of dopamine synthesis, in calcium-free medium, is due to an increase in cyclic AMP concentration. These results indicate that cyclic AMP might play an important role in the short-term regulation of catecholamine synthesis.

7. THE METABOLIC INACTIVATION OF CATECHOLAMINES

The major metabolites of noradrenaline injected or synthesized in brain are O-methylated deaminated compounds, suggesting that both methylation and deamination play an important role in the inactivation of catecholamines in the brain and in the peripheral sympathetic nervous system (Glowinski et al., 1965).

The distribution of the metabolites in the cerebrospinal fluid or in the urine varies considerably with the animal species. For example, in man the essential urinary catabolites are vanilmandelic acid (VMA) (Armstrong et al., 1957) and homovanillic acid (HVA) while in the rat the 3-methoxy-4-hydroxyphenylglycol (MOPEG) is quantitatively the most important (Figure 3).

Two enzymes, monoamine oxidase and catechol-O-methyltransferase, which are widely distributed in various brain regions, contribute to the inactivation of catecholamines and the production of their metabolites (Bogdanski et al., 1957; Axelrod et al., 1959a).

Monoamine oxidase (MAO) and catechol-O-methyltransferase (COMT) can act either separately or successively (Figure 4).

COMT can produce O-methylated but not deaminated compounds:

1. normetanephrine formed from norepinephrine, metanephrine from adrenaline;
2. 4-hydroxy-3-methoxyphenylethylamine from dopamine and HVA from dihydroxyphenylacetic acid.

MAO produces deaminated but not methylated compounds:

1. 3,4-dihydroxyphenylacetaldehyde which can form 3,4-dihydroxyphenylacetic acid (DOPAC) or 3,4-dihydroxyphenylethanol (DOPET) (from dopamine);
2. 3,4-dihydroxyphenylglycolaldehyde which can form 3,4-dihydroxy-D-mandelic acid (DOMA) and 3,4-dihydroxyphenylglycol (DOPEG) (from norepinephrine).

The action of both enzymes produces deaminated and O-methylated compounds, methylation generally preceding deamination:

1. 4-hydroxy-3-methoxyphenylglycolaldehyde which can form VMA or MOPEG (from norepinephrine);
2. 4-hydroxy-3-methoxyphenylacetaldehyde which can form HVA or 4-hydroxy-3-methoxyphenylethanol (MOPET) (from dopamine).

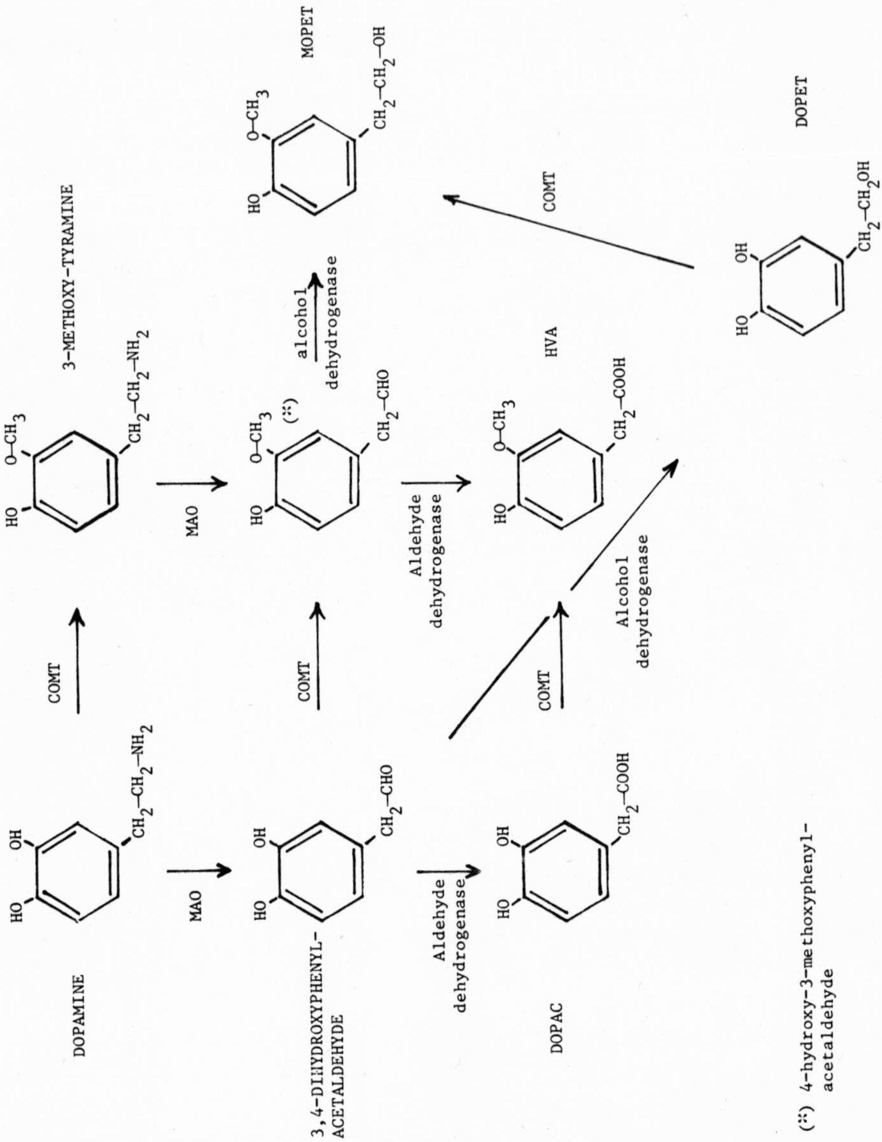

Figure 3. Catabolism of norepinephrine.

(*) 4-hydroxy-3-methoxyphenyl-acetaldehyde

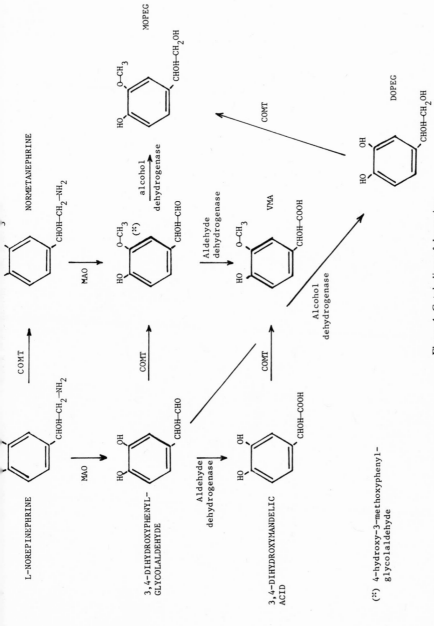

Figure 4. Catabolism of dopamine.

After oxidative deamination by MAO, two minor enzymes react with the resulting catecholaldehydes:

1. Alcohol dehydrogenase or aldehyde reductase (forming the corresponding alcohol);
2. Aldehyde oxidase or aldehyde dehydrogenase (forming the corresponding acid).

Finally, a phenylsulfotransferase and perhaps a glycuronyltransferase form sulfo- or glycuronyl conjugates from the ethanolic or glycolic derivatives.

7.1 Catechol-*O*-Methyltransferase (COMT, EC 2.11.6)

This enzyme of catecholamine catabolism was discovered by Axelrod and Tomchick (1958) following the observation by Armstrong *et al.*, (1957) showing that VMA was the major catabolite of adrenaline in man. The enzyme is not located exclusively in the nervous system being also found in the liver, kidney, and erythrocytes.

In the nervous system the location of COMT is neuronal and glial, the enzyme being found in neuronal fractions and in cultures of both gliomas and astrocytes (Katz *et al.*, 1969; Silberstein *et al.*, 1972). The enzyme has been purified from rat liver. It is soluble but partially associated with the microsomal fractions. The purified enzyme is very labile and sensitive to oxidants. The molecular weight of the enzyme is about 23,000, but electrophoresis of the preparations shows some heterogeneity suggesting the presence of isoenzymes (Bohuon and Assicot, 1973).

Catechol-*O*-methyltransferase *O*-methylates the catecholamines in the presence of *S*-adenosylmethionine and Mg^{++} but does not *O*-methylate monohydroxy derivates of phenylethylamines. Hence, norepinephrine, epinephrine, dopamine, dopa, 3,4-dihydroxymandelic acid, and 3,4-dihydroxyphenylacetic acid can be methylated as can certain exogenous catecholamines like 3,4-dihydroxyamphetamines or 3,4-dihydroxyephedrines.

O-Methylation of 3,4-dihydroxy catechols occurs preferentially in the *meta* position (Masri *et al.*, 1962). However, both *in vitro* (Senoh *et al.*, 1959; Masri *et al.*, 1964; Creveling *et al.*, 1970, 1972; Katz and Jacobson, 1972) and *in vivo* (Daly *et al.*, 1960), some action on the *p*-hydroxyl group may exist. Small amounts of 4-*O*-methylated dihydroxyphenylacetic acid (isohomovanillic acid) were found in urine (Assicot and Bohuon, 1971) and the cerebrospinal fluid (Mathieu and Revol, 1970). It was claimed by

Mathieu and Revol (1970) that as much as 10 to 20% of urinary homovanillic acid is composed of this isomer.

Moreover it was suggested that p-methylation of dopamine may be of importance in certain psychiatric disorders (pink spot). Friedhoff and Van Winkle (1962) reported that 3,4-dimethoxyphenylethylamine (DMPEA or homoveratrylamine or "pink spot") was present in the urine of a majority of schizophrenic patients but was not excreted by normal subjects. Sen and McGeer (1964) using another chromatographic method found DMPEA in urine of 50% of schizophrenic patients. Other authors (Kuehl et al., 1966; Wagner et al., 1966) found this compound both in normal controls and in schizophrenics and suggested an exogenous dietary source (Stabenan et al., 1970; Perry et al., 1964). More recently, Friedhoff et al., (1972a) reported that dopamine can be converted into DMPEA in vivo; thus, even if it is absent in urine small amounts could be present in brain.

The same authors (Friedhoff et al., 1972b) found in rat and human livers an enzymatic system able to form 3,4,5-trimethoxyphenylethylamine. Neither the dimethoxy compound nor mescalin seem to be formed through COMT which requires that substrates have an adjacent free hydroxyl group (Axelrod and Tomchick, 1958).

The physiological role of catechol-O-methyltransferase is the inactivation of norepinephrine and dopamine since normetanephrine has for example only $\frac{1}{1000}$ of the potency of norepinephrine on the cardiac β-receptor (Kukovets et al., 1959). The enzyme has a similar role at the synaptic level in the central nervous system (Katz et al., 1969).

Inhibition in vitro is easily caused by dichloromercuribenzoate, pyrogallol, or its derivatives, such as propylgallate or butylgallate. These last two substances are equally good inhibitors in vivo but are toxic (Ericsson, 1971). Dihydroxyphenylacetamide, a substrate for the enzyme is an excellent inhibitor in vivo (Ross and Haljasmaa, 1964).

7.2. Monoamine Oxidase

Monoamine oxidase (monoamine:O_2 oxidoreductase, deaminating, EC 1.4.3.4) was discovered as tyramine oxidase (Hare, 1928). Later Blaschko et al. (1937a,b) established that adrenaline, noradrenaline, and dopamine are also substrates for this enzyme. MAO also deaminates phenylethylamines, indolamines, methylhistamine, and benzylamine but is without effect on aliphatic amines and histamine. However, N-methylation and β-hydroxylation of phenylethylamines reduce their susceptibility to attack by MAO (Blaschko, 1952).

This deamination which requires molecular oxygen and FAD gives rise to an aldehyde, H_2O_2 and NH_3. The enzyme is widely distributed as an integral part of mitochondrial outer membranes, particularly in those from synaptosomal mitochondria. The active enzyme molecule is a flavoprotein containing copper (Gabay and Valcourt, 1968). Its special characteristics and high molecular weight (290,000 daltons) make its isolation and purification difficult (Youdim, 1972).

In fact, both *in vivo* and in crude enzyme preparations, at least two different MAO activities can be detected, but extensive purification procedures result in a loss in this distinction (Houslay and Tipton, 1973). However, by taking into account: (i) pharmacological evidence (Johnston, 1968; Hall *et al.*, 1969; Squires, 1972; Neff *et al.*, 1973); (ii) enzymological evidence from substrate specificity and kinetics; and (iii) structural evidence such as electrophoretic behavior (Youdim, 1972) and sedimentation coefficients (Neff *et al.*, 1973), we know that there are two forms of the enzyme, *A* and *B*, with the following properties:

1. The *A* form is inhibited *in vitro* and *in vivo* by low concentrations of clorgyline or harmaline, is relatively thermostable, is totally inactivated by trypsin, has a K_m of 0.1 mM for tyramine and uses norepinephrine and 5-hydroxy-tryptamine as natural substrates;
2. The *B* form is inhibited by low concentrations of deprenyl or pargyline, is thermolabile, is totally inactivated by trypsin, has a K_m of 0.8 mM for tyramine and uses the β-phenylethylamines as natural substrates. It should be noted that both the *A* and *B* forms deaminate dopamine, tyramine, and tryptamine.

The pharmacological inhibitors of MAO are numerous. They include hydrazine derivatives such as iproniazid (Zeller and Barsky, 1952), amines carrying an acetylenic group such as cyclopropylamine (pargyline), and alkaloids such as harmaline, these compounds being bound irreversibly and covalently to the enzyme or to its flavin moiety (Zeller and Hsu, 1973).

7.3. Oxidative-Reductive Pathways for Metabolism of Biogenic Aldehyde

The β-hydroxycatecholaldehydes formed during oxidative deamination of phenylethylamines by MAO are generally reduced to alcohols, whereas those which are not β-substituted are normally oxidized to acids. Thus, norepinephrine and normetanephrine are essentially metabolized to alcohol derivatives, whereas dopamine is mainly transformed into HVA (Goldstein and Gerber, 1963; Glowinski *et al.*, 1965; Rutledge and Jonasson, 1967).

The transformation of the catecholaldehydes to the corresponding acid is catalyzed by an NAD-dependent aldehyde dehydrogenase (EC 1.2.1.3) (Erwin and Deitrich, 1966). This enzyme is localized on mitochondria external membrane (Duncan and Tipton, 1961) and is inhibited by disulfiram and other reactives of thiol groups.

The transformation of the aldehydes to the corresponding alcohols is catalyzed by aldehyde reductases or alcohol dehydrogenases. Two aldehyde reductases isolated from brain have been described (Tabakoff and Erwin, 1970; Erwin *et al.*, 1972; Turner and Tipton, 1972). One of these is NADH-dependent and the other is NADPH-linked, but only the latter enzyme is able to reduce the catecholaldehydes. It is inhibited by barbiturates, hydantoins, phenothiazines, and oxazolidinediones. There also exists in the brain a "classical" NAD-linked alcohol dehydrogenase which acts on the same substrates as the NADPH-linked enzyme, but this former is specifically inhibited by pyrazole (Raskin and Sokoloff, 1970).

7.4. Sulfate Conjugate in the Brain

MOPEG-SO_4 was the first endogenous sulfurylated biogenic metabolite to be identified in the central nervous system (Schanberg *et al.*, 1968). Earlier Goldstein and Gerber (1963) found that conjugated methoxyhydroxyphenylethanol was found in brain after peripheral injection of labeled dopa.

After intraventricular injection of labeled tyramine, dopamine, norepinephrine, and normetanephrine, conjugation of the amines and their acidic and neutral metabolites occurred in brain (Sugden and Eccleston, 1971; Goldstein *et al.*, 1970; Taylor and Laverty, 1969).

Meek and Neff (1973) confirmed in *in vitro* studies the occurrence of the phenolsulfotransferase in brain. This enzyme has been recently purified (Foldes and Meek, 1973). Phosphoadenosine-5-phosphosulfate is the sulfate donor. The highest activity occurs in hypothalamus, but is not restricted to adrenergic neurons since its activity in spinal cord does not diminish after axonal section (Meek and Foldes, 1973). Phenolsulfotransferase might be preferentially located postsynaptically to neurons whose transmitters are phenols.

8. TURNOVER OF CATECHOLAMINES

Noradrenaline in the central and peripheral nervous systems turns over continuously. This turnover gives some idea of the intensity with which the transmitter is used and synthesized. Several methods have been applied to measure turnover, in particular in studies on the effects of pharmacolocical agents. The turnover of catecholamines can be determined either by administering precursors of noradrenaline and dopamine such as labeled tyrosine and dopa, and by measuring the amount of noradrenaline synthesized and diluted in the total pool, or by injecting labeled noradrenaline and following the loss of label. The rapid decline of specific activity of the catecholamines indicates a rapid turnover rate. Since dopamine as well as noradrenaline fail to penetrate the blood–brain barrier, these catecholamines are injected directly into the lateral ventricle of the brain. Under these conditions, injected dopamine was rapidly converted into noradrenaline (Glowinski and Iversen, 1966). Other methods are based on the inhibition of catecholamine biosynthesis by α-methyl-p-tyrosine and follow the decrease in levels in the central nervous system, or the increased levels after inhibition of degradation with monoamine oxidase inhibitors are measured. Naturally, these drugs perturb the system and the results have to be interpreted with caution. In fact the average half-lives for dopamine and noradrenaline in mammalian brain are respectively, 2 hr and 4 hr (Udenfriend and Zaltzman-Nirenberg, 1963; Burack and Draskoczy, 1964). However, great differences in the rate of turnover of noradrenaline exist among the various brain regions. The turnover varies from 2–4 hr (2 hr in the cerebellum, 3 hr in the cortex and hippocampus to 4 hr in hypothalamus and medulla oblongata (Fuxe, 1966: Iversen and Glowinski, 1966).

9. THE RELEASE OF NORADRENALINE

A variety of experimental approaches has been used to investigate the release of noradrenaline from nerve terminals, and diffusion to adjacent effector cells and target sites. Small amounts of noradrenaline overflowing into the blood from a stimulated organ have been detected (Cannon and Uridil, 1921). Under certain conditions the noradrenaline released by nerve stimulation accumulates in the effector tissue and may overflow into the circulation. Release of noradrenaline from isolated perfused organs subject to direct stimulation of their sympathetic nerves was observed (Loewi, 1921; Gaddum and Kwiatkowski, 1939; Eliasson *et al.,* 1955). The transmitter was also detected in the venous effluent of organs, such as the heart, liver, or spleen during direct stimulation of their sympathetic nerve supply (Mirkin and Bonnycastle, 1954; Brown and Gillespie, 1957). Quantitative studies of the release of noradrenaline in response to nerve stimulation have been recently made (Brown, 1960, 1965).

The release of labeled noradrenaline after previous administration in response to nerve stimulation indicates that it is present in the same store as the endogenous catecholamines (Hertting and Axelrod, 1961; Gillespie and Kirpekar, 1965). It was also shown that the rate of disappearance of labeled noradrenaline from sympathetic innervated tissues was dependent on sympathetic nerve activity (Hertting et al., 1962).

Frequency of stimulation of sympathetic nerves plays an important role in the release of noradrenaline. Great quantitative differences may be elicited by minute changes in stimulation frequency. The normal rate of discharge of postganglionic sympathetic fibers rarely exceeds 10/sec and is generally in the range 1–2/sec. In the cat spleen the amount of noradrenaline liberated per stimulus was constant at frequencies of 1–8/sec but was less at very low frequencies (0.5/sec) (Haefely et al., 1965).

At physiological frequencies of stimulation only small amounts of noradrenaline overflow into the circulation (Celander, 1954). It may increase under certain conditions. Relatively large amounts of noradrenaline metabolites are excreted in the urine (5–10 mg noradrenaline/day in man) and appreciable levels of noradrenaline are found in plasma. The origin of urinary noradrenaline is under discussion. The majority of this noradrenaline seems to be derived from neuronal structures, since the urinary excretion of noradrenaline and its metabolites is not significantly lowered after adrenalectomy (von Euler et al., 1954), while increased adrenergic activity is correlated with rises in urinary excretion of noradrenaline (von Euler et al., 1955) and ganglionic blocking agents decrease the urinary excretion of noradrenaline (Sundin, 1958). It seems that only 20% of the total urinary catecholamine metabolites derive from adrenal medulla adrenaline. Although appreciable amounts of released transmitter overflow into the circulation from peripheral adrenergic synapses, most of the released noradrenaline from nerve endings is inactivated locally in peripheral tissues. Thus the urinary excretion of noradrenaline is markedly increased after inhibition of this inactivation with certain drugs (Benfey et al., 1959).

The primary event that leads to transmitter release is depolarization of the presynaptic terminal during the action potential of the invading nerve impulse. The mechanism by which noradrenaline is released from noradrenergic nerves seems similar to that of acetylcholine at cholinergic synapses (Eccles, 1964). Both noradrenaline and acetylcholine are stored in synaptic vesicles in the presynaptic nerve terminals. The output of noradrenaline per stimulus decreases with increasing stimulation frequencies (Brown and Gillespie, 1957). As for acetylcholine, the release is dependent on calcium ions and promoted by depolarizing concentrations of extracellular potassium (Douglas and Rubin, 1963). It was suggested that the release occurs through an attachment of storage vesicles to the inner surface of the presynaptic fiber, followed by exocytosis with discharge of the contents of vesicles into the synaptic cleft. The secretion of catecholamines is accompanied by release of adenine nucleotides and dopamine-β-hydroxylase (Viveros *et al.*, 1968).

9.1. The Uptake of Catecholamines

The uptake of exogenous catecholamines into storage sites by sympathetic nerves in peripheral tissues has been demonstrated either after administration of large doses of adrenaline or noradrenaline *in vivo* (Raab and Humphreys, 1947; Nickerson *et al.*, 1950; Raab and Gigee, 1953, 1955), or of ^{14}C- or ^{3}H-labeled adrenaline or noradrenaline (Schayer, 1951; Udenfriend and Wyngaarden, 1956; Axelrod *et al.*, 1959b; De Schaepdryver and Kirshner, 1961; Whitby *et al.*, 1961).

Slices of cat cerebral cortex (Dengler *et al.*, 1962) and of mice cerebral cortex or brain stem are able to take up and accumulate exogenous labeled noradrenaline when incubated with the labeled amine *in vitro* by a high affinity uptake (Ross and Renyi, 1964) similar to that of peripheral catecholamine neurons. Cocaine, phenoxybenzamine, imipramine, desmethylimipramine, amphetamine, and other sympathomimetic amines inhibit the uptake (Dengler *et al.*, 1961; Ross and Renyi, 1964). The blood–brain barrier prevents catecholamine uptake in brain tissue *in vivo*, but uptake and storage of tritiated noradrenaline were observed in catecholamine-containing neurons after intraventricular administration (Glowinski *et al.*, 1965; Glowinski and Axelrod, 1966; Glowinski and Iversen, 1966). Large amounts of labeled amine could be found in the striatum, suggesting that exogenous catecholamines may be taken up and retained indiscriminately by noradrenaline or dopamine-containing neurons.

There is a significant correlation between the amount of tritiated noradrenaline taken up by a tissue and the endogenous content of noradrenaline (Crout, 1964). The uptake of ^{3}H-noradrenaline is markedly reduced in various tissues after surgical sympathectomy or immunosympathectomy (Hertting *et al.*, 1961; Iversen, 1965; Iversen *et al.*, 1966). Evidence for the localization of noradrenaline uptake in sympathetic nerves and in preterminal axons was obtained by histochemical methods (Hamberger *et al.*, 1964), by conventional autoradiography techniques, and optical microscopy in the brain, spleen, and heart (Marks *et al.*, 1962; Samorajski and Marks, 1962).

The uptake process of catecholamines proceeds against a high concentration gradient (Axelrod *et al.*, 1961; Dengler *et al.*, 1961; Whitby *et al.*, 1961) in various tissues as well as in brain slices, and has a remarkable ability to concentrate catecholamines up to several times the normal content. Dengler *et al.* (1961, 1962) were the first to suggest that the uptake of noradrenaline was mediated by a saturable membrane process, which agrees with the classical Michaelis–Menten equation used to describe saturable enzyme/substrate interactions. Values for the maximum rates of noradrenaline uptake (V_{max}) and the dissociation constant for the interaction between noradrenaline and the uptake site (K_m) were calculated. Kinetic studies could show the existence of a high and a low affinity uptake of noradrenaline (Iversen, 1965). Similarly two kinds of uptake processes have been demonstrated in nerve storage particles (von Euler and Lishajko, 1963). The initial uptake of catecholamines is mediated by a membrane carrier system in the axonal membrane (Iversen, 1963), and then the amines rapidly enter the intraneuronal storage particles.

There is a marked preference for the uptake of the L-isomers of noradrenaline (Iversen, 1963) compared to that of D-noradrenaline. However, the demonstration of a stereospecific uptake depends on the use of small doses of catecholamines since at high perfusion concentrations, the uptake of D-noradrenaline may be equal to that of L-noradrenaline. The uptake of noradrenaline was quantitatively more important than that of adrenaline in different tissues (Axelrod *et al.*, 1959b; Whitby *et al.*, 1961; Iversen and Whitby, 1962; Hertting, 1964, and many others). Also adrenaline and noradrenaline compete for the uptake into common sites in tissues.

Many structurally related amines may be taken up by the catecholamine uptake process in sympathetic nerves.

The accumulated catecholamines do not mix freely with the endogenous noradrenaline store and the accumulated amine exchanges slowly with the endogenous store. Chidsey and Harrison (1963) found that at short times after the administration of ^{3}H-noradrenaline the labeled amine was preferentially released from the dog heart by nerve stimulation. Furthermore, it was suggested that the exogeneous noradrenaline is released from two or three intraneuronal pools and the fate of the release from these pools is different (Axelrod *et al.*, 1961; Kopin and Gordon, 1962, 1963a).

When sympathetic postganglionic nerves are stimulated, noradrenaline which is released is "'inactivated" locally, even when catechol-O-methyltransferase or monoamine oxidase or both enzymes are inhibited (Brown and Gillespie, 1957; Stinson, 1961). Thus the nonmetabolic inactivation of catecholamines by tissue redistribution may be more important than metabolic degradation (Burn and Rand, 1958; Koelle, 1959). The efficient specific noradrenaline uptake process in sympathetic nerve terminals had led to the view that it is this process which is primarily responsible for the termination of the actions of liberated transmitter at adrenergic nerve terminals. Thus a very high amount of the noradrenaline released from nerve terminals in the cat spleen is inactivated by tissue-binding (Brown, 1965), although some doubt remains about the exact proportion of the released noradrenaline which is inactivated by reuptake into sympathetic nerves. The efficiency of the reuptake may depend on the rate of blood flow through the tissue. Since the released noradrenaline tends to cause a local vasoconstriction it may be supposed that under normal conditions, reuptake will be favored (Rosell *et al.*, 1963). Although sympathetically innervated tissues are able to accumulate circulating catecholamines, sympathetic nerve terminals are able to synthesize noradrenaline sufficiently rapidly to maintain a constant level of noradrenaline under most conditions (Kopin and Gordon, 1963*b*; Kopin *et al.*, 1965).

10. SOME ASPECTS OF THE PHARMACOLOGY OF BRAIN CATECHOLAMINES

Advances in knowledge of monoamines greatly stimulated investigation of new drugs acting on catecholamine metabolism. On the other hand, the use of drugs as tools was very helpful in the elucidation of basic metabolic mechanisms. Two drugs have played a fundamental role in pharmacology of brain catecholamines: reserpine (Holzbauer and Vogt, 1956; Carlsson *et al.*, 1957), which causes a long-lasting depletion of catecholamines and 5-hydroxytryptamine, and the monoamine oxidase inhibitor, iproniazid (Zeller *et al.*, 1952), which counteracts the amine-depleting effects of reserpine and which causes an increase in monoamines. Since then, many other drugs acting on brain catecholamines with correlated changes in behavior have been discovered.

Since, in general, the mode of action of drugs on peripheral and central catecholaminergic neurons is similar, many of studies on the action of drugs were performed on peripheral sympathetic nerves, where the approach is easier, as well as on brain. Recently the effects of drugs acting on catecholaminergic neurons were investigated in cell cultures (Mandel *et al.*, 1974).

10.1. Drugs Acting on Biosynthetic and Inactivating Enzymes

Several drugs act on the biosynthetic enzymes of catecholamines. Several inhibitors derived from tyrosine, like α-methyltyrosine (Spector *et al.*, 1965), iodotyrosine (Goldstein and Weiss, 1965), reversibly inhibit tyrosine hydroxylase, the rate-limiting enzyme in the biosynthesis of catecholamines. As a consequence, a considerable decrease in endogenous nora-drenaline and dopamine levels occurs after repeated administration of these drugs. Some of these drugs, like α-methyl-p-tyrosine, lower elevated blood pressure in patients with pheochromocytoma (Sjoerdsma, 1966).

Inhibitors of aromatic amino acid decarboxylase have been found and used as antihypertension or psychotropic drugs. Some of these dopa decarboxylase inhibitors inhibit the peripheral enzyme and enhance thus the conversion of administered L-dopa into dopamine in the central nervous system (Bartholini and Pletscher, 1968; Porter, 1971).

Various compounds like benzylhydrazines, benzyloxyamines, and de-rivatives of picolinic acid, as well as substances which act probably by copper chelation, like disulfiram and tropolone, have been found to be inhibitors *in vitro* and/or *in vivo* of dopamine-β-hydroxylase. Some of them have been used to treat hypertension and patients with Parkinson's syndrome (Mena *et al.*, 1971). Several dopamine-β-hydroxylase inhibitors decrease the nor-epinephrine and raise the dopamine levels in brain (Goldstein, 1966; Sulser and Sanders-Busch, 1971; Hidaka, 1973).

Catecholamines, like other transmitters, barely pass the blood–brain barrier in adults. In contrast, the immediate precursors of the amines like L-dopa, due probably to the presence of specific transport systems, penetrate into the brain where decarboxylation produces the amines. Thus with high doses of L-dopa, dopamine accumulates in dopaminergic and noradrenergic neurons. However, dopamine, under these conditions, can also accumulate in 5-hydroxytryptaminergic neurons (Carlsson, 1972; Shore, 1972).

The increase of transmitter levels by application of the immediate precursors as is the case for L-dopa, is widely used in Parkinson's syndrome. Thus the combination of L-dopa with decarboxylase inhibitors shows ad-vantages in the treatment of Parkinson's syndrome with L-dopa (see Bar-beau, 1974).

There are several groups of monoamine oxidase inhibitors with long-lasting effects on the enzyme *in vivo*. There is a good correlation between changes in monoamine metabolism and the clinical action of monoamine oxi-dase inhibitors. Some inhibitors may also enhance or inhibit monoamine release (Pletscher *et al.*, 1966).

The exact mechanism of action of monoamine oxidase inhibitors is not entirely clarified. Several possibilities have been suggested: an "overflow" of monoamines which may explain psychostimulation, an inhibition of monoamine release as well as an accumulation of false transmitters (Pletscher *et al.*, 1966; Kopin, 1968).

Monoamine oxidase inhibitors have been often used as a tool for re-search in monoamines. Recently, due to specific inhibitory effects, two types of monoamine oxidase isoenzymes have been detected (Neff *et al.,* 1973) (see Section 7.2).

Some pharmacological effects have been observed with various substances: inhibitors of catechol-*O*-methyl transferase (COMT) like polyphenols: pyrogallol, catechol derivatives, tropolones, etc. They may act by competing with the catecholamine substrate or by noncompetitive inhibition (Udenfriend *et al.,* 1959; Belleau and Burba, 1961). However, no COMT inhibitors have been used routinely up to now in medical therapy.

10.2. Drugs Acting on the Active Uptake

The antidepressant action of drugs which inhibit the active uptake of monoamines leading to an increased concentration of amines in the synaptic cleft, i.e., in the vicinity of the amine receptors, was largely used in the search for further antidepressant drugs. Several compounds like imipramine, desmethylimipramine, nortriptyline, protryptyline, are widely used in the treatment of mental depression. Some of them are more potent with regard to the inhibition of the uptake of a specific amine transmitter (Sulser and Sanders-Bush, 1971). The uptake of dopamine of the striatum does not seem to be affected appreciably by tricyclic antidepressants like desmethylimipramine. In contrast, the neuronal uptake of dopamine as well as norepinephrine was found to be inhibited by certain anticholinergic and antihistamine drugs used in the treatment of Parkinson's disease (Shore, 1972).

Lithium, used in manic-depressive illness, seems to enhance the uptake of norepinephrine into nerve terminals (Himwich and Alpers, 1970; Shore, 1972).

10.3. Drugs Acting on Storage of Catecholamines

Rauwolfia alkaloids, among which the most frequently used is reserpine, and similar drugs, deserpidine and rescinnamine, inhibit the uptake of noradrenaline and dopamine into storage organelles. Since they are no longer protected, these amines are degraded by intraneuronal monoamine oxidase. Whether or not the drug interferes with the intragranular binding remains to be investigated. Reserpine has also been used as a tool for research into the differentiation of various amine pools, and for elucidating monoamine metabolism and its functional role in various organs.

Several compounds deriving from benzo(a)quinolizine with a similar effect to reserpine, are less potent than reserpine, of shorter duration of action and are probably more selective for the brain (Pletscher *et al.,* 1962). Various phenylethylamine derivatives seem to decrease tissue monoamines by a reserpinelike mechanism.

Some compounds act by displacing intraneuronal norepinephrine from its storage sites. Thus, tyramine liberates amines which are not degraded by intraneuronal MAO and therefore remain physiologically active, stimulating noradrenergic receptors. It seems that tyramine probably acts mainly on a relatively small pool of newly synthesized norepinephrine (Kopin, 1964; Weiner, 1970).

Similarly, amphetamine displaces endogenous norepinephrine and probably dopamine. Some effects of amphetamine locomotor stimulation and increased aggressiveness are probably due to displaced norepinephrine, while stereotyped activity may be related to dopamine liberation (Sulser and Sanders-Bush, 1971). Amphetamine also inhibits catecholamine uptake and when absorbed may act as a false transmitter. This type of compound accumulates in the same storage sites as the physiological transmitter, is released by nerve stimulation and depleted by agents that also deplete the physiological transmitter (Fuxe and Ungerstedt, 1970; Sulser and Sanders-Bush, 1971).

Various amines fulfill the criteria of a false transmitter: octopamine, α-methyloctopamine, *m*-octopamine, metaraminol, α-methylnoradrenaline, etc. Some of these amines are metabolically formed from precursors like α-methyldopamine and α-methyl-noradrenaline from α-methyldopa, α-methyl-*m*-tyramine from α-methyl-*m*-tyrosine, and so on.

The functional effects of a false transmitter is related to its interaction with the receptor and/or its action on the release and reuptake of the physiological transmitter. The functional effects of false transmitters are inferior to those of the physiological transmitter which may explain their pharmacological effects. The false transmitters are valuable tools for developing new psychotropic drugs.

10.4. Drugs Acting on Monoamine Release and Catabolism

Certain drugs are taken up into adrenergic neurons and may have a stabilizing action on the neuronal membrane. This is the case of drugs like bretylium, bethanidine, guanethidine, guanisoquine, and debrisoquine. These drugs inhibit the ability of a nerve impulse to release norepinephrine, some of them (debrisoquine) also have a monoamine oxidase inhibitory effect, some others without monoamine oxidase inhibitory effect (guanethidine) which acts also as an uptake inhibitor, cause a depletion of neuronal norepinephrine (Shore, 1972).

10.5. Drugs Acting on Monoamine Receptors

Some drugs interfere with monoamine receptors. Among the receptor-blocking drugs, neuroleptics, like phenothiazines, butyrophenones, clozapine, block dopamine and to some extent also block noradrenaline receptors, especially in the central nervous system. The turnover of cerebral noradrenaline and dopamine may be increased under these conditions (see Bartholini *et al.*, 1972). Blockade of dopamine receptors produces catalepsy in animals and disturbance of extrapyramidal functions in man. Some drugs stimulate catecholamine receptors. Apomorphine is the prototype of a dopamine receptor agonist. It lowers symptoms in Parkinson's disease and concomitantly decreases dopamine turnover in the striatum (Pletscher, 1973). Clonidine seems to act as a noradrenaline receptor agonist, and reduces the turnover of cerebral noradrenaline (Andén *et al.*, 1970). It is obvious that these various drugs may facilitate research on receptor active drugs.

11. CONCLUSIONS

Since von Euler developed the hypothesis that norepinephrine was the transmitter for mediation of the nerve impulse within the sympathetic nervous system, further studies have shown the fundamental role of catecholamines in the peripheral and the central nervous system. There is good evidence for the involvement of catecholamines in a number of affective states. Thus knowledge about the distribution—biosynthesis and inactivation, storage, and release—is fundamental for the understanding of basic phenomena like arousal and emotion and of the effects of drugs on behavioral alterations. However, the mechanism by which catecholamines intervene in active states and mental diseases needs to be better clarified. Several hypotheses concerning the involvement of catecholamines in neurological and mental diseases are under investigation, and one may expect rapid progress regarding the possible functions of catecholamines in the biochemical processes that underlie normal and abnormal behavior.

12. REFERENCES

Alousi, A., and Weiner, N., 1966, *Proc. Natl. Acad. Sci. (U.S.)* **56**:1491.
Anden, N. E., Corrodi, H., Fuxe, K., Hökfelt, T., Rydin, C., and Svensson, T., 1970, *Life-Sci.* **9**:513–523.

Armstrong, M. D., McMillan, A., and Shaw, K. N. F., 1957, *Biochim. Biophys. Acta* **25**:422.
Assicot, M., and Bohuon, C., 1971, *Biochimie* **53**:871.
Aunis, D., Miras-Portugal, M. T., and Mandel, P., 1973*a*, *Biochim. Biophys. Acta* **327**:313.
Aunis, D., Miras-Portugal, M. T., and Mandel, P., 1973*b*, *Biochem. Pharmacol.* **22**:2581.
Aunis, D., Miras-Portugal, M. T., and Mandel, P., 1974, *Biochim. Biophys. Acta* **365**:259.
Aunis, D., Allard, D., Miras-Portugal, M. T., and Mandel, P., 1975, *Biochim. Biophys. Acta,* (in press).
Axelrod, J., 1962*a*, *J. Biol. Chem.* **237**:1657–1660.
Axelrod, J., 1962*b*, *J. Pharmacol. Exptl. Therap.* **138**:28.
Axelrod, J., 1963, *Science* **140**:499.
Axelrod, J., and Tomchick, R. 1958, *J. Biol. Chem.* **233**:702.
Axelrod, J. and Vessell, E. S., 1970, *Mol. Pharmacol.* **6**:78.
Axelrod, J., and Weinshilboum, R., 1972, *New Engl. J. Med.* **287**:237.
Axelrod, J., Albers, R. W., and Clemente, C. D., 1959*a*, *J. Neurochem.* **5**:68.
Axelrod, J., Weil-Malherbe, H., and Tomchick, R., 1959*b*, *J. Pharmacol. Exptl. Therap.* **127**:251–256.
Axelrod, J., Hertting, G., and Patrick, R. W., 1961, *J. Pharmacol. Exptl. Therap.* **134**:325.
Bagchi, S. P., and McGeer, P. L., 1964, *Life Sci.* **3**:1195.
Barbeau, A., 1961, *Proc. 7th Int. Congr. Neurol.,* vol. 2, p. 925, Societa Grafica Romana, Rome.
Barbeau, A., 1974, *Ann. Rev. Pharmacol.* **14**:91.
Bartholini, G., and Pletscher, A., 1968, *J. Pharmacol. Exptl. Therap.* **161**:14.
Bartholini, G., Haefely, W., Jalfre, M., Keller, H. H., and Pletscher, A. 1972, *Brit. J. Pharmacol.* **46**:736.
Belleau, B., and Burba, J. 1961, *Biochim. Biophys. Acta* **54**:195.
Bender, D. A., and Coulson, W. F., 1972, *J. Neurochem.* **19**:2801.
Benfey, B. G., Ledoux, G., and Melville, K. I., 1959, *Brit. J. Pharmacol.* **14**:142.
Bertler, Å., 1961, *Acta Physiol. Scand.* **51**:97–107.
Bertler, Å., and Rosengren, E., 1959*a*, *Acta Physiol. Scand.* **47**:350.
Bertler, Å., and Rosengren, E., 1959*b*, *Acta Physiol. Scand.* **47**:362.
Birkmayer, W., and Hornykiewicz, O., 1961, *Wien. Klin. Wochschr.* **73**:787.
Bisby, M. A., Fillenz, M., and Smith, A. D., 1973, *J. Neurochem.* **20**:245.
Blaschko, H., 1939, *J. Physiol. (Lond.)* **96**:50p.
Blaschko, H., 1952 *Pharmacol. Rev.* **4**:415.
Blaschko, H., Richter, D., and Schlossmann, H., 1937*a*, *J. Physiol. (Lond.)* **90**:1.
Blaschko, H., Richter, D., and Schlossmann, H., 1937*b*, *Biochem. J.* **31**:2187.
Bloom, F. E., 1972, Catecholamines, in *Handbook of Experimental Pharmacology,* Vol. 33, H. Blaschko, and E. Muscholl, eds., pp. 46–78, Springer-Verlag, Heidelberg.
Bogdanski, D. F., Weissbach, H., and Udenfriend, S., 1957, *J. Neurochem.* **1**:272.
Bohuon, C., and Assicot, M., 1973, In: *Frontiers in Catecholamine Research* (E. Usdin and S. Snyder, eds.), pp. 107–112, Pergamon Press, Oxford.
Brandau, K., and Axelrod, J., 1973, In: *Frontiers in Catecholamine Research* (E. Usdin and S. Snyder, eds.), pp. 129–131, Pergamon Press, Oxford.
Brown, G. L., 1960, In: *Adrenergic Mechanisms,* pp. 116–124, Ciba, Churchill, London.
Brown, G. L., 1965, *Proc. Roy. Soc. London Ser. B.* **162**:1.
Brown, G. L., and Gillespie, J. S., 1957, *J. Physiol. (London)* **138**:81.
Burack, W. R., and Draskoczy, P. R. 1964, *J. Pharmacol. Exptl. Therap.* **144**:66.
Burn, J. H., and Rand, M. J., 1958, *J. Physiol. (London)* **144**:314.
Cannon, W. B., and Uridil, J. E., 1921, *Am. J. Physiol.* **58**:353.
Carlsson, A., 1972, *Acta Neurol. Scand. Suppl.* **51**:11.

Carlsson, A., Rosengren, E., Bertler, Å., and Nilsson, J. 1957, In: *Psychotropic Drugs* (S. Garattini and V. Ghetti eds.), pp. 363–372, Elsevier, Amsterdam.

Carlsson, A., Lindqvist, M., Magnusson, T., and Waldeck, B., 1958, *Science* 127:417.

Carlsson, A., Falck, B., and Hillarp, N.-Å., 1962a, *Acta Physiol. Scand. Suppl.* 196:28.

Carlsson, A., Falck, B., Hillarp, N.-Å. 1962b, *Acta Physiol. Scand.* 54:385.

Cattabeni, F., Koslow, S. H., and Costa, E. 1972, *Science* 178:166.

Celander, O., 1954, *Acta Physiol. Scand. Suppl.* 116:128.

Chidsey, C. A., and Harrison, D. C., 1963, *J. Pharmacol. Exptl. Therap.* 140:217.

Christenson, J. G., Dairman, W. D., and Udenfriend, S., 1970, *Arch. Biochem. Biophys.* 141:356.

Chrusciel, T. L., 1960, In: *Adrenergic Mechanisms* (J. R. Vane, G. E. W. Wolstenholme, and M. O'Connor, eds.), pp. 539, Churchill, London.

Chubb, I. W., Preston, B. N., and Austin, L., 1969, *Biochem. J.* 111:243.

Ciaranello, R. D., 1973, In: *Frontiers in Catecholamine Research* (E. Usdin and S. Snyder, eds.), pp. 101–105, Pergamon Press, Oxford.

Ciaranello, R. D., Jacobowitz, D., and Axelrod, J. 1973, *J. Neurochem.* 20:799.

Costa, E., Green, A. R., Koslow, S. H., Lefevre, H. J. Revuelta. A. V., and Wang, C. 1972, *Pharmacol. Rev.* 24:167.

Costa, E., and Neff, N. H. 1966, In: *Biochemistry and Pharmacology of the Basal Ganglia* (E. Costa, L. T. Côte, and M. D. Yahr, eds.), pp. 141–155, Raven Press, New York.

Cotzias, G. C., Papavasiliou, P. S., Ginos, J., Steck, A., and Düby, S., 1971, *Ann. Rev. Med.* 22:305.

Coyle, J. T., 1972, *Biochem. Pharmacol.* 21:1935.

Creveling, C. R., Dalgard, N., Shimizu, H., and Daly, J. W., 1970, *Mol. Pharmacol.* 6:691.

Creveling, C. R., Morris, N., Shimizu, H., Ong, H. H., and Daly, J. W., 1972, *Mol. Pharmacol.* 8:398.

Crout, J. R., 1964, *Proc. Soc. Expt. Biol. Med.* 108:482.

Cuello, A. C., Hiley, R., and Iversen, L. L., 1973, *J. Neurochem.* 21:1337.

Dahlström, A., 1965, *J. Anat. (London)* 99:677.

Dahlström, A., 1971, *Phil. Trans. Roy. Soc. London B* 261:325.

Dahlström, A., and Fuxe, K., 1965, *Acta Physiol. Scand. Suppl.* 247:36.

Dahlström, A., Fuxe, K., and Hillarp, N.-Å., 1965, *Acta Pharmacol. Toxicol.* 22:277.

Dairman, W., Christenson, J. G., and Udenfriend, S., 1971, *Proc. Natl. Acad. Sci. (U.S.)* 68:2117.

Dairman, W., Christenson, J. G., and Udenfriend, S., 1972, *Pharmacol. Rev.* 24:269.

Dairman, W., Christenson, J. G., and Udenfriend, S., 1973, In: *Frontiers in Catecholamine Research* (E. Usdin and S. Snyder, eds.), pp. 61–67, Pergamon Press, Oxford.

Daly, J. W., Axelrod, J., and Witkop, B., 1960, *J. Biol. Chem.* 235:1155.

Demis, D. J., Blaschko, H., and Welch, A. D., 1955, *J. Pharmacol. Exptl. Therap.* 113:14.

Dengler, H. J., Michaelson, I. A., Spiegel, H. E., and Titus, E. O. 1962, *Intern. J. Pharmacol.* 1:23.

Dengler, H. J., Spiegel, H. E., and Titus, E. O. 1961, *Science* 133:1072.

De Potter, W. P., Smith, D. A., and De Schaepdryver, A. F., 1970, *Tissue and Cell* 2:529.

De Robertis, E., and Bennett, H. S., 1954, *Federation Proc.* 13:35.

De Robertis, E., and Pellegrino De Iraldi, A., 1961a, *Experientia* 17:122.

De Robertis, E., and Pellegrino De Iraldi, A., 1961b, *J. Biophys. Biochem. Cytol.* 10:361.

De Schaepdryver, A. F., and Kirshner, N., 1961, *Arch. Intern. Pharmacodyn. Therap.* 131:433.

Diliberto, E. J., Jr., and DiStefano, V., 1969, *Anal. Biochem.* 32:281.

Douglas, W. W., and Rubin, R. P. 1963, *J. Physiol.* (*London*) **167**:288.

Duncan, R. J. S., and Tipton, K. F., 1971, *European J. Biochem.* **22**:257.

Eagles, P. A. M., and Iqbal, M., 1974, *Brain Res.* **80**:177.

Eccles, J. C., 1964, *The Physiology of Synapses* Springer-Verlag, Berlin.

Ehringer, H., and Hornykiewicz, O., 1960, Wien. Klin. Wochschr. **38**:1236.

Eliasson, R., von Euler, U. S., and Stjärne, L., 1955, *Acta Physiol. Scand. Suppl.* **118**:69.

Eränko, O., 1952, *Acta Anat.* (*Basel*) **16**(Suppl. 16):60.

Ericsson, A. D., 1971, *J. Neurol. Sci.,* **14**:L93.

Erwin, V. G., and Deitrich, R. A., 1966, *J. Biol. Chem.* **241**:3533.

Erwin, V. G., Heston, W. D., and Tabakoff, B., 1972, *J. Neurochem.* **19**:2269.

Euler, U. S. von, 1946, *Acta Physiol. Scand.* **12**:73.

Euler, U. S. von, 1956, Noradrenaline American Lecture Series (Physiology), (R. F. Pitts, ed.), Charles C. Thomas, Springfield.

Euler, U. S. von, and Lishajko, F., 1963, *Acta Physiol. Scand.* **57**:468.

Euler, U. S. von, Franksson, C., and Hellström J., 1954, *Acta Physiol. Scand.* **31**:1.

Euler, U. S. von, Björkman, S., and Orwen, I., 1955, *Acta Physiol. Scand. Suppl.* **118**:10.

Falck, B., 1962, *Acta Physiol. Scand. Suppl.* **197**:26.

Falck, B., and Hillarp, N.-A., 1959, *Acta Anat.* **38**:277.

Falck, B., and Owman, C., 1965, *Acta Univ.* (*Lund.*) Section II, **7**:1–23.

Falck, B., and Torp, A., 1961, *Med. Exp.* **5**:428.

Falck, B., Hillarp, N.-A., Thieme G., and Torp, A., 1962, *J. Histochem. Cytochem.* **10**:348.

Fillenz, M., 1971, *Phil. Trans. Roy. Soc. London Ser B* **261**:319.

Foldes, A., and Meek, J. L., 1973, *Federation Proc.* **32**:797.

Friedhoff, A. J., and Van Winkle, E., 1962, *Nature* **194**:897.

Friedhoff, A. J., Schweitzer, J. W., and Miller, J., 1972*a*, *Res. Commun. Pharmacol. Pharm. Pathol.* **3**:293.

Friedhoff, A. J., Schweitzer, J. W., and Miller, J., 1972*b*, *Nature* **237**:454.

Fuller, R. W., and Hunt, J. M., 1967, *Life Sci.* **6**:1107.

Fuller, R. W., Warren, B. J., and Molloy, B. B. 1970, *Biochim. Biophys. Acta* **222**:210.

Fuxe, K. 1966, *Pharmacol. Rev.* **18**:641.

Fuxe, K., and Ungerstedt, U., 1970, *Symposium on Amphetamine and Related Compounds* (E. Costa and S. Garattini, eds.), pp. 257–288, Raven Press, New York.

Fuxe, K., Goldstein, M., Hökfelt, T., Freedman, L., and Anagnoste, B., 1971, *Acta Pharmacol. Toxicol.* **29**(Suppl. 4):15.

Fuxe, K., Goldstein, M., Hökfelt, T., Joh, T. H., Freedman, L. S., and Anagnoste, B., 1972, *Federation Proc.* **31**:544.

Gabay, S., and Valcourt, A. J., 1968, *Biochim. Biophys. Acta* **159**:440.

Gaddum, J. H., and Kwiatkowski, H., 1939, *J. Physiol.* (*London*) **96**:385.

Geffen, L., 1974, *Life Sci.* **14**:1593.

Geffen, L. B., and Ostberg, A., 1969, *J. Physiol.* (*London*) **204**:583.

Geffen, L. B., and Rush, R. A. 1973, In: *Frontiers in Catecholamine Research* (E. Usdin and S. Snyder, eds.), pp. 483–489, Pergamon Press, Oxford.

Gillespie, J. S., and Kirpekar, S. M., 1965, *J. Physiol.* (*London*) **178**:44p.

Glowinski, J., and Axelrod, J., 1966, *Pharmacol. Rev.* **18**:775.

Glowinski, J., and Iversen, L. L. 1966, *J. Neurochem.* **13**:655.

Glowinski, J., Kopin, I. J., and Axelrod, J., 1965, *J. Neurochem.* **12**:25.

Goldstein, M., 1966, *Pharmacol. Rev.* **18**:77.

Goldstein, M., 1972, In: *Research Methods in Neurochemistry* (N. Marks and R. Rodnight, eds.), pp. 317–340, Plenum Press, New York.

Goldstein, M., and Gerber, H., 1963, *Life Sci.* **2**:97.

Goldstein, M., Anagnoste, B., Yamamoto, H., and Felch, W. C., 1970, *J. Pharmacol. Exptl. Therap.* **171**:196.

Goldstein, M., Ohi, Y., and Backstrom, T., 1970a, *J. Pharmacol. Exptl. Therap.* **174**:77.

Goldstein, M., Freedman, L. S., and Backstrom, T., 1970b, *J. Pharm. Pharmacol.* **22**:715.

Goldstein, M., Anagnoste, B., Freedman, L. S., Roffman, M., Ebstein, R. P., Park, D. H., Fuxe, K., and Hökfelt, T., 1973, In: *Frontiers in Catecholamine Research* (E. Usdin and S. Snyder, eds.), pp. 69–78, Pergamon Press, Oxford.

Goldstein, M., and Weiss, Z. 1965, *Life Sci.* **4**:261.

Gray, E. G., and Whittaker, V. P., 1962, *J. Anat.* **96**:79.

Haefely, W., Hürlimann, A., and Thoenen, H., 1965, *J. Physiol.* (*London*) **181**:48.

Hagen, P., 1956, *J. Pharmacol. Exptl. Therap.* **116**:26.

Hall, D. W. R., Logan, B. W., and Parsons, G. H., 1969, *Biochem. Pharmacol.* **18**:1447.

Hamberger, B., Malmfors, T., Norberg, K. A., and Sachs, C., 1964, *Biochem. Pharmacol.* **13**:841.

Hare, M. L. C., 1928, *Biochem. J.* **22**:968.

Harris, J. E., and Roth, R. H., 1971, *Mol. Pharmacol.* **7**:593.

Hertting, G., 1964, *Biochem. Pharmacol.* **13**:1119.

Hertting, G., and Axelrod, J., 1961, *Nature* **192**:172.

Hertting, G., Axelrod, J., Kopin, I. J., and Whitby, L. G., 1961, *Nature* **189**:66.

Herrting, G., Potter, L. T., and Axelrod, J. 1962, *J. Pharmacol. Exptl. Therap.* **136**:289.

Hess, S. M., Connamacher, R. H., Ozaki, M., and Udenfriend, S., 1961, *J. Pharmacol. Exptl. Therap.* **134**:129.

Idaka, H., 1973, In: *Frontiers in Catecholamine Research*, (E. Usdin and S. Snyder, eds.,), pp. 87–90, Pergamon Press, Oxford.

Hillarp, N.-Å., and Hökfelt, T., 1953, *Acta Physiol. Scand.* **30**:55.

Himwich, H. E., and Alpers, H. S., 1970, *Ann. Rev. Pharmacol.* **10**:213.

Hökfelt, T., 1968, *Z. Zellforsch.* **91**:1.

Hökfelt, T., 1969, *Acta Physiol. Scand.* **76**:427.

Hökfelt, T., 1973, In: *Frontiers in Catecholamine Research* (E. Usdin and S. Snyder, eds.), pp. 439–446, Pergamon Press, Oxford.

Holtz, P., 1950, *Acta Physiol. Scand.* **20**:354.

Holtz, P., Heise, R., and Ludtke, K., 1938, *Arch. Exptl. Pathol. Pharmakol.* **191**:87.

Holzbauer, M. and Vogt, M., 1956, *J. Neurochem.* **1**:8.

Houslay, M. D., and Tipton, K. E., 1973, In: *Frontiers in Catecholamine Research* (E. Usdin and S. Snyder, eds.), pp. 147–149, Pergamon Press, Oxford.

Ikeda, M., Fahien, L. A., and Udenfriend, S., 1966, *J. Biol. Chem.* **241**:4452.

Ikeda, M., Levitt, M., and Udenfriend, S., 1965, *Biochem. Biophys. Res. Commun.* **18**:482.

Iversen, L. L., 1963, *Brit. J. Pharmacol. Chemother.* **21**:523.

Iversen, L. L., 1965, *Brit. J. Pharmacol. Chemother.* **25**:18.

Iversen, L. L., and Glowinski, J., 1966, *J. Neurochem.* **13**:671.

Iversen, L. L., Glowinski, J., and Axelrod, J., 1966, *J. Pharmacol. Exptl. Therap.* **151**:273.

Iversen, L. L., and Whitby, L. G., 1962, *Brit. J. Pharmacol. Chemother.* **19**:355.

Joh, T. H., and Goldstein, M., 1973, *Mol. Pharmacol.* **9**:117.

Johnston, J. P., 1968, *Biochem. Pharmacol.* **17**:1285.

Joyce, D., 1962, *Brit. J. Pharmacol.* **18**:370.

Kapeller, K., and Major, D., 1967, *Proc. Roy. Soc. London Ser B* **167**:282.

Katz, R. I., Goodwin, J. S., and Kopin, I. J., 1969, *Life Sci.* (Part II)**8**:561.

Katz, R. I., and Jacobson, A. E., 1972, *Mol. Pharmacol.* **8**:594.

Kaufman, S. 1973, In: *Frontiers in Catecholamine Research* (E. Usdin and S. Snyder, eds.), pp. 53–60, Pergamon Press, Oxford.

Kehr, W., Carlsson, A., Lindqvist, M., Magnusson, T., and Attack, C. (1972) *J. Pharm. Pharmacol.* **24**:744.

Kirshner, N., and Goodall, McC. 1956, *Federation Proc.* **15**:110.

Kirshner, N., and Goodall, McC., 1957, *Biochim. Biophys. Acta* **24**:658.

Kitabchi, A. E., and Williams, R. H., 1969, *Biochim. Biophys. Acta* **178**:181.

Koelle, G. B., 1959, *Pharmacol. Rev.* **11**:381.

Kopin, I. J., 1964, *Pharmacol. Rev.* **16**:179.

Kopin, I. J., 1968, *Ann. Rev. Pharmacol.* **8**:377.

Kopin, I. J., and Gordon, E. K., 1962, *J. Pharmacol. Exptl. Therap.* **138**:351.

Kopin, I. J., and Gordon, E. K., 1963a, *J. Pharmacol. Exptl. Therap.* **140**:207.

Kopin, I. J., and Gordon, E. K., 1963b, *Nature* **199**:1289.

Kopin, I. J., Gordon, E. K., and Horst, W. D. 1965, *Biochem. Pharmacol.* **14**:753.

Kopin, I. J., Weise, V. K., and Sedvall, G. C. 1969, *J. Pharmacol. Exptl. Therap.* **170**:246.

Koslow, S. H., Cattabeni, F., and Costa, E., 1972, *Science* **176**:177.

Krakoff, L. R., and Axelrod, J., 1967, *Biochem. Pharmacol.* **16**:1384.

Kuczenski, R. T., and Mandell, A. J., 1972, *J. Biol. Chem.* **247**:3114.

Kuehl, F. A., Jr., Ormond, R. E., and Vandenheuvel, W. J. A., 1966, *Nature* **211**:606.

Kukovetz, W. R., Hess, M. E., Shanfield, J., and Haugaard, N., 1959, *J. Pharmacol. Exptl. Therap.* **127**:122.

Laduron, P., 1973, In: *Frontiers in Catecholamine Research* (E. Usdin and S. Snyder, eds.), pp. 121–128, Pergamon Press, Oxford.

Lancaster, G. A., and Sourkes, T. L., 1972, *Can. J. Biochem.* **50**:791.

Lapetina, E. G., Soto, E. F., and De Robertis, E., 1968, *J. Neurochem.* **15**:437.

Laverty, R., Michaelson, I. A., Sharman, D. F., and Whittaker, V. P., 1963, *Brit. J. Pharmacol. Chemother.* **21**:482.

Leeper, L. C., and Udenfriend, S., 1956, *Federation Proc.* **15**:298.

Lever, J. D., and Esterhuizen, A. C., 1961, *Nature* **192**:566.

Levin, E. Y., and Kaufman, S., 1961, *J. Biol. Chem.* **236**:2043.

Lindvall, O., Björklund, A., and Falck, B., 1973, In: *Frontiers in Catecholamine Research* (E. Usdin and S. Snyder, eds.), pp. 683–687, Pergamon Press, Oxford.

Loewi, O. 1921, *Pflüegers Arch. Ges. Physiol.* **189**:239.

Lovenberg, W., Weissbach, H., and Udenfriend, S., 1962, *J. Biol. Chem.* **237**:89.

Lund, A., 1949, *Acta Pharmacol. Toxicol.* **5**:75, 121, 231.

Mandel, P., Ciesielski-Treska, J., Hermetet, J. C., Hertz, L., Nissen, C., Tholey, G. and Warter, F., 1974, In: *Central Nervous System. Studies on Metabolic Regulation and Function* (E. Genazzani and H. Herken, eds.), pp. 223–230, Springer-Verlag, Berlin.

Marks, B. H., Samorajski, T., and Webster, E. J., 1962, *J. Pharmacol. Exptl. Therap.* **138**:376.

Masri, M. S., Booth, A. N., and Deeds, F., 1962, *Biochim. Biophys. Acta* **65**:495.

Masri, M. S., Robbins, D. J., Emerson, O. H., and Deeds, F., 1964, *Nature* **202**:878.

Masuoka, D. T., Clark, W. G., and Schott, H. F., 1961, *Rev. Canad. Biol.* **20**:1.

Masuoka, D. T., Schott, H. F., Akawie, R. I., and Clark, W. G., 1956, *Proc. Soc. Exptl. Biol. Med.* **93**:5.

Masuoka, D. T., Schott, H. F., and Petriello, L., 1963, *J. Pharmacol. Exptl. Therap.* **139**:73.

Mathieu, P., and Revol, L., 1970, *Bull. Soc. Chim. Biol.* **52**:1039.

McGeer, E. G., and McGeer, P. L. 1962, *Can. J. Biochem. Physiol.* **40**:1141.

Meek, J. L., and Foldes, A., 1973, In: *Frontiers in Catecholamine Research* (E. Usdin and S. Snyder, eds.), pp. 167–171, Pergamon Press, Oxford.

38 Paul Mandel et al.

Meek, J. L., and Neff, N. H., 1973, *J. Neurochem.* **21**:1.

Mena, I., Crout, J., and Cotzias, G. C., 1971, *J. Am. Med. Assoc.* **218**:1829-1830.

Miras-Portugal, M. T., Aunis, D., and Mandel, P. 1975*a, Biochimie* (in press).

Miras-Portugal, M. T., Aunis, D., Mandel, P., Warter, J. M., Coquillat, G., and Kurtz, D., 1975*b, Psychopharmacologia* **41**:75.

Mirkin, B. L., and Bonnycastle, D. D., 1954, *Am. J. Physiol.* **178**:529.

Molinoff, P. B., and Axelrod, J., 1971, *Ann. Rev. Biochem.* **40**:465.

Montagu, K. A. 1957, *Nature* **180**:244.

Montagu, K. A., 1963, *Biochem. J.* **86**:9.

Moore, R. Y. 1973, In: *Frontiers in Catecholamine Research* (E. Usdin and S. Snyder, eds.), pp. 767-769, Pergamon Press, Oxford.

Mueller, R. A., Thoenen, H., and Axelrod, J., 1969*a, J. Pharmacol. Exptl. Therap.* **169**:74.

Mueller, R. A., Thoenen, H., and Axelrod, J., 1969*b, Mol. Pharmacol.* **5**:463.

Musacchio, J. M., d'Angelo, G. L., and McQueen, C. A., 1971*a, Proc. Natl. Acad. Sci. (U.S.)* **68**:2087.

Musacchio, J. M., and Craviso, G. L., 1973, In: *Frontiers in Catecholamine Research* (E. Usdin and S. Snyder, eds.), pp. 47-52, Pergamon Press, Oxford.

Musacchio, J. M., McQueen, C. A., and Craviso, G. L., 1973, In: *New Concepts in Neurotransmitter Regulation* (A. J. Mandell, ed.), pp. 69-88, Plenum Press, New York.

Musacchio, J. M., Wurzburger, R. J., and d'Angelo, G. L., 1971*b, Mol. Pharmacol.* **7**:136.

Nagatsu, T., Kato, T., Kuzuya, H., Umezawa, H. and Takenchi, T. 1973, In: *Frontiers in Catecholamine Research* (E. Usdin and S. Snyder, eds.), pp. 83-86, Pergamon Press, Oxford.

Nagatsu, T., Levitt, M., and Udenfriend, S., 1964, *Biochem. Biophys. Res. Commun.* **14**:543.

Nagatsu, T., Mizutani, K., Nagatsu, I., Matsuura, S., and Sugimoto, T. 1972, *Biochem. Pharmacol.* **21**:1945.

Nakashima, Y., Suzue, R., Sanada, H., and Kowada, S., 1972, *Arch. Biochem. Biophys.* **152**:515.

Neff, N. H., Yang, H. Y. T., and Goridis, C. (1973) In: *Frontiers in Catecholamine Research* (E. Usdin and S. Snyder, eds.), pp. 133-138, Pergamon Press, Oxford.

Neri, R., Hayano, M., Stone, D., Dorfman, R. I., and Elmanjian, F., 1956, *Arch. Biochem. Biophys.* **60**:297.

Nickerson, M., Berghout, J., and Hammerström, R. N., 1950, *Am. J. Physiol.* **160**:479.

Nikodijevik B., Daly, J., and Creveling, C. R., 1969, *Biochem. Pharmacol.* **18**:1577.

Nobin, A., and Björklund, A., 1973, In: *Frontiers in Catecholamine Research* (E. Usdin and S. Snyder, eds.), pp. 677-681, Pergamon Press, Oxford.

Palade, G. E., and Palay, S. L. 1954, *Anat. Rec.* **188**, 335.

Pellerin, J., and d'Iorio, A., 1957, *Can. J. Biochem. Physiol.* **35**:151.

Perry, T. L., Hansen, S., and Macintyre, L., 1964, *Nature* **202**:519.

Petrak, B., Fetzer, V., and Altiere, R. 1973, In: *Frontiers in Catecholamine Research* (E. Usdin and S. Snyder, eds.), pp. 97-100, Pergamon Press, Oxford.

Pletscher, A., 1973, In: *Frontiers in Catecholamine Research* (E. Usdin and S. Snyder, eds.), pp. 27-37, Pergamon Press, Oxford.

Pletscher, A., Brossi, A., and Gey, K. F., 1962, *Intern. Rev. Neurobiol.* **4**:275.

Pletscher, A., Gey, K. F., and Burkard, W. P., 1966, In: *Handbook of Experimental Pharmacology* Vol. 19, (O. Eichler and A. Farah, eds.), pp. 593-735, Springer-Verlag, Berlin.

Pohorecky, L. A., Zigmond, M., Karten, H., and Wurtman, R. J., 1969, *J. Pharmacol. Exptl. Therap.* **165**:190.

Porter, C. C., 1971, *Federation Proc.* **30**:871.

Potter, T. L., and Axelrod, J., 1963, *J. Pharmacol. Exptl. Therap.* **142**:291.
Raab, W., and Gigee, W., 1953, *Arch. Exptl. Pathol. Pharmak.* **219**:248.
Raab, W., and Gigee, W., 1955, *Circulation Res.* **3**:553.
Raab, W., and Humphreys, R. J., 1947, *J. Pharmacol. Exptl. Therap.* **89**:64.
Raskin, N. H., and Sokoloff, L., 1970, *J. Neurochem.* **17**:1677.
Richardson, K. C., 1962, *J. Anat.* (London) **96**:427.
Roffman, M., Freedman, L. S., and Goldstein, M., 1973, *Life Sci.* (Part II) **12**:369.
Rosell, S., Kopin, I. J., and Axelrod, J., 1963, *Am. J. Physiol.* **205**:317.
Ross, S. B., and Haljasmaa, O., 1964, *Acta Pharmacol. Toxicol. Scand.* **21**:215.
Ross, S. B., and Renyi, A. L., 1964, *Acta Pharmacol. Toxicol. Scand.* **21**:226.
Rutledge, C. O., and Jonason, J., 1967, *J. Pharmacol. Exptl. Therap.* **157**:493.
Saelens, J. K., Schoen, M. S., and Kovacsics, G. B., 1967, *Biochem. Pharmacol.* **16**:1043.
Samorajski, T., and Marks, B. H. 1962, *J. Histochem. Cytochem.* **10**:392.
Sano, I., Gamo T., Kakimoto, Y., Taniguchi, K., Takesada, M., and Nishinuma, K., 1959, *Biochim. Biophys. Acta* **32**:586.
Schanberg, S. M., Breese, G. R., Schildkraut, J. J., Gordon, E. K., and Kopin, I., 1968, *Biochem. Pharmacol.* **17**:2006.
Schayer, R. W., 1951, *J. Biol. Chem.* **189**:301.
Seiler, N., and Wiechmann, M. 1967, *J. Chromatog.* **28**:351.
Sen, N. P., and McGeer, P. L., 1964, *Biochem. Biophys. Res. Commun.* **14**:227.
Senoh, S., Daly, J., Axelrod, J., and Witkop, B., 1959, *J. Am. Chem. Soc.* **81**:6240.
Shiman, R., Akino, M., and Kaufman, S. 1971, *J. Biol. Chem.* **246**:1330.
Shiman, R., and Kaufman, S., 1970, *Methods in Enzymology Vol. 17A*, pp. 609–615.
Shimizu, H., and Daly, J. W., 1972, *European J. Pharmacol.* **17**:240.
Shore, P. A., 1972, *Ann. Rev. Pharmacol.* **12**:209.
Silberstein, S. D., Shein, H. M., and Ber, K. R., 1972, *Brain Res.* **41**:245.
Sims, K. L., and Bloom, F. E., 1973, *Brain Res.* **49**:165.
Sims, K. L., Davis, G. A., and Bloom, F. E., 1973, *J. Neurochem.* **20**:449.
Sjoerdsma, A., 1961, *Circulation Res.* **9**:734.
Sjoerdsma, A., 1966, *Pharmacol. Rev.* **18**:673.
Sjöstrand, F. S., 1954, *Z. Wiss. Mikroskopie.* **62**:65.
Smith, A. D., 1968, In: *A Symposium on the Interaction of Drugs and Subcellular Components in Animal Cells* (P. N. Campbell, ed.), pp. 239–292, J. & A. Churchill, London.
Smith, A. D., 1971, *Phil. Trans. Roy. Soc. London Ser B* **261**:363.
Smith, D. S., Järlfors, U., and Beraneck, R., 1970, *J. Cell Biol.* **46**:199.
Sourkes, T. L., 1954, *Arch. Biochem. Biophys.* **51**:444.
Spector, S., Gordon, R., Sjoerdsma, A., and Udenfriend, S., 1967, *Mol. Pharmacol.* **3**:549.
Spector, S., Sjoerdsma, A., and Udenfriend, S., 1965, *J. Pharmacol. Exptl. Therap.* **147**:86.
Squires, R. F. 1972, In: *Advances in Biochemical Psychopharmacology Vol. 5,* (E. Costa, ed.), pp. 355–370, Raven Press, New York.
Stabenan, J. R., Creveling, C. R., and Daly, J., 1970, *Am. J. Psychiat.* **127**:611.
Stinson, R. H., 1961, *Can. J. Biochem. Physiol.* **39**:309.
Sugden, R. F., and Eccleston, D. J., 1971, *J. Neurochem.* **18**:2461.
Sulser, F., and Sanders-Bush, E., 1971, *Ann. Rev. Pharmacol.* **11**:209.
Sundin, T., 1958, *Acta Med. Scand.* (Suppl. 336):59.
Tabakoff, B., and Erwin, V. G., 1970, *J. Biol. Chem.* **245**:3263.
Taylor, K. M., and Laverty, R., 1969, *J. Neurochem.* **16**:1367.
Thoenen, H., Kettler, R., Burkard, W., and Saner, A., 1971, *Naunyn-Schmiedebergs Arch. Exptl. Pathol. Pharmak.* **270**:146.

Thomas, J. A., Van Orden, L. S., III, Redick, J. A., and Kopin, I. J., 1973, In: *Frontiers in Catecholamine Research* (E. Usdin and S. Snyder, eds.), pp. 79–81, Pergamon Press, Oxford.

Thureson-Klein, A., Klein, R. L., Lagercrantz, H., and Stjärne, L., 1970, *Experientia* **26**:994.

Tranzer, J. P., 1973, In: *Frontiers in Catecholamine Research* (E. Usdin and S. Snyder, eds.), pp. 453–458, Pergamon Press, Oxford.

Tranzer, J. P., and Thoenen, H., 1967, *Experientia* **23**:123.

Tranzer, J. P., and Thoenen, H., 1968, *Experientia* **24**:484.

Tranzer, J. P., Thoenen, H., Snipes, R. L., and Richards, J. G., 1969, *Mechanisms of synaptic transmission, Progr. Brain Res.* **31**:33.

Turner, A. J., and Tipton, K. F. 1972, *European J. Biochem.* **30**:361.

Udenfriend, S., 1962, *Fluorescence Assay in Biology and Medicine* Academic Press, New York.

Udenfriend, S., 1966, *Pharmacol. Rev. (Part I)* **18**:43.

Udenfriend, S., and Wyngaarden, J. B., 1956, *Biochim. Biophys. Acta* **20**:48.

Udenfriend, S., and Zaltzman-Nirenberg, P., 1963, *Science* **142**:394.

Udenfriend, S., Creveling, C. R., Ozaki, M., Daly, J. W., and Witkop, B., 1959, *Arch. Biochem. Biophys.* **84**:249.

Udenfriend, S., Zaltzman-Nirenberg, P., and Nagatsu, T., 1965, *Biochem. Pharmacol.* **14**:837.

Ungerstedt, U., 1968, *European J. Pharmacol.* **5**:107.

Ungerstedt, U., 1971*a*, *Acta Physiol. Scand. Suppl.* **367**:1.

Ungerstedt, U., 1971*b*, *Acta Physiol. Scand. Suppl.* **367**:49.

Ungerstedt, U., 1971*c*, *Acta Physiol. Scand. Suppl.* **367**:69.

Ungerstedt, U., 1971*d*, *Acta Physiol. Scand. Suppl.* **367**:95.

Ungerstedt, U., and Ljungberg, T., 1973, In: *Frontiers in Catecholamine Research* (E. Usdin and S. Snyder, eds.), pp. 689–693, Pergamon Press, Oxford.

Viveros, O. H., Arqueros, L., and Kirshner, N., 1968, *Life Sci.* **7**:609.

Vogt, M., 1954, *J. Physiol. (London)* **123**:451.

Wagner, A. F., Cirillo, V. J., Meisinger, M. A. P., Ormond, R. E., Kuehl, F., Jr., and Brink, N. G., 1966, *Nature* **211**:604.

Weil-Malherbe, H., 1961, In: *Methods in Medical Research* Vol. IX (Quastel, ed.), pp. 130–146.

Weil-Malherbe, H., and Bone, A. D., 1952, *Biochem. J.* **51**:311.

Weiner, N. 1970, *Ann. Rev. Pharmacol.* **10**:273.

Weiner, N., and Selvaratnam, I., 1968, *J. Pharmacol. Exptl. Therap.* **161**:21.

Whitby, L. G., Axelrod, J., and Weil-Malherbe, H., 1961, *J. Pharmacol. Exptl. Therap.* **132**:193.

Whitsett, T. L., McKinney, A. S., and Goldberg, L. I., 1970, *Clin. Res.* **18**:28.

Whittaker, V. P., 1966, *Ann. N.Y. Acad. Sci.* **137**:982.

Wolfe, D. E., Potter, L. T., Richardson, K. C., and Axelrod, J., 1962 *Science* **138**:440.

Woods, R. I., 1970, *Proc. Roy. Soc. London Ser B* **176**:63.

Yahr, M. D., Duvoisin, R. C., Shear, M. J., Barrett, R. E., and Hoeln, M. M., 1969, *Arch. Neurol.* **21**:343.

Youdim, M. B. H., 1972, Monoamine oxidases: New vistas in: *Advances in Biochemical Psychopharmacology*, *Vol. 5* (E. Costa and M. Sandler, eds.), pp. 67–77, Raven Press, New York.

Zeller, E. A., and Barsky, J., 1952, *Proc. Soc. Exptl. Biol.* **81**:459.

Zeller, E. A., and Hsu, M., 1973, In: *Frontiers in Catecholamine Research*, (E. Usdin and S. Snyder, eds.), pp. 153–155, Pergamon Press, Oxford.

Zeller, E. A., Barsky, J., Berman, E. R., and Fouts, J. R., 1952, *J. Lab. Clin. Med.* **40**:965.

Chapter 2

Catecholamines in Regulation of Motor Function

K. G. Lloyd
and
O. Hornykiewicz

Department of Pharmacology
University of Toronto
and
Department of Psychopharmacology
Clarke Institute of Psychiatry
Toronto, Ontario, Canada

1. INTRODUCTION

The function of the catecholamines, dopamine (DA) and noradrenaline (NA), in the control of movement encompasses a large field of physiology and pathology. However, in the examination of CNS function direct investigation of the "normal" state is difficult, if not impossible, and the information available is often the result of the examination of pathological or drug-induced conditions. In the study of movement disorders, two syndromes are prominent: Parkinson's disease and Huntington's disease. It is from the study of these two syndromes (with emphasis on the former) that the present concepts of catecholamines and motor behavior have evolved. From these studies animal models for the central control of movement have been developed.

2. CLINICAL EVIDENCE FOR THE INVOLVEMENT OF CATECHOLAMINES IN THE CONTROL OF MOVEMENT

2.1. Parkinson's Syndrome

2.1.1. Parkinson's Disease

2.1.1a. Symptomatology. The cardinal symptoms of Parkinson's disease, namely, akinesia, rigidity, and tremor, are primarily those of motor dysfunction. Parkinsonian rigidity results in a physical impediment of the limbs to perform movements and may be related to a decrease of γ-efferent activity from the motoneurons (Steg, 1972). The control of the γ-efferent activity by higher nervous system structures is associated with both pyramidal and extrapyramidal pathways (cf. Calne, 1970; Granit, 1970).

The study of Parkinsonian akinesia (the inability to initiate movement) indicates that the initiation of movement is controlled separately from its perpetuation. This can be seen from the clinical observation that in some Parkinsonian patients once the movement has begun (e.g., by rocking on the feet) the motor pattern can be maintained but not restarted without external aid. Associated with the initiation of movement is the acceleration or alteration of ongoing movements. Thus, akinetic patients suffer not only from an inability to start, but also changes in speed and direction are impaired. In Parkinsonian patients akinesia and rigidity are not necessarily coexistent. The significance of Parkinsonian tremor in relation to the control of motor function is at present obscure.

2.1.1b. Neuropathology and Chemistry. The outstanding neuropathology of Parkinson's disease is a depigmentation and loss of the melanin-containing cell bodies of the pars compacta of the substantia nigra and other pigmented areas of the brain (e.g., the locus coeruleus). There is also a consistent chemical pathology involving notably DA and to a lesser extent NA and 5-hydroxytryptamine (5-HT) (cf. Hornykiewicz, 1966a). The decrease in DA is highly significant and is specific for the caudate nucleus, putamen, and substantia nigra. On the average the DA content of the striatum is less than 10% of normal; in idiopathic Parkinson's disease this decrease is significantly more severe in the putamen than in the caudate (Bernheimer *et al.,* 1973; Lloyd *et al.,* 1973). Associated with the loss in DA is a parallel deficiency in its synthetic enzymes (tyrosine hydroxylase and dopa decarboxylase) (Lloyd *et al.,* 1973, 1975), the specific uptake system for DA (Lloyd and Hornykiewicz, 1972) and the level of homovanillic acid (HVA), the major metabolite of DA in the brain (cf. Hornykiewicz, 1966a; Bernheimer *et al.,* 1973). From these findings and especially from biochemical and histofluorescent studies on animal models it is now widely accepted that there is a neuronal pathway with cell bodies in the pars compacta of the substantia nigra, and terminals in the striatum, which utilizes DA as a putative neurotransmitter. It is presently thought that it is this ...hway that is specifically degenerated in Parkinson's disease. NA and ...ns are also decreased in Parkinson's disease to ap-... control values (cf. Hornykiewicz, 1966b). The func-... changes is not clear at present; possibly they are ...dence of severe depression in patients suffering ...juriaguerra et al., 1972).

...of Neuropathological with the Clinical Findings of ...Relation to Control of Motor Function. Upon the dis-...ific destruction of the nigrostriatal DA pathway in ...se, it was proposed that this was the neuropathological ...nical symptomatology of this disorder. That this may be so ...by the observations that (i) the degree of DA deficiency corre-...e cell loss in the substantia nigra but not with changes found in ...l ganglia nuclei (Bernheimer et al., 1973); (ii) in a patient with ...kinsonism there was a more severe loss of DA in the striatum in ...isphere contralateral to the side of symptoms (Barolin et al., 1964); ...e immediate precursor of DA, L-dopa, was found to be a very effica-...agent for the treatment of Parkinsonian akinesia and rigidity (for ...nces see Calne, 1970); and (iv) in the brains of Parkinsonian patients ...ted with L-dopa, the DA concentrations of the striatum were severalfold ...se of the non-dopa-treated patients and in some cases approached ...rmal levels (Davidson et al., 1971). In these studies the DA levels were ...ound to be dependent upon the time before death of the last dose of L-dopa ...(Lloyd et al., 1973).

The above may be considered as circumstantial evidence that the decrease in striatal DA is the causative factor for the akinesia and rigidity in Parkinson's disease. In this context, it has recently been demonstrated that the repletion, by L-dopa, of DA levels in the striatum is directly correlated with the amelioration of Parkinsonian symptoms. Thus, in a group of patients with similar initial severity of akinesia and rigidity, and all receiving a similar dose of L-dopa, the striatal levels of DA were elevated only in those patients who showed a good clinical response to the drug (Lloyd et al., 1973).

Therefore, it appears that in Parkinson's disease a deficiency of DA in the striatum is correlated with rigidity and akinesia, and that repletion of this loss reverses these movement disorders. However, as stated above, akinesia and rigidity can be considered to be two different phenomena. From

an extensive study of the neurochemistry and morphology of Parkinson's
syndromes of different etiology (Bernheimer *et al.*, 1973) it has been concluded that the cell bodies of the rostral zona compacta of the substantia
nigra project to the caudate nucleus, and those of the caudal portion project
to the putamen. In addition, the severity of the akinesia in Par
disease was found to correlate significantly with the loss o
the caudate nucleus. Thus, it would appear that the
volved with striatal initiation of locomotor ac
neurotransmitter and to a large extent has its c
tion of pars compacta of the substantia nigra a
date nucleus.

2.1.2. Drug-Induced Parkinsonism

In addition to Parkinson's disease proper, Parkinsonian
pear as a side effect of many psychotropic (neuroleptic) drugs.
of these drugs on the brain's catecholamine systems may be
directly in animals, it is possible with this model to gain some in
the role played by brain catecholamines in motor function. Drug
Parkinsonism may be caused by two types of drugs: drugs which dep
brain of catecholamines and drugs which block catecholamine recepto

2.1.2a. Drugs Which Lower Brain Catecholamine Concentra
Those drugs which typically lower brain catecholamine concentrations
either by interference with storage (e.g., reserpine which depletes DA,
and 5-HT) or by blockade of synthesis (e.g., α-methyl-*p*-tyrosine) of ca
cholamines. Reserpine treatment of both animals and humans results in
syndrome of severe catalepsy (including rigidity and akinesia) which may b
clinically indistinguishable from Parkinson's disease. These symptoms are
reversed by L-dopa but not by L-5-HTP (Carlsson *et al.*, 1957), indicating
that it is the loss of catecholamines and not 5-HT which is important for the
extrapyramidal effects. Like the rigidity of Parkinson's disease, in the rat,
the rigidity due to reserpine is associated with decreased γ-efferent activity
to the muscle spindles and an increased α-motoneuron activity (Arvidsson *et
al.*, 1966).

In laboratory animals the reversal of the reserpine syndrome by L-dopa
is correlated with a large increase in brain DA concentrations. Several
observations suggest that formation of NA from L-dopa may play a role
auxiliary to that of DA in the anti-Parkinson effects of the drug (cf.
Hornykiewicz, 1974). Thus, in mice and rats, drugs with both DA-mimetic
and NA-mimetic properties (e.g., amphetamine) exert locomotor effects
quantitatively comparable to those of L-dopa; in contrast, compounds with
predominantly DA-mimetic activity (e.g., apomorphine) are considerably

weaker in stimulating locomotor activity in experimental animals and as anti-Parkinson agents (cf. Hornykiewicz, 1974).

2.1.2b. Drugs Which Block Catecholamine Receptors. In addition to reserpine, many other drugs used in the treatment of psychotic states produce Parkinsonian side effects in man and catelepsy in animals. These are the neuroleptics of the phenothiazine and butyrophenone series. However, rather than depleting brain catecholamine stores, these compounds are thought to interfere with the brain's catecholaminergic mechanisms by blockade of the postsynaptic receptor sites. The extrapyramidal effects of these drugs can be partially reversed by substances which increase catecholamine synthesis or release (e.g., L-dopa, amphetamine) or directly stimulate the catecholamine receptors (e.g., apomorphine). As a consequence of the receptor blockade the above neuroleptics trigger a (probably receptor-mediated) feedback activation of the catecholamine neurons. The evidence for this is: (i) these compounds induce an increase in the levels of the metabolites of DA (i.e., HVA) and NA (i.e., 3-methoxy-4-hydroxyphenylethyleneglycol) without changing the amine levels themselves (Andén *et al.,* 1964; DaPrada and Pletscher, 1966; Keller *et al.,* 1973); (ii) the rate of firing of DA neurons in the substantia nigra is increased by these drugs (Bunney *et al.,* 1973); and (iii) the conversion of tyrosine to DA and NA is increased by these drugs (Nybäck and Sedvall, 1970; Bartholini and Pletscher, 1969).

Although some of these neuroleptic compounds block both NA and DA receptors, the evidence indicates that it is primarily the DA-blocking ability which is responsible for the catalepsy. Thus, those compounds which are markedly cataleptogenic (haloperidol, chlorpromazine) are extremely potent in increasing DA turnover, whereas the less cataleptogenic compounds (e.g., clozapine) are less effective on DA turnover (Andén and Stock, 1973; Bartholini and Pletscher, 1972; Bartholini *et al.,* 1972). In addition, the NA-receptor blocking potency of the neuroleptic compounds in question does not seem to parallel their cataleptogenic potencies (Keller *et al.,* 1973).

2.2. Huntington's Disease

Huntington's disease in many aspects is the clinical opposite of Parkinson's disease. The neurological picture of muscle hypotonia with involuntary hyperactivity results in facial grimacing, writhing, and twisting of the trunk and limbs. These symptoms are in obvious contrast to the lack of facial expression, rigidity, and akinesia observed in Parkinson's disease.

Neuropathologically, Huntington's disease is characterized by a severe atrophy of the striatum (small- and medium-sized cells) as well as cortical atrophy. The substantia nigra is apparently morphologically intact. Neurochemically, there is a mild loss of DA and HVA in the caudate nucleus but not the putamen or substantia nigra (Bernheimer and Hornykiewicz, 1973). This had led to the speculation that in Huntington's disease the DA system of the putamen may be hyperactive as compared with that of the caudate (i.e., DA imbalance between caudate and putamen in favor of the latter) possibly resulting in some of the characteristic extrapyramidal symptoms of this disease. This is in contrast to idiopathic Parkinson's disease in which the decrease of DA is more severe in the putamen than in the caudate nucleus (Bernheimer et al., 1973). (For a comprehensive survey of the varied aspects of Huntington's disease, see Barbeau et al., 1973.)

Pharmacologically there is some support for the hypothesis that a hyperactivity of catecholaminergic neurons is responsible for the hyperkinesias of Huntington's chorea. Thus, drugs which deplete catecholamine levels, e.g., reserpine or tetrabenzamine (Birkmayer, 1969; Ringel et al., 1973), or block catecholamine, notably DA, receptors, e.g., haloperidol (Duvoisin, 1972) or inhibit DA and NA synthesis, e.g., α-methyl-p-tyrosine (Birkmayer, 1969) reduce the choreatic hyperactivity. In contrast to the above observations L-dopa exacerbates or precipitates the dyskinesias (Gerstenbrand et al., 1963; Ringel et al., 1973).

2.3. Other Dyskinetic Syndromes

2.3.1 L-Dopa-Induced Dyskinesias

As outlined above, L-dopa reverses the rigidity and akinesia of Parkinson's disease by being transformed to DA specifically in the striatum. In addition to its ameliorative effects, L-dopa has other effects on motor function of Parkinsonian patients. In many patients (40–60%), after several months of L-dopa therapy, an array of hyperkinetic symptoms may occur; these are termed the L-dopa dyskinesias and consist most frequently of oral-buccal-facial dyskinesias (grimacing, tongue-protrusion, lip-smacking, chewing, and head-rolling) as well as choreoathetotic movements of the extremities (cf. Barbeau, 1969). That these symptoms are due to overstimulation of the DA receptors in the striatum is indicated by: (i) the dyskinesias disappear with a decrement in L-dopa dose (cf. Calne, 1970; Barbeau, 1969); (ii) they may be reversed by treatment with DA-receptor blocking agents (cf. Barbeau, 1969; Postma, 1972); (iii) their reversal is frequently accompanied by a worsening of the underlying Parkinsonism (Barbeau, 1969); (iv) the dyskinesias occur more severely on the affected side in hemi-Parkinsonian patients (Duvoisin *et al.*, 1969; Klawans, 1973); (v) lesioning of the striatum in man results in athetoid or choreiform movements (cf. Duvoisin, 1972; Korczyn, 1972); (vi) there appears to be a parallelism between the beneficial responses of the Parkinsonian symptoms to L-dopa therapy and the severity of the resultant dyskinesias (Markham, 1971; Mones *et al.*, 1971); and (vii) L-dopa-induced dyskinesias resemble in many aspects the stereotyped behavior produced by high doses of amphetamine (Rubovits *et al.*, 1973).

Supplementing the above evidence that it is the striatal DA receptor that are responsible for the dyskinesias is the observation that both naive laboratory animals (rats, monkeys) (Sassin *et al.*, 1972; Bieger and Hornykiewicz, unpublished observations) and animals with specific lesions of the nigrostriatal tract (Goldstein *et al.*, 1973), will also develop dyskinesias on L-dopa therapy. Thus, in monkeys with tegmental lesions, high doses of L-dopa, L-dopa plus a peripheral decarboxylase inhibitor, or DA-receptor stimulating agents (piribedil) result in a dose-dependent oral-buccal syndrome and chorea while simultaneously producing relief of the experimental Parkinsonism. These effects of L-dopa are blocked by haloperidol but not by the inhibition of NA formation (Goldstein *et al.*, 1973). Also, in cats, unilateral injection of L-dopa, DA, methoxytyramine, or *d*-amphetamine (but not NA) into the rostromedial caudate nucleus results in a choreoathetosis-like syndrome (Cools, 1973). In this respect it is important to keep in mind that the striatum deprived of its DA innervation can be expected to develop the phenomenon of "denervation supersensitivity" to DA. This is likely for animal models of Parkinson's disease (substantia nigra lesions; Ungerstedt, 1971), and it also appears to apply to Parkinson's disease. Thus (i) therapeutic doses of L-dopa do not produce noticeable dyskinesias in non-Parkinsonian human controls (Barbeau, 1969), and (ii) Parkinsonian patients with a higher degree of striatal DA deficiency (i.e., higher degree of nigral degeneration) have been noted to react more sensitively to single iv test doses of L-dopa than patients with less severe DA decreases (Bernheimer *et al.*, 1973).

2.3.2. Tardive Dyskinesias

The chronic use of antipsychotic drugs which block catecholaminergic neurons (e.g., haloperidol, chlorpromazine, etc.) may result in an array of often practically irreversible dyskinetic symptoms. These symptoms are most commonly oral-buccal-facial dyskinesias and chorea- and athetosis-like conditions, and are in marked contrast to the initial Parkinsonism which most of these drugs provoke. These dyskinesias are termed "tardive" because of the long latency of their onset (cf. Crane, 1972).

At present the most attractive explanation for the occurrence of the tardive dyskinesias is that they are a manifestation of the brain's (notably the striatum) homeostatic response to the Parkinsonism normally induced by these neuroleptic drugs. The proposed mechanism for this homeostasis is that: (i) blockade of catecholamine receptors is known to produce an increase in the turnover of the corresponding transmitter in the synpatic terminals (Nybäck and Sedvall, 1970), and (ii) after prolonged blockade, the receptors may eventually become supersensitive to the respective transmitters (Ungerstedt, 1971). The view that tardive dyskinesias are an expression of compensatory nervous overactivity to the neuroleptics is supported by the observations that: (i) they most commonly become worse upon cessation or reduction of neuroleptic therapy, and (ii) they can be reversed by reinstating or increasing the neuroleptic dosage (cf. Crane, 1972; Degwitz, 1969; Greenblatt et al., 1970).

A large body of indirect evidence seems to suggest that the tardive dyskinesias are due to a hyperreactivity of the striatal DA system: (i) the incidence of dyskinesias in response to a given neuroleptic drug appears to parallel its Parkinsonism-producing ability in man (Klawans, 1973) and DA-receptor blockade in animals; (ii) patients initially exhibiting drug-induced Parkinsonism are more likely to develop tardive dyskinesias that those without the Parkinsonism (Crane, 1972; Klawans, 1973); (iii) L-dopa worsens the dyskinetic symptoms present and may precipitate others (Klawans, 1973); (iv) the remarkable resemblance between the tardive dyskinesias and the L-dopa-induced dyskinesias in patients with Parkinson's disease (Calne and Reid, 1972); (v) in patients with concurrent Parkinsonism and tardive dyskinesias there is an inverse relation between the severity of the two sets of symptoms i.e., treatments which alleviate the Parkinsonism exacerbate the dyskinesias and vice versa (Crane, 1972).

3. ANIMAL MODELS FOR THE STUDY OF CATECHOLAMINES AND MOTOR FUNCTION

3.1. Drugs Which Mimic Catecholaminergic Mechanisms

Drugs which mimic the action of catecholaminergic neurons may do so by two different mechanisms, namely, presynaptic (release of catecholamines from the stores by, e.g., amphetamine) or postsynaptic (by direct action on the receptors, e.g., apomorphine, clonidine).

3.1.1. Drugs Which Release Catecholamines

The mechanism of action of amphetamine on catecholamine neurons appears to be mainly presynaptic and dependent upon ongoing catecholamine synthesis. The presence of normal catecholamine levels in the stores is not necessary for its action, as in reserpinized animals amphetamine still exerts its effect. If, in addition to reserpine, the animals are pretreated with a catecholamine synthesis inhibitor (α-methyl-p-tyrosine), amphetamine becomes ineffective (Carlsson, 1970). Behaviorally, amphetamine's effects can be separated into at least two different motor components: locomotor activity and stereotyped behavior.

3.1.1a. Locomotor Activity. In untreated animals, amphetamine usually increases locomotion. This effect is competitive with the cataleptic effect of reserpine, and to a lesser extent, other neuroleptic drugs. The stimulating effect of amphetamine on motor activity appears to be dependent upon release of both NA and DA stores inasmuch as blockers of NA synthesis as well as DA-blocking agents in addition to α-methyl-p-tyrosine antagonize the amphetamine-induced activity (cf. Carlsson, 1970).

3.1.1b. Stereotyped Behavior. In addition to increased motor activity in many species, amphetamine also induces a series of highly consistent repetitive movements which are termed "stereotyped behavior." These movements typically include sniffing, licking, chewing, and rubbing of the face and snout with the forepaws. These activities appear to depend largely upon the presence of DA in the brain, as they are blocked by α-methyl-p-tyrosine but not by disulfiram, and are also effectively reversed by agents blocking DA-but not NA-receptors (cf. Fog, 1972; Randrup and Munkvad, 1970).

3.1.2. Compounds Which Directly Stimulate Catecholamine Receptors

3.1.2a. Apomorphine. In contrast to amphetamine, the site of apomorphine's action appears to be a postsynaptic stimulation of the DA receptor. The effects of apomorphine administration on motor activity resemble most notably the stereotyped behavior induced by amphetamine. Also, because of its postsynaptic actions, apomorphine is still active in animals with lesions of their catecholaminergic pathways (see below) (Ungerstedt, 1971) or animals which have been treated with reserpine and α-methyl-p-tyrosine (Andén, 1970). Haloperidol, pimozide, and other DA-receptor blocking agents antagonize the apomorphine behavior. In accord with its DA receptor stimulant activity, apomorphine reverses the reserpine syndrome in rats (Andén *et al.*, 1967).

3.1.2b. L-Dopa. In most laboratory animals, L-dopa produces increased motor activity as compared to untreated animals. Similarly, L-dopa reverses completely or partially the catalepsy following reserpine (Carlsson *et al.,* 1957), α-methl-*p*-tyrosine (Bedard *et al.,* 1970), phenothiazines (Klawans, 1968), or lesions of the nigrostriatal tract (Ungerstedt, 1971). That it is not L-dopa itself but an amine metabolite which is active is shown by the fact that central decarboxylase inhibition blocks the effect of L-dopa (Butcher and Engel, 1969), but inhibition of MAO enhances its activity (Blaschko and Chrusciel, 1960). Like amphetamine, it appears that L-dopa exerts its locomotor activity utilizing both DA and NA, as blockade of its conversion to NA (by inhibition of DA-β-hydroxylase) partially blocks the locomotor effects of L-dopa (references see Hornykiewicz, 1974).

3.1.2c. Clonidine. Per se, clonidine does not have any major effects on locomotor activity in laboratory animals such as mice and rats. However, clonidine restores the maximal activity of L-dopa and amphetamine in animals pretreated with an inhibitor of DA-β-hydroxylase. Similarly, clonidine greatly increases the locomotor stimulant effectiveness of the predominantly DA-mimetic apomorphine. These observations have been taken as evidence for the auxiliary role of central noradrenergic mechanisms for the dopaminergic control of locomotor activity (cf. Hornykiewicz, 1974).

3.2. Destruction of Specific Brain Regions and Fiber Tracts

The demonstration that DA was severely reduced in the striatum of Parkinsonian patients and that this decrease was likely a result of destruction of cell bodies in the pars compacta of the substantia nigra led to the proposal of a nigrostriatal pathway utilizing DA as the neurotransmitter. These findings together with the subsequent elucidation of the NA pathways laid the groundwork for animal models of Parkinson's disease. In early studies, monkeys receiving unilateral lesions of the ventromedial tegmentum displayed tremor and hypokinesia of the contralateral limbs. Concomitant with these symptoms was a loss of DA, HVA, and the related DA-synthesizing enzymes in the striatum homolateral to the nigral lesion. In contrast to the DA loss, the less severe decreases of 5-HT and NA did not parallel the degree of destruction of the substantia nigra, but rather the intrusion of the lesion into the median region of the ventromedial tegmentum (involving damage to the medial forebrain bundle) (Sourkes and Poirier, 1966; Goldstein *et al.,* 1966). Animals which had received lesions of similar magnitude but which did not involve the nigrostriatal tract were without effect on both the motor behavior and the catecholamine levels (Sourkes and Poirier, 1966; Goldstein *et al.,* 1966).

In addition to the monkey, the albino rat has frequently been used for the study of motor function. In these experiments bilateral or unilateral lesions were placed in the brain and the pharmacological and physiological responses observed.

3.2.1 Bilateral Lesions

Bilateral lesions of the substantia nigra by local stereotaxic injection of 6-hydroxy-DA (6-OH-DA) results in an initial hyperactivity for 1–2 days postoperatively, followed by a period of akinetic behavior and catalepsy. The animals are also adipsic and aphagic. After 3–4 weeks the animals recover autonomic functions, and their motor behavior is indistinguishable from unoperated animals (Ungerstedt, 1971). The initial phase of hyperactivity seems to be associated with the release of DA from degenerating striatal terminals, as there is first an increase and then a slow decline of DA levels for 48 hr after lesion of the nigrostriatal DA tracts (Andén et al., 1972). The NA neurons are unaltered by the nigral injection of 6-OH-DA (Hökfelt and Ungerstedt, 1973). In addition to the development of supersensitivity of DA receptors there likely takes place a readjustment of compensatory noncatecholaminergic mechanisms (e.g., cholinergic) which also modulate striatal activity.

In spite of the apparently normal motor behavior of these animals, their response to catecholaminergic drugs is distinctly abnormal. Thus, after either bilateral nigral destruction or intraventricular 6-OH-DA injection (which destroys not only nigrostriatal DA neurons but also NA neurons in the brain) amphetamine does not cause the increase in locomotor activity seen in unoperated animals (Fibiger, 1973; Iversen, 1971).

However, if in contrast to removing only the nigrostriatal DA neurons, the striatal DA receptors are also destroyed (by bilateral lesion of the striatum) the animal exhibits a different response to pharmacological treatment. Thus, the effects of L-dopa and amphetamine (which have a presynaptic mechanism) on stereotyped behavior are abolished, as is the cataleptogenic effect of perphenazine (Fog et al., 1970; Naylor and Olley, 1972).

3.2.2. Unilateral Lesions

Following unilateral lesion of the substantia nigra (or of the striatopetal fibers originating from the substantia nigra) the animals (rats) may have an initial transient asymmetry or else appear normal. There is a lack of asymmetry of posture or rotation movements, and there is no difference in the α- or γ-motoneuron activity between the two sides. However, these animals respond to pharmacological treatment in a manner different from either unoperated or bilaterally lesioned animals. Thus, reserpine treatment results in an asymmetric rigidity related to an increased motor unit activity (both at rest and in motion) on the side contralateral to the lesion. This is accompanied by an increase in α-motoneuron and decrease in γ-motoneuron activity. That these effects of reserpine are due to catecholamine depletion are implied by their reversal by L-dopa (cf. Andén et al., 1971).

Amphetamine treatment of unilaterally nigral-lesioned animals results in a turning of the animal to the lesioned side (Andén et al., 1971; Ungerstedt et al., 1973). This amphetamine-induced rotation does not occur in animals with unilateral raphe lesions. The effect of amphetamine is prevented by α-methyl-p-tyrosine but not by FLA-63 (a DA-β-hydroxylase inhibitor), indicating a specific DA component in the rotation (Andén, 1967; Marsden and Guldberg, 1973).

In these nigrally lesioned animals, injection of apomorphine results in turning behavior toward the unlesioned side (i.e., the opposite of the amphetamine effect). This response to apomorphine is enhanced as the duration of the postoperative period lengthens (cf. "denervation supersensitivity") (Ungerstedt, 1971).

If instead of the substantia nigra, the striatum is unilaterally lesioned (i.e., in addition to the neurons the receptors are also removed) the results of pharmacological treatment are in some ways quite different. Reserpine induces a turning to the side opposite the lesion with an abduction of the limbs of the operated side and adduction of those of the opposite side. Like the nigrally lesioned animal there is a rigidity of the limbs contralateral to the lesion which is reversed by L-dopa. In these striatally lesioned animals haloperidol or chlorpromazine results in a contralateral rotation, whereas phenoxybenzamine and propranalol do not induce asymmetries. If L-dopa, apomorphine, or amphetamine is injected in the lesioned animal the animals turn to the operated side, effects which are blocked by haloperidol (Andén, 1967).

The interpretation of these experiments has been commonly related to the disturbed balance between the nigrostriatal mechanisms of the hemispheres induced by such unilateral lesions. In animals receiving a unilateral lesion there may be an initial transient period of abnormal motor behavior which is soon eliminated by compensatory mechanisms of the brain. However, this compensation is unilateral, and thus the two sides of the brain will react differently to "stressful" situations (including drugs). If the lesion is placed in the substantia nigra the DA neurons and terminals degenerate, but the striatal receptors remain intact. In fact, it is believed that these receptors become supersensitive (as indicated by the increasing postoperative response to apomorphine) (Ungerstedt, 1971). Thus, in these animals, presynaptically acting agents (e.g., amphetamine) will affect the

DA terminals only on the unlesioned side with a resultant turning toward the lesion. In contrast, drugs which directly affect the receptors (apomorphine) will have a greater effect on the striatum of the lesioned hemisphere, because the denervated receptors have become supersensitive; thus, the result is a turning away from the lesioned side (Ungerstedt, 1971). If the striatum is unilaterally destroyed, both terminals and receptors are removed. Therefore, in these animals drugs which act presynaptically have the same effect as in an animal with a nigral lesion; in addition, in the striatally lesioned animal postsynaptically acting drugs will have the same effect as the presynaptically acting agents.

   3.2.2a. Spinal Cord Noradrenaline. The above considerations have dealt solely with the catecholamines present in the brain (excluding cerebellum). However, NA is also present in nerve terminals in the spinal cord. From histofluorescence and biochemical studies it appears that NA fibers (originating in the pons) terminate in the ventral and dorsal horns, the sympathetic lateral column, and the substantia gelatinosa (Dahlstrom and Fuxe, 1965) of the spinal cord. The normal physiological function of these neurons is at present not completely understood; however in the spinal animal L-dopa (or clonidine) increases flexor activity evoked by either pinching the hindlimb or by a tetanic stimulation of the flexor reflex afferents (cf. Andén, 1970). Similarly, stimulation of noradrenergic spinal mechanisms (with iv clonidine) promotes locomotion (on the treadmill) of the acute spinal cat (Forssberg and Grillner, 1973). Further insight into this problem may be obtained from the observation that stimulation of the VIIIth cranial nerve produces negative dorsal root potentials which are blocked or depressed by reserpine, tetrabenazine, or phenoxybenzamine and potentiated by nialamide (Barnes and Pompeiano, 1971). From the above observations it would appear that NA is involved at the spinal and lower brain stem levels in the control of locomotion and postural adjustments. As a matter of fact, these findings might be interpreted as supporting the pharmacologically demonstrable (see above) interdependence of central dopaminergic and noradrenergic mechanisms for locomotor activity.

4. CONCLUSION

   Both clinical and experimental studies indicate that the brain catecholamines are involved in the central control of motor function. If the locomotor aspects are considered, both dopamine and noradrenaline are important for the normal performance of motor activity. Dopaminergic neurons alone will sustain a basal motor behavior, whereas noradrenaline neurons will not. Stereotyped behavior is a motor behavior not involving locomotion as such and for which hyperactivity of the striatal dopaminergic neurons may be the underlying mechanism.

5. REFERENCES

Ajuriaguerra, J. de, Constantinidis, J., Eisenring, J. J., Yanniotis, G., and Tissot, R., 1972, Behavior disorders and L-dopa therapy in parkinson's Syndrome, in: *Parkinson's Disease, Vol. 1* (J. Siegfried, ed.), pp. 201–217, Hans Huber, Bern.

Andén, N.-E., 1967, Physiology and pharmacology of the nigro-neostriatal dopamine neurons, in: *Progress in Neurogenetics* (A. Barbeau and J. R. Brunette, eds.), pp. 265–271, Excerpta Med., Amsterdam.

Andén, N.-E., 1970, Effects of amphetamine and some other drugs on central catecholamine mechanism, in: *Amphetamines and Related Compounds* (E. Costa and S. Garattini, eds.), pp. 447–462, Raven Press.

Andén, N.-E., and Stock, G., 1973, Effect of clozapine on the turnover of dopamine in the corpus striatum and in the limbic system, *J. Pharm. Pharmacol.* **25**:346.

Andén, N.-E., Roos, B.-E., and Werdinius, B., 1964, Effects of chlorpromazine, haloperidol and reserpine on the levels of phenolic acids in rabbit corpus striatum, *Life Sci.* **3**:149.

Andén, N.-E., Rubenson, A., Fuxe, K., and Hökfelt, T., 1967, Evidence for dopamine receptor stimulation by Apomorphine, *J. Pharm. Pharmacol.* **19**:627.

Andén, N.-E., Larsson, K., and Steg, G., 1971, The influence of the nigro-neostriatal dopamine pathway on spinal motoneuron activity, *Acta Physiol. Scand.* **82**:268.

Andén, N.-E., Bédard, P., Fuxe, K., and Ungerstedt, U., 1972, Early and selective increase in brain dopamine levels after axotomy, *Experientia* **28**:300.

Arvidsson, J., Roos, B.-E., and Steg, G., 1966, Reciprocal effects on α- and γ-motoneurons of drugs influencing monoaminergic and cholinergic transmission, *Acta Physiol. Scand.* **67**:298.

Barbeau, A., 1969, L-Dopa therapy in parkinson's disease: A critical review of nine years experience. *Can. Med. Assoc. J.* **101**:791.

Barbeau, A., Chase, T. N., and Paulson, G. W., (eds.), 1973, Huntington's chorea, in: *Advances in Neurology, Vol. 1,* Raven Press, New York.

Barnes, C. D., and Pompeiano, 1971, The interaction of brain stem adrenergic systems with VIIIth nerve stimulation of the spinal cord, *Neuropharmacology* **19**:437.

Barolin, G. S., Bernheimer, H., and Hornykiewicz, O., 1964, Seitenverschiedenes Verhalten des Dopamin (3-Hydroxytyramin) in Gehirn eines Falles von Hemiparkinson. *Schweiz. Arch. Neurol. Psychiat.* **94**:241.

Bartholini, G., and Pletscher, A., 1969, Enhancement of tyrosine hydroxylation within the brain by cholorpromazine, *Experientia* **25**:919.

Bartholini, G., and Pletscher, A., 1972, Drugs affecting monoamines in the basal ganglia in: *Advances in Biochemical Psychopharmacology, Vol. 6,* (E. Costa, L. L. Iverson, and R. Paoletti, eds.), pp. 135–148, Raven Press, New York.

Bartholini, G., Haefely, W., Jalfre, M., Keller, H. H., and Pletscher, A., 1972, Effects of clozapine on cerebral catecholaminergic neuronal systems, *Brit. J. Pharmacol.* **46**:736.

Bédard, P., Larochelle, L., Poirier, L. J., and Sourkes, T. L., 1970, Reversible effect of L-dopa on tremor and catatonia induced by α-Methyl-p-tyrosine, *Can. J. Physiol. Pharmacol.* **48**:82.

Bernheimer, H., and Hornykiewicz, O., 1973, Brain amines in Huntington's chorea, in: *Advances in Neurology, Vol. 1* (A. Barbeau, T. N. Chase, and G. W. Paulson, eds.), pp. 525–531, Raven Press, New York.

Bernheimer, H., Birkmayer, W., Hornykiewicz, O., Jellinger, K., and Seitelberger, F., 1973, Brain dopamine and the syndromes of Parkinson and Huntington, *J. Neurol. Sci.* **20**:415.

Birkmayer, W., 1969, The Alpha-methyl-*p*-tyrosine effect in extrapyramidal disorders. *Wien. Klin. Wochschr.* **81**:10.

Blasckho, H., and Chrusciel, T. L., 1969, The decarboxylation of amino acids related to tyrosine and their awakening action in reserpine-treated mice, *J. Physiol.* **151**:272.

Bunney, B. S., Walters, J. R., Roth, R. H. and Aghajanian, G. K., 1973, Dopaminergic neurons: Effects of antipsychotic drugs and amphetamines on single cell activity, *J. Pharm. Pharmacol.* **185**:560.

Butcher, L. L., and Engel, J., 1969, Peripheral factors in the mediation of the effects of L-dopa on locomotor activity, *J. Pharm. Pharmacol.* **26**:614.

Calne, D. B., 1970, *Parkinsonism,* Arnold, London.

Calne, D. B., and Reid, J. L., 1972, Antiparkinsonian drugs: Pharmacological and therapeutic aspects, *Drugs* **4**:49.

Carlsson, A., 1970, Amphetamine and brain catecholamines, in: *Amphetamines and Related Compounds* (E. Costa and S. Garattini, eds.), pp. 289–300, Raven Press, New York.

Carlsson, A., Lindquist, M., and Magnusson, T., 1957, 3,4-Dihydroxyphenylalanine and 5-hydroxytryptophan as reserpine antagonists, *Nature* **180**:1200.

Cools, A. R., 1973, *The Caudate Nucleus and Neurochemical Control of Behavior,* Brakkenstein, Nijmegen.

Crane, G. E., 1972, Pseudoparkinsonism and tardive dyskinesia, *Arch. Neurol.* **27**:426.

Dahlström, A., and Fuxe, K., 1965, Evidence for the existence of monoamine neurons in the central nervous system. II. Experimentally induced changes in the intraneuronal amine levels of bulbospinal neurone systems, *Acta Physiol. Scand. Suppl.* **247**:1.

DaPrada, M., and Pletscher, A., 1966, On the mechanism of chlorpromazine-induced changes of cerebral homovanillic acid, *J. Pharm. Pharmacol.* **18**:628.

Davidson, L., Lloyd, K. G., Dankova, J., and Hornykiewicz, O., 1971, L-dopa treatment in Parkinson's disease: Effect on dopamine and related substances in discrete brain regions, *Experientia* **27**:1048.

Degwitz, R., 1969, Extrapyramidal motor disorders following long-term treatment with neuroleptic drugs, in: *Psychotropic Drugs and Dysfunctions of the Basal Ganglia* (G. E. Crane and R. Gardner, eds.), Public Health Service Publ. 1938, U.S. Govt. Printing Office, Washington, D.C.

Duvoisin, R., 1972, Clinical diagnosis of the dyskinesias, *Med. Clin. N. Am.* **56**:1321.

Duvoisin, R., Barrett, R., Schear, M., Hoehn, M. and Yahr, M., 1969, The use of L-dopa in Parkinsonism, in: *Third Symposium on Parkinson's Disease* (F. J. Gillingham and I. M. L. Donaldson, eds.), pp. 185–192, Livingstone, Edinburgh.

Fibiger, H. C., 1973, Behavioral pharmacology of *d*-amphetamine: Some metabolic and pharmacological considerations, in: *Frontiers in Catecholamine Research* (F. Usdin and S. H. Snyder, eds.), pp. 933–937, Pergamon Press, New York.

Fog, R., 1972, *On Stereotype and Catalepsy: Studies on the Effect of Amphetamines and Neuroleptics in Rats,* Munksgaard, Copenhagen.

Fog, R., Randrup, A., and Pakkenberg, H., 1970, Lesions in corpus striatum and cortex of rat brains and the effect of pharmacologically induced stereotyped, aggressive and cataleptic behavior, *Psychopharmacologia* **18**:246.

Forssberg, H., and Grillner, S., 1973, The locomotion of the acute spinal cat injected with clonidine iv, *Brain Res.* **50**:184.

Gerstenbrand, F., Pateisky, K., and Prosenz, P., 1963, Erfahrungen mit L-dopa in der Therapie des Parkinsonismus, *Psychiat. Neurol.* **146**:246.

Goldstein, M., Anagnoste, B., Owen, W. S., and Battista, A. S., 1966, The effects of ventromedial tegmental lesions on the biosynthesis of catecholamines in the striatum, *Life Sci.* **5**:2171.

Goldstein, M., Battista, A. F., Ohmoto, T., Anagnoste, B., and Fuxe, K., 1973, Tremor and involuntary movements in monkeys: Effects of L-dopa and of a dopamine receptor stimulating agent, *Science* **179**:816.

Granit, R., 1970, *The Basis of Motor Control,* Academic Press, London and New York.

Greenblatt, D. J., Shader, R. I., and DiMascio, A., 1970, Extrapyramidal effects, in: *Psychotropic Drug Side Effects* (R. I. Shader and A. DiMascio, eds.), pp. 92–106, Williams and Wilkins, Baltimore.

Hökfelt, T., and Ungerstedt, U., 1973, Specificity of 6-hydroxydopamine induced degeneration of central monoamine neurones: An electron and fluorescent microscopic study with special reference to intracerebral injection and the striatal dopamine system, *Brain Res.* **60**:269.

Hornykiewicz, O., 1966a, Dopamine and brain function, *Pharmacol. Rev.* **18**:925.

Hornykiewicz, O., 1966b, Metabolism of brain dopamine in human Parkinsonism: Neurochemical and clinical aspects, in: *Biochemistry and Pharmacology of the Basal Ganglia,* (E. Costa, L. J. Côté, and M. D. Yahr, eds.) pp. 171–181, Raven Press, New York.

Hornykiewicz, O., 1974, The mechanisms of action of L-dopa in Parkinson's disease, *Life Sci.* **15**:1249.

Iversen, S. D., 1971, The effect of surgical lesions to frontal cortex and substantia nigra on amphetamine responses in rats, *Brain Res.* **31**:295.

Keller, H. H., Bartholini, G., and Pletscher, A., 1973, Increase of 3-methoxy-4-hydroxyphenylethyleneglycol in rat brain by neuroleptic drugs, *European J. Pharmacol.* **23**:183.

Klawans, H. L., 1968, The pharmacology of Parkinsonism, *Diseases Nervous System* **29**:805.

Klawans, H. L., 1973, The pharmacology of tardive dyskinesias, *Am. J. Psychiat.* **130**:82.

Korczyn, A. D., 1973, pathophysiology of drug-induced dyskinesias, *Neuropharmacology* **11**:601.

Lloyd, K. G., and Hornykiewicz, O., 1972, Dopamine uptake into striatal synaptosomes of normal and Parkinsonian patients, *Fifth Intern. Cong. Pharmacol.* (abstr.).

Lloyd, K. G., Davidson, L., and Hornykiewicz, O., 1973, Metabolism of levodopa in the human brain, in: *Advances in Neurology, Vol. 3* (D. B. Calne, eds.), pp. 173–188, Raven Press, New York.

Lloyd, K. G., Davidson, L., and Hornykiewicz, O., 1974, The biochemistry of parkinsonism: Effects of levodopa treatment, (in preparation).

Markham, C. H., 1971, The choreoathetoid movement disorders induced by L-dopa, in: *Monoamines Noyaux Gris Centraux et Syndrome de Parkinson* (J. de Ajuriaguerra and G. Gauthier, eds.), pp. 485–490, Masson, Paris.

Marsden, C. A., and Guldberg, H. C., 1973, The role of monoamines in rotation induced by amphetamine after nigral, raphe and mesencephalic reticular lesions in the rat brain, *Neuropharmacology* **12**:195.

Mones, R. J., Elizan, T. S. and Siegel, G. J., 1971, Analysis of L-dopa-induced dyskinesias in 51 patients with parkinsonism, *J. Neurol. Neurosurg.* **34**: 668.

Naylor, R. J., and Olley, J. E., 1972, Modification of the behavioral changes induced by amphetamine in the rat by lesions in the caudate nucleus, the caudate-putamen and globus pallidus, *Neuropharmacology* **11**:91.

Nyback, H., and Sedvall, G., 1970, Further studies on the accumulation and disappearance of catecholamines formed from tyrosine-^{14}C in mouse brain. Effect of some phenothiazine analogues, *European J. Pharmacol.* **10**:193.

Postma, J. U., 1972, Haloperidol in dopa-induced chorea-athetosis, *Psychiat. Neurol. Neurochir.* **75**:69.

Randrup, A., and Munkvad, I., 1970, Biochemical, anatomical and psychological investigations of stereotyped behavior induced by amphetamine, in: *Amphetamines and Related Compounds* (E. Costa and S. Garattini, eds.), pp. 695–713, Raven Press, New York.

Ringel, S. P., Guthrie, M., and Klawans, H. L., Jr., 1973, Current treatment of Huntington's chorea, in: *Advances in Neurology, Vol. 1* (A. Barbeau, T. N. Chase, and G. W. Paulson, eds.), pp. 797–801, Raven Press, New York.

Rubovits, R., Patel, B. C., and Klawans, H. L., 1973, Effect of prolonged chlorpromazine pretreatment on the threshold for amphetamine stereotype: A model for tardive dyskinesias, in: *Advances in Neurology, Vol. 1* (A. Barbeau, T. N. Chase, and G. W. Paulson, eds.), pp. 671–679, Raven Press, New York.

Sassin, J. F., Taub, S., and Weitzman, E. D., 1972, Hyperkinesia and changes in behavior produced in normal monkeys by L-dopa, *Neurology* **22**:1122.

Sourkes, T. L., and Poirier, L. J., 1966, Neurochemical basis of tremor and other disorders of movement, *Can. Med. Assoc. J.* **94**:53.

Steg, G., 1972, Pathophysiological aspects in Parkinson's syndrome, *Acta Neurol. Scand.* **48**: Suppl. 51, pp. 139–150.

Ungerstedt, U., 1971, Use of intracerebral injections of 6-hydroxydopamine as a tool for morphological and functional studies on central catecholamine neurons, in: *6-Hydroxydopamine and Catecholamine Neurons* (T. Malmfors and H. Thoenen, eds.), pp. 315–332, North-Holland, Amsterdam.

Ungerstedt, U., Avemo, A., Ljungberg, T. and Ranje, C., 1973, Animal models of Parkinsonism, in: *Advances in Neurology, Vol. 3* (D. B. Calne, ed.), pp. 257–271, Raven Press, New York.

Chapter 3

Catecholamines in Behavior and Sensorimotor Integration: The Neostriatal System

George M. Krauthamer

College of Medicine and Dentistry of New Jersey
Rutgers Medical School
New Brunswick, New Jersey

1. INTRODUCTION

The basal ganglia and their significance for behavior and brain function continue to provide major challenges to neurobiology. Indeed, the enormous progress of the past 15 years in the neurochemistry and neuropharmacology of the corpus striatum has not simply solved old problems; it has recast many of them in a new light and added quite a few new ones of its own.

The demonstration that the neostriatum is the largest catecholamine-containing area of the brain and that its dopamine concentration is among the highest of all brain regions has acted as a powerful catalyst to neurobiological research. The evidence linking Parkinson's disease to a reduction in striatal dopamine and the dramatic results of L-dopa therapy have underscored the importance of dopamine for brain function. Since the maintenance of a normal catecholamine metabolism in the neostriatum is dependent upon the dopaminergic pathway linking some neurons of the substantia nigra with those of the caudate nucleus and putamen, the nigrostriatal projection system has come to occupy a key position in the currently widely accepted concept of the function of the basal ganglia (Bartholini and Pletscher, 1972; Hornykiewicz, 1972a; Van Rossum, 1970; Bloom and Giarman, 1968; Crane and Gardner, 1968).

It is perhaps natural that these recent discoveries should have overshadowed other aspects of neostriatal structure and function, but it would be premature to conclude that these have ceased to be of importance. In its simplest form, the dopamine view of striatal function directly and causally associates the nigrostriatal system and the dopamine concentration of the neostriatum with neuronal inhibition, phasic behavioral arousal, and the control of motor and postural activity by the extrapyramidal motor system. It has, in fact, been termed variously the hemi-Parkinsonian model system or dopamine deficiency syndrome (Bolme et al., 1972; Brimblecombe and Pinder, 1972; Hornykiewicz, 1972b; Snyder et al., 1972; Shellenberger, 1971). Despite the wealth of data correlating catecholamine levels, drug effects, and motor behavior, one may question the heuristic value of this model as one designed to increase specifically our understanding of striatal neurophysiology and its morphological basis. It is the author's viewpoint that this model is unsatisfactory in its present form because it fails to integrate much of the catecholamine data with important aspects of neostriatal structure and function. In short, the model tends to bypass these two variables intervening between neurochemistry and behavior. The present chapter makes no attempt to present an alternative model; it will merely try to highlight those issues which need to be reexamined in terms of the catecholamine-related findings. Its aim is to broaden our perspective and, hopefully, balance our view of dopamine in terms of neostriatal functions as they are presently known.

The neostriatum is a large aggregate of neurons with very extensive afferent and efferent connections enmeshed in an elaborate intrinsic neuropil; it is a brain region not only rich in dopamine but also in acetylcholine, γ-aminobutyric acid, serotonin, and their enzyme systems (McGeer et al., 1971; Okady et al., 1971; Hassler and Bak, 1969; Portig and Vogt, 1969; Shute and Lewis, 1967). There is evidence that the basal ganglia in general, and the corpus striatum, neostriatum, or caudate-putamen in particular, are implicated in a range of functions which are more appropriately viewed in terms of central neuronal modulation, sensorimotor integration and complex behavioral and perceptual alterations. This evidence has been contributed by a wide array of techniques: clinical observation, behavioral studies, neurophysiological experiments, and anatomical analysis.

2. CLINICAL CONSIDERATIONS

Speculations and suggestions that the striatum is implicated in the etiology of schizophrenia go back to the turn of the century when attention was first drawn to a possible relationship between the corpus striatum and the bizarre posturing and catatonic stance seen in schizophrenia (Warburton, 1967). More recently, Mettler and Crandall (1959) have reemphasized this possibility as have other authors at various times (Klawans *et al.*, 1972; Kline and Mettler, 1961; Hopf, 1954). The fact that the antipsychotic phenothiazines have the induction of dyskinesia as their major side effect is common knowledge. Since these neuroleptics change *inter alia* the dopaminergic functions of the striatum, the suggested participation of the corpus striatum in the genesis of emotional disorders is not particularly far-fetched (MacLean, 1972; Schildkraut and Kety, 1967; Kety, 1959). Similarly, the restitution of striatal dopamine by the administration of L-dopa in therapeutic doses has led to a wide variety of behavioral and psychiatric side effects (Murphy *et al.*, 1972, 1973; Malitz, 1972; Celesia and Barr, 1970). Conversely, there are a good many clinical reports about behavioral and psychiatric symptoms seen in patients whose primary disorder is paralysis agitans (Warburton, 1967).

Observations such as these are merely suggestive of a striatal involvement in certain emotional disturbances. They can provide no information as to the possible morphological and functional correlates, but they do emphasize that to approach the study of striatal functions exclusively in terms of extrapyramidal motor mechanisms may be an oversimplication (Divac, 1968a; Krauthamer and Albe-Fessard, 1964).

3. BEHAVIORAL OBSERVATIONS

Experimental studies of behavior which indicate that the corpus striatum is of importance in the performance of acts other than postural or motor are of two kinds. One set of data deals with the alteration of performances which were not acquired in specifically structured learning situations; that is, essentially "unlearned" behavior and complex sequential acts of adaptive value. The other set of data deals with the alterations seen in a variety of specifically learned tasks. The advantage of the latter is their ease of quantification and replication, the advantage of the former is their intrinsic value to the organism and their adaptive significance for the organism's interplay with its environment.

In a careful study of cats with small unilateral and bilateral caudate lesions Gybels *et al.* (1967) observed an array of disturbances outside the motor or sensory spheres proper. Visually guided and tactually guided behavior, attack–defense reactions, and a variety of complex performances such as eating, prey-catching, and playing were altered. According to the authors "a peculiar discrepancy between the integrity of the elementary motor and sensory functions and the appearance of severe motor and sensory disturbances as soon as the animal finds itself in a behavioral situation" represented the most striking feature of the syndrome. Similar conclusions have been arrived at by other investigators (Wang and Akert, 1962; Mettler, 1955; Mettler et al., 1939). All modalities of sensorimotor integration were involved but not to the same extent. Visuomotor integration was most severely affected; in cats with unilateral caudate lesions, a contralateral visual field neglect could be demonstrated and differentiated from true hemianopsia. These results bear a close resemblance to the more restricted observations of Wang and Akert (1962). Based on a behavioral comparison of decorticate cats with and without intact neostriatum (striatal vs. thalamic cats) the authors concluded that the corpus striatum had additional functions quite apart from the previously described "motor inactivation syndrome" (Akert and Andersson, 1951). These other functions were characterized as the maintenance of the proper sequential occurrence of reflexes in the performance of complex acts. Thus, intactness of the striatum was required for the proper performance of spontaneous eating, grooming, and mating behavior. The effective performance of such organized behavioral sequences is definable neither as an exclusively motor sequence nor as a sensory processing; more appropriately, it is thought of as a function of central modulation essential to sensorimotor integration.

Quantifiable disturbances of visuomotor integration have been described in the monkey on a visuomotor tracking task (Bowen, 1969) and in Parkinsonian patients on the "Aubert task," a test of visual–postural performance (Teuber and Proctor, 1964). The deficit on the Aubert task is noteworthy for two reasons. It may implicate the vestibular system (Potegal et al., 1971) but, more significantly, abnormal performance on the Aubert task is also characteristic of patients with frontal lobe injury (Teuber and Mishkin, 1954). This relationship in man between frontal lobes, caudate nucleus, and deficit on a specific behavioral task is most intriguing because of the analogous situation presented by the delayed alternation and delayed response performance of primates and cats.

In monkeys, ablation of the dorsolateral frontal cortex causes a selective impairment of delayed alternation performance but not of other learned tasks such as visual discrimination or object reversal (Dean and Davis, 1959; Rosvold et al., 1958). Lesions limited to the head of the caudate nucleus similarly impair performance on delayed-response type tasks (Rosvold and Szwarcbart, 1964) as do other methods of interfering with striatal functions such as electrical stimulation (Rosvold and Delgado, 1956) and localized but reversible cooling of the caudate nucleus (Krauthamer et al., 1967b).

Qualitatively analogous deficits have been reported in cats (Kitsikis et *al.*, 1972; Kitsikis and Roberge, 1973; Divac, 1968*b*) and in rats (Schmaltz and Isaacson, 1968; Gross *et al.*, 1965). In their recent studies, Kitsikis *et al.*, (1972; Kitsikis and Roberge, 1973) have been able to demonstrate for the first time a functional relationship between striatal dopamine levels and delayed-response performance. Such a relationship is also suggested by the earlier results of Cianci (1965) who noted impaired performance following electrical stimulation of the substantia nigra.

Delayed-response tasks represent very complex types of behavior, and it is likely that delayed-response impairment can not be attributed to a single or "simple" behavioral variable (Gross and Weiskrantz, 1964; Teuber, 1964). Whatever its cause, it is a deficit which cannot be readily explained within the traditional concept of extrapyramidal motor functions. The critical cortical area, the dorsolateral prefrontal convexity surrounding the sulcus principalis, lies well rostral to motor and premotor cortex (areas 4 and 6) or the frontal eye field (area 8), and it does not receive thalamic projections from the ventrolateral nucleus which is implicated in the extrapyramidal functions of the basal ganglia. The specificity of the delayed-response deficit is striking because it is restricted to this portion of cortex and its caudate projection territory only. The other major subcortical projection zone of the dorsolateral cortex is the dorsomedial nucleus of the thalamus. Attempts to interfere with delayed-response tasks by lesions restricted to the dorsomedial nucleus have been inconclusive or negative (Schulman, 1964; Rosvold *et al.*, 1958; Chow, 1954). However, reminiscent of the contralateral visual neglect observed by Gybels *et al.* (1967) to follow small caudate lesions, Orem *et al.* (1973) have reported a seemingly similar visual neglect following dorsomedial thalamic lesions. Although there is no conclusive evidence that dorsomedial thalamic lesions or stimulation can reproduce the delayed-response deficit associated with striatal or frontal cortical sites (Schulman, 1964; Rosvold *et al.*, 1958), conditioned avoidance and bar-press behavior are altered by lesions or stimulation of nucleus dorsalis medialis (Means *et al.*, 1973; Delacour, 1971; Rougeul *et al.*, 1967). It appears therefore, that some behavioral functions are susceptible to striatal as well as thalamic lesions, whereas others are selectively susceptible to lesions of one subcortical projection zone but not to lesions of the other.

A further complicating note is introduced by ontogenetic studies. These have shown that there is recovery from the effects of dorsolateral cortical ablation on delayed alternation performance when the lesion is made in young monkeys, but that no such recovery of function is observed following early caudate lesions (Goldman and Rosvold, 1972). These results indicate that the two structures are not functionally equivalent and that the difference in impairment of delayed alternation is more than a simple quantitative one.

Other disturbances of learned behavior have been linked to striatal functions. Impaired maze learning has been demonstrated in rats with striatal lesions or following electrical stimulation at various phases of maze learning (Peeke and Herz, 1971; Gross *et al.*, 1965). Classical and instrumental conditioned responses can be transiently blocked in cats by the intracaudate injection of potassium chloride (Prado-Alcala *et al.*, 1973). Passive avoidance, which requires the inhibition of a previously learned response in order to avoid punishment, has been impaired by striatal lesions and electrical stimulation (Gold and King, 1972; Kirkby and Kimble, 1968; Wyers *et al.*, 1968; Fox *et al.*, 1964). Analogous results have been observed in tasks of active avoidance or escape which require a specific response such as bar-pressing or hurdle-jumping to avoid punishment (Allen and Davison, 1973; Green *et al.*, 1967; Fox *et al.*, 1964).

The impairment of avoidance conditioning is not the result of interference with the requisite motor or sensory activities nor is it related to any resultant generalized hyperactivity (Allen and Davison, 1973). Since a deficit in passive avoidance learning could be observed when the caudate stimulation was delayed as long as 30 sec, Wyers *et al.*, (1968) believe that perceptual disorganization cannot explain the impairment, and that interference with memory storage processes is a more probable hypothesis, as it is for similar effects observed after thalamic stimulation (Mahut, 1964).

Bar-pressing behavior on various schedules of positive reinforcement or reward can also be arrested by caudate stimulation (Schoenfeld and Seiden, 1969). Liebman and Butcher (1973) noted that rats pressing a lever to receive electrical self-stimulation of the lateral hypothalamus would reduce the lever-pressing rate following pharmacological manipulations of predominantly dopaminergic transmission mechanisms, thus suggesting that the effects of rewarding self-stimulation may not be entirely attributable to noradrenergic mechanisms of the hypothalamus as is commonly assumed. This observation is, perhaps, of wider significance in view of the reported dopaminergic nature of the lateral hypothalamic syndrome involving alimentary behavior (Fibiger *et al.*, 1973; Ungerstedt, 1971).

Striatal dopamine has been implicated in the maintenance and acquisition of conditioned avoidance behavior (Cooper *et al.*, 1973; Fuxe and Hanson, 1967), but serotonergic (Cools, 1972) and cholinergic mechanisms have also been implicated (Haycock *et al.*, 1973; Deadwyler *et al.*, 1971; Hull *et al.*, 1967; Stevens *et al.*, 1961). The fact that the manipulation of dopaminergic and cholinergic mechanisms, electrical stimulation, lesions, cooling, and functional depression by KCl all result in a disturbed performance and, at times, the impaired acquisition of complex learned behavior sequences does not lend itself to a simple unimodal interpretation. Rather, it strengthens the concept of the striatum as an integrative structure with mutually interdependent cholinergic and dopaminergic mechanisms in which a variety of neurotransmitters may be critically implicated (Keller *et al.*, 1973; Bak *et al.*, 1972; Lalley *et al.*, 1970; Barbeau, 1962).

The alteration of complex learned behaviors as evidenced on conditioned-avoidance and delayed-response tasks cannot be fitted into the classical schema of basal ganglia circuitry (Jung and Hassler, 1960). These observations are clearly set apart from the ipsiversive and contraversive circling and the various forms of "arrest reaction" or striatal inactivation syndrome which result from interference with normal striatal functions and which can be more readily understood in terms of the anatomical connections between the basal ganglia, motor cortex, ventrolateral thalamus, and other "extrapyramidal" structures. However, even these reactions are not simply effects on posture and movement since gross interference with the execution of movements by capsular stimulation is ineffective (Buser *et al.*, 1964). Furthermore, autonomic, alimentary, psychomotor, and other affective responses are also elicited (Liles and Davis, 1969*a*; Dieckmann and Hassler, 1967; Lewin *et al.*, 1967; Rubinstein and Delgado, 1963). Moreover, the effect of striatal stimulation on learned and unlearned movements depends upon the type of movement and effort required, degree of motivation, intensity and frequency of stimulation, and site of stimulation within the neostriatum (Kitsikis, 1968; Hassler and Dieckman, 1967; Buchwald *et al.*, 1964; Mettler, 1955).

Abnormal movements and alterations of postural tone can also be produced by chemical stimulation, analogous to that used for the impairment of conditioned behavior. Direct involvement of dopaminergic mechanisms has been suggested as the primary cause (Cools, 1972, 1973; Frigyesi *et al.*, 1971; Ungerstedt *et al.*, 1969). Others have reported similar effects following the intrastriatal application of KCl (Weiss and Fifkova, 1963), or cholinergic and anticholinergic drugs (Keller *et al.*, 1973; Costall *et al.*, 1972: Lalley *et al.*, 1970).

There is evidence of a definite organization of functions within the neostriatum. Divac *et al.* (1967) have shown that different portions of the caudate nucleus subserve different behavioral functions. Similarly, Liles and Davis (1969*a*) have delineated neostriatal zones which when stimulated or lesioned, are either excitatory or inhibitory for cortically evoked movements. Finally, Hassler and Dieckman (1967) have emphasized the difference in motor effects obtained upon stimulation of the putamen or caudate nucleus, and Cools (1973) has provided evidence that a differentiation of function within the neostriatum can also be demonstrated pharmacologically.

This regional functional differentiation of the neostriatum is matched by the recent anatomical evidence which has demonstrated an orderly, topographically organized system of afferent and efferent neostriatal projections.

Whether the functionally differentiated regions of the neostriatum have their exact counterpart in the anatomical projection topography remains to be demonstrated. As far as the dopaminergic mechanisms are concerned, they presumably operate in all regions of the neostriatum since there is no consistent evidence for local differences in concentration or local aggregates of dopamine-sensitive neurons.

4. ANATOMICAL STUDIES

Like much of the behavioral data, the afferent and efferent anatomical projections of the striatum are not readily compressed within the classical extrapyramidal motor system, but they are more readily correlated with the available neurophysiological evidence of widespread striatal influences on central neuronal mechanisms.

The neostriatum receives its major direct inputs from three different sources: the neocortex, the thalamus, and the substantia nigra; it thus entertains direct synaptic relations with the telencephalon, diencephalon, and mesencephalon. In primates and subprimates there exists an orderly and precise topographic projection of practically the entire neocortical mantle upon the whole of the corpus striatum (Kemp and Powell, 1970; Johnson et al., 1968; Webster, 1965). These findings, based upon silver impregnation methods of orthograde terminal degeneration, Golgi studies, and electron microscopy have been comprehensively presented and summarized by Kemp and Powell (1971e). The evidence forces a major revision of the earlier notion of a nontopographic projection largely restricted to the precentral gyrus or motor and premotor cortex (Jung and Hassler, 1960).

Basically, the topographic organization of the cortical projections proceeds in a dorsoventral and rostrocaudal direction so that the frontal lobe projects anteriorly and the occipital lobe posteriorly, with temporal projections passing ventrally; similarly the medial, lateral, and orbital aspects of the frontal lobe project dorsally, laterally, and medially upon the caudate nucleus and putamen. The existence of an orderly topographic projection does not, however, imply strict point-to-point projection. On the contrary, there is an extensive overlap from adjacent cortical regions, and this overlap of functionally heterogeneous cortical zones may constitute part of the morphological substrate for the considerable functional convergence observed in the caudate nucleus.

The motor cortex provides a large contribution to the corticostriatal projection but, as Kemp and Powell (1970) have pointed out, an equally substantial projection is derived from the somatosensory cortex.

Phylogenetic differences are reflected in the increased contribution of the frontal and parieto-temporal granular or "association" cortex to the striatal projections. Thus, in the cat, the projection of the sensorimotor cortex leads to degeneration in a very large area of the striatum, but in the monkey the increase in cortical "association" areas is reflected in the proportionately larger volume of striatum given over to projections from association cortex as compared to sensorimotor cortex (Kemp and Powell, 1970; Webster, 1965). The fact that the corticostriatal connections are not only definable in structural terms but that they also correspond to a functional topography defined in terms of complex learned behaviors has been strongly emphasized by Johnson et al., (1968).

The thalamic projections to the striatum originate in the intralaminar nuclei (Mehler, 1966; Powell and Cowan, 1956). Centralis lateralis, centralis medialis, and paracentralis project to the head of the caudate nucleus; centrum medianum and parafascicularis project largely or exclusively to the putamen. Comparable to the corticostriate input, the projections of the intralaminar thalamus are topographically organized in an anteroposterior dimension, but unlike the corticostriate projections which have a dorsoventral orientation, the thalamic ones follow a mediolateral distribution pattern. The potential significance of the dorsoventral and mediolateral distribution of cortical and thalamic afferent fibers lies in the further increase of convergence due to the resulting grid pattern of termination. Thus, fibers originating in centrum medianum would be in synaptic contact with projections emanating from medial, lateral, and ventral cortex. Indeed, Kemp and Powell (1971c,d) have concluded that cortical and thalamic fibers terminate on the same striatal neurons, both almost exclusively on dendritic spines. Such an arrangement, in a crossed register, should expose all portions of the striatum to a functionally and structurally organized dual input. Cortical motor, somatosensory, auditory, visual, and association activity would thus interact with the largely nonspecific, polysensory, and arousal-related diencephalic input.

On the other hand, there is no convincing evidence for striatal projections from the principal thalamic nuclei, including nucleus ventralis anterior and nucleus ventralis lateralis (Strick, 1973; Johnson, 1961; Powell and Cowan, 1956). Thus, it is evident that the direct thalamostriatal input, even more than the corticostriatal one, is not from nuclei related predominantly to extrapyramidal structures and motor cortex or sensory cortex but from nonspecific regions of the thalamus.

Projections from the mesencephalic tegmentum, exclusive of substantia nigra, are relatively sparse and can hardly be of great significance as a striatal input in contrast to the cortical and thalamic influx (Nauta and Kuypers, 1958). On the other hand, the projection from the substantia nigra, long-denied and disputed by neuroanatomists (Mettler, 1970; Carpenter and Strominger, 1967; Cole *et al.*, 1964) has turned out to be an input of absolutely primary importance since it is the only one responsible for the dopaminergic functions of the neostriatum.

The ascending projection is essential for the maintenance of normal striatal dopamine and tyrosine hydroxylase levels since lesions of the medial substantia nigra, pars compacta, lead to a marked reduction of striatal dopamine within a few days (Bédard *et al.*, 1969a; Faull and Laverty, 1969; Goldstein *et al.*, 1967, 1969; Poirier *et al.*, 1967a, 1969). Lesions of the thalamus or cortex are not followed by changes in striatal dopamine biosynthesis (Battista *et al.*, 1969; Bédard *et al.*, 1969b; Poirier *et al.*, 1967b). The postulation of a single dopaminergic input is made most plausible by these findings.

The initial histofluorescent demonstrations (Andén *et al.*, 1964; Dahlström and Fuxe, 1964) of the nigrostriatal pathway have since been substantiated by conventional neuroanatomical methods and autoradiography (Hattori *et al.*, 1973; Maler *et al.*, 1973; Carpenter and Peter, 1972; Hedreen, 1971; Mettler, 1970). Like the cortical and thalamic projections, the nigrostriatal projection is topographically organized and is reciprocally linked with caudate and putamen (Niimi *et al.*, 1970; Szabo, 1970, 1967; Voneida, 1960).

The efferent projections of the striatum reach only two structures, the substantia nigra and the globus pallidus (Szabo, 1962, 1967, 1970; Adinolfi, 1969; Cowan and Powell, 1966; Voneida, 1960). Claims for striatocortical projection have at times been entertained on neurophysiological and anatomical grounds but these have not found wide acceptance (Ermolaeva and Ermolenko, 1972; Ermolenko, 1971; Li, 1966; Spehlmann *et al.*, 1960; Purpura *et al.*, 1958).

The pallidal projection is unquestionably the major efferent pathway for the neostriatum so that the external and internal segments of the globus pallidus, or entopeduncular nucleus in subprimates, can be regarded as a veritable funnel for the striatal outflow.

Since neither the cortex nor the thalamus nor the midbrain, exclusive of substantia nigra, seem to be the recipients of direct striatal efferent projections, it is to the globus pallidus that one must turn to understand the pathways by which the striatum and its dopaminergic nigral input can exert their action on other portions of the brain and, eventually, on behavior. Leaving aside the reciprocal loop joining the pallidum with the subthalamic nucleus of Luys (Nakamura and Sutin, 1972; Carpenter *et al.*, 1968; Carpenter and Strominger, 1967) the pallidal outflow is predominantly directed toward the thalamus. Reaching the thalamus via the fasciculus lenticularis and the ansalenticularis, forming a continuous, anteroposteriorly directed curved sheet of fibers, the terminations are most dense in portions of the lateral and anterior ventral nuclei, the intralaminar nuclei, including centrum medianum and perhaps the parvocellular portion of the dorsomedial nucleus (Kuo and Carpenter, 1973; Kaelber, 1967; Nauta and Mehler, 1966; Khalifeh et al., 1965; Johnson, 1961; Nauta and Whitlock, 1954). In the ventrolateral nucleus there is a considerable overlap with fibers from the brachium conjunctivum which have originated in the deep cerebellar nuclei. The thalamocortical projection of this region is primarily to the motor and premotor cortex and thus in a position to exert a rather direct influence on the corticospinal and corticobulbar pathways. It is that portion of the striatal output most directly identifiable with the postural and motor functions of the striatum both in terms of the functional specialization as well as in terms of the massiveness of the fiber projection. Presumably, the lesser projections terminating in the fields of Forel and the perirubral region of the midbrain have a similar functional significance (Nauta and Mehler, 1966).

The intralaminar projections involve a fundamentally different anatomic and functional organization. These nuclei receive an equally important contingent of the pallidal output as the ventrolateral nucleus, perhaps by collaterals of the same pallidal axons or by independent fibers. However, with the exception of centrum medianum, they do not enter into the same close or predominant association with cerebellum and motor cortex. Instead, they are intimately related to the ascending reticular system and the spinothalamic tract (Boivie, 1971; Scheibel and Scheibel, 1970; Mehler, 1966; Bowsher, 1965). The functional significance of these connections must be sought in the ascending arousal mechanisms and the polysensory or sensory convergence features which, by means of the intralaminar thalamus, are directly linked with the neostriatum. A special position must be assigned to the centrum medianum. Defined in its large sense, as the centrum medianum–parafascicular complex, it can be considered jointly with the other intralaminar nuclei, indeed it becomes an important component of the intralaminar system. But, defined in the strictest sense, the centrum medianum occupies a unique place among the thalamic recipients of striopallidal projections (Bowsher, 1966; Mehler, 1966). It is generally conceded that the centrum medianum receives projections from the motor cortex but there is some question as to its afferent projections from other cortical areas and, more importantly, its efferent projections to the cortex (Rasminsky et al., 1973; Albe-Fessard et al., 1971; Benita and Condé, 1971; Murray, 1966). Its intrathalamic connections are poorly known, though perhaps no less so than those of any other thalamic nuclei (Scheibel and Scheibel, 1972).

Among the intrathalamic connections it is important to underline the reciprocal relationships between the centrum medianum and the anterior and lateral ventral nuclear group; it not only provides a thalamic integrative circuit between the sensory nonspecific medial thalamus and the motor regulatory functions of the ventrolateral thalamus, but it also provides both thalamic regions with two separate striatal feedback systems. Impulses arising in centrum medianum can return to the striatum directly, or via a cortical detour by first engaging neurons of the ventrolateral thalamus. Similarly, activity generated in the ventrolateral thalamus can reach the striatum via a cortical route or subcortically through centrum medianum. A circumscribed portion of the centrum medianum–parafascicular complex thus seems to sit astride a plexus of connections involving, in a fairly direct fashion, motor cortex, ventrolateral thalamus and cerebellum, spinothalamic tract, ascending reticular formation, neostriatum, and globus pallidus. Whether or not the centrum medianum is, in fact, an important thalamic nodal point, as suggested above, remains to be established.

To appreciate the structural basis of the system upon which the nigral dopaminergic influences are apparently exclusively exerted one must not only consider the afferent and efferent projections of the striatum but also the nature of its intrinsic organization. From all the available evidence, it is quite apparent that the neostriatum does not function like a relay structure but rather like an integrator, though it may be questioned whether the discrete informational content of the input is retained during the striatal processing.

The neuronal composition of the neostriatum consists of three major cell types: some large neurons, a great number of Golgi type II neurons, and some small neurons (Kemp and Powell, 1971a,b). Approximately 95% of the cells are stellate cells of medium size, their dendrites with spines, their axons with collaterals. The processes of these neurons are limited entirely to intrastriatal connections and few seem to extend beyond a radius of 450 μm. According to Kemp and Powell (1971a) the efferent output is mediated by axons of the large cells so that less than 5% of the neuron population can be directly implicated in the neostriatal output. Most cells must therefore be exclusively involved in intrastriatal mechanisms and can, presumably, act upon the transformation of the striatal input from cortex, thalamus, and substantia nigra, prior to its exit from the striatum. The integrative nature of the transformations is suggested by a number of structural and functional clues. Cortical and thalamic terminals coexist on the same striatal neurons; many if not most afferent terminals are *en passant* so that any one afferent axon spreads its synaptic influence over many striatal neurons, and finally, the neostriatum consists of a homogeneous neuropil. Although the neurons form clusters in a dense plexus of axons, axon collaterals, and dendrites, these clusters are randomly distributed throughout the neostriatum (Tennyson and Marco, 1973). The structural homogeneity is further enhanced by the absence of orientation of dendritic fields most of which tend to be spherical or ovoid.

The synaptic organization has revealed an overwhelming preponderance of synapses on dendritic spines and few axosomatic or other synapses. The great majority of synapses are asymmetrical and most importantly, all of the afferent fibers form asymmetric synapses on striatal neurons. Generally, asymmetrical synapses are considered to be excitatory, hence, according to morphological criteria the dopaminergic nigral input should be classified as excitatory along with the cortical and thalamic ones. Symmetrical and presumably inhibitory synapses are made by many intrinsic striatal neurons as well as by all the large efferent axons projecting to the substantia nigra and the globus pallidus (Kemp and Powell, 1971e; Adinolfi, 1969).

Structurally and regionally, there is little basis for a differentiation of function unless it is imposed by extrastriatal influences which, in turn, modify the intrinsic and efferent actions of the neostriatum. It is doubtful if anatomical studies can resolve this problem or reconcile the seeming contradiction between the claimed inhibitory action of dopamine and the synaptic morphology, which suggests an excitatory nigral input, as do most electrophysiological studies.

5. FUNCTIONAL ASPECTS

Considerably more is known about the functional properties of the caudate nucleus than the putamen. The two components of the neostriatum are morphologically identical and have correspondingly organized afferent and efferent connections; it is therefore commonly accepted that they constitute a single nucleus merely separated by the fibers of the internal capsule (Kemp and Powell, 1970).

Functionally, however, this is an oversimplication. The results of behavioral experiments (Divac et al., 1967), of evoked potential and single unit recordings (Marco et al., 1973a,b; Feltz and Albe-Fessard, 1972, Herz and Zieglgänsberger, 1968; Malliani and Purpura, 1967; Segundo and Machne, 1956), or observing the effects of striatal stimulation on neuronal activity elsewhere in the brain (Liles and Davis, 1969b; Siegel and Lineberry, 1968; Krauthamer and Albe-Fessard, 1965), and of noting the effects of striatal lesions and stimulation on posture and movements (Cools, 1973; Liles and Davis, 1969a; Dieckmann and Hassler, 1967; Hassler and Dieckmann, 1967) all demonstrate the existence of functional localization and differentiation within the neostriatum. Caution is therefore called for when data obtained from the caudate nucleus are extrapolated to the putamen or, for that matter, when generalizations are made about caudate functions which are derived from studies of only a restricted portion of the caudate nucleus.

The peripheral, cortical, thalamic, and nigral inputs to the neostriatum have been studied intracellularly at the unit level as well as with gross electrodes. The caudate nucleus and putamen are clearly structures with sensory convergence properties. Evoked potential and single unit recordings have revealed that somesthetic, visual, auditory, and vestibular stimuli activate striatal neurons in a largely nonspecific manner (Potegal et al., 1971; Sedgewick and Williams, 1967; Albe-Fessard, et al., 1960a,b; Segundo and Machne, 1956). The neostriatum shares the property of polysensory convergence with the centrum medianum–parafascicular complex and adjacent intralaminar thalamic neurons (Albe-Fessard, 1967; Kruger and Albe-Fessard, 1960), the association cortex (Albe-Fessard and Fessard, 1963; Bental and Bihari, 1963; Thompson et al., 1963), and portions of the bulbar and mesencephalic reticular formation (Lindsley et al., 1973; Robertson et al., 1973; Bowsher et al., 1968; Bell et al., 1964). The central afferent pathways by which these sensory inputs are conveyed to the neostriatum are not completely known but a corticofugal route can be ruled out since polysensory responses persist in the caudate nucleus following chronic cortical ablations (Albe-Fessard et al., 1960a).

Fully confirming the anatomical findings, stimulation of all accessible portions of the neocortex generates excitatory responses in caudate neurons. However, latencies and firing pattern are quite complex and no simple pattern has emerged (Buchwald et al., 1973; Rocha-Miranda, 1965). Most probably, the complexity of the response pattern reflects varying effects of intracaudate transmission and processing, and the sampling bias in favor of large neuron recordings introduced by the microelectrode technique (Marco et al., 1973a,b). When intracellular records of caudate neurons have been obtained, the initial response to cortical stimulation or to intracaudate stimulation is one of excitatory postsynaptic depolarization. The initial excitatory phase is variably followed by prolonged periods of hyperpolarization or inhibition. (Buchwald et al., 1973; Marco et al., 1973a).

The thalamic input from the medial thalamus follows a direct anatomical route and, like the cortical one, is excitatory. Its excitatory action is, however, weaker than the cortical one and frequently remains below firing threshold. (Buchwald et al., 1973; Purpura and Malliani, 1967; Purpura et al., 1967). Consequently, the thalamic input is primarily an input which raises the striatal threshold of excitability, thus rendering its neurons more responsive to other, presumably cortical impulses. The direct excitatory influx from the intralaminar thalamus stands in contrast to the inconstant and very weak action exerted by the ventrolateral nucleus, an input which occurs polysynaptically via cortical or thalamic detours. Thus, the two major thalamic receiving zones for the striatal output, ventrolateral–ventral anterior nucleus and centrum medianum–intralaminar nuclei, have different feedback actions on the neostriatum. One must add to this the yet poorly understood reciprocal connections between centrum medianum and the ventrolateral nucleus which, undoubtedly, provide a further important area for the interplay of neurons influenced by the neostriatum (Purpura, 1970; Scheibel and Scheibel, 1970).

It becomes, therefore, of some importance to appreciate the properties of the thalamic projection zones and the striatal influences playing upon them. The extensive studies of Frigyesi and Machek (1970, 1971) have provided the evidence for the directly and indirectly exerted synaptic actions on thalamic neurons. By way of the pallidal outflow over ansa lenticularis and via the substantia nigra, the striatum exerts a powerful excitatory–inhibitory regulatory action on thalamic neurons. Because of the partial but considerable overlap of cerebellofugal, pallidofugal, and nigrofugal projections, the ventrolateral nucleus plays a readily appreciated key role in the extrapyramidal control of motor functions (Desiraju and Purpura, 1969; Purpura et al., 1967; Mehler et al., 1958). Much of the striatal influence on the diencephalon is funneled through the globus pallidus which, itself, is subjected to a predominantly inhibitory striatal influence (Noda et al., 1968; Malliani and Purpura, 1967). It has been postulated that the globus pallidus may exert an important gating effect on the striopallidal output (Frigyesi and Rabin, 1971).

It is more difficult to integrate the intralaminar thalamic complex into the extrapyramidal schema. An appreciation of the reciprocal action between neostriatum and intralaminar thalamus is important because both the caudate nucleus and the centrum medianum–parafascicular complex are components of the polysensory convergence system or systems. Their response properties to sensory stimulation in any modality are entirely comparable to those of the nonspecific association cortex, nucleus gigantocellularis of the bulbar reticular formation and portions of the mesencephalic reticular formation: complete or partial convergence of auditory, visual, and somesthetic inputs; response latencies in the range of 12 to 20 msec, that is, longer than for the primary sensory specific structures; inability to follow fast repetitive stimulation; enhanced responsivity under chloralose anesthesia or during deep slow wave sleep and wakeful relaxation (Thompson and Shaw, 1965; Albe-Fessard et al., 1964). The anatomical and functional connections linking these polysensory convergence regions remain a subject of some dispute and are, unquestionably, quite complex, consisting of oligosynaptic long axon projections as well as short axon polysynaptic chains (Nelson and Bignall, 1973; Robertson and Thompson, 1973; Albe-Fessard *et al.*, 1971; Buser and Bignall, 1967).

The caudate nucleus plays a key role in the sensory convergence system. Caudate stimulation exerts a powerful inhibitory and some excitatory action on the polysensory neurons of centrum medianum–parafascicular complex, centralis lateralis, lateral portions of dorsomedial nucleus, and a zone just ventral to centrum medianum (Frigyesi and Machek, 1971; Feltz *et al.*, 1967; Krauthamer *et al.*, 1967a). The inhibition, which lasts up to 300 msec is blocked by subconvulsive doses of strychnine, a characteristic of postsynaptic inhibition (Krauthamer and Yamaguchi, 1964; Krauthamer, 1963) but it is also altered by picrotoxin (Collins and Simonton, 1967). While the entire intralaminar thalamus is affected, there are definite quantitative differences in the striatal actions so that this thalamic area can be divided into domains of polysensory neurons subject to differentially exerted caudate influences (Feltz *et al.*, 1967; Krauthamer *et al.*, 1967a). As a result of the modulating action occurring at the level of the intralaminar thalamus and, perhaps at several other levels extending as far caudally as the nucleus gigantocellularis of the bulbar reticular formation, the polysensory responses of the entire "association" cortex are blocked (Krauthamer and Albe-Fessard, 1965, 1961; Krauthamer and Bagshaw, 1963). The duration of the inhibition observed on the association cortex parallels in time and intensity the inhibition of thalamic neurons. The concurrent absence of cortical responses to the inhibitory caudate stimulation and the results of acute and chronic cortical ablations indicate that the altered response of the nonspecific cortex must be regarded as a passive reflection of the subcortical events produced by caudate stimulation.

The inhibitory action of the caudate nucleus is selectively exerted on the polysensory response system. The responsivity of lemniscal neurons and of the primary sensory cortical areas remains unaffected. Such a differential action on polysensory and modality-specific sensory cortex could, in turn, profoundly modify the corticostriatal input from sensory and association cortex. The ultimate behavioral significance of this modulation of sensory integrative mechanisms remains to be determined (Krauthamer and Albe-Fessard, 1965; 1964), as does its relationship to the more diffusely organized arousal mechanisms (Dieckmann and Sasaki, 1970; Demetrescu and Demetrescu, 1965).

The studies of Thompson and Shaw (1965) and Thompson and Bettinger (1970) have linked the polysensory convergence system to the orienting response to novel stimuli and the habituation of this response upon stimulus repetition. Such a function is supported by the observation that caudate stimulation also blocks the ventral root discharges associated with the startle reflex caused by sudden sensory stimuli (Lamarche and Buser, 1968).

The caudate inhibition of subcortical polysensory neurons provides evidence for a functional differentiation within the neostriatum. The inhibitory effects are limited, rostrally, to the anterior dorsomedial and dorsolateral caudate nucleus just beneath the third ventricle. More caudally, the inhibitory zones tend to lie ventrolaterally and invade the internal capsule. A very powerful inhibition by extremely low intensity stimulation is obtained from the globus pallidus and entopeduncular nucleus, but the presence of large numbers of fibers of passage makes selective stimulus effects difficult to achieve. No inhibitory effects have been observed after stimulation of the putamen. The rostrocaudal and dorsal to ventral progression of the inhibitory caudate zones can be demonstrated by selectively cooling restricted portions of these zones to $+5°C$ and blocking the inhibitory outflow. Cooling rostral to the caudate stimulus site was ineffective, but when the cooling probe was inserted caudal to the stimulus point or in the globus pallidus, the polysensory inhibition was blocked until the cooled zone was allowed to recover its normal temperature (Benita and Krauthamer, 1966). Nigral lesions did not block the inhibition but nigral stimulation does exert a similar though not identical effect (Krauthamer and Dalsass, 1972). Whether inhibitory nigral stimulation operates indirectly via the nigrostriatal pathway or directly via a nigrothalamic output has yet not been determined.

In this complex multiplicity of striatal functions the precise role of the dopaminergic nigrostriatal projection system remains unclear. There is a large and growing body of evidence which has clearly demonstrated the almost total dependence of neostriatal dopamine on the intactness of the substantia nigra. There is also evidence that the iontophoretic application of dopamine in close proximity to caudate neurons has a predominantly depressing effect on these neurons (Connor, 1970; Herz and Zieglgänsberger, 1968; McLennan and York, 1967; Bloom et al., 1965). Since the striatal dopamine is not contained in striatal cells but in the terminal processes of neurons whose cell bodies lie in the substantia nigra, the natural release of dopamine by nigral stimulation should, logically, inhibit the striatal neurons, just as does its iontophoretic application. According to Connor (1970), this is indeed the case; however, mixed results were obtained by McLennan and York (1967) who reported that iontophoretically applied dopamine inhibited caudate neurons which were excited by nigral stimulation. Electrophysiological studies have, likewise, given equivocal results. Both excitatory and inhibitory effects have been observed to follow electrical stimulation of the substantia nigra (Feltz and Albe-Fessard, 1972; Hull et al., 1970; Albe-Fessard et al., 1967; Frigyesi and Purpura, 1967), and it has been postulated that there may be a dopaminergic as well as a nondopaminergic nigrostriatal input (Feltz and De Champlain, 1972a; 1972b). Several complications make an interpretation of these studies very difficult. There is, first, the complexity of the nigral system itself. According to Olivier *et al.* (1970) the striatonigral projection is cholinergic and excitatory, but according to Precht and Yoshida (1971) the pathway is inhibitory and mediated by γ-aminobutyric acid. Within the substantia nigra itself there exists a complex synaptic organization closely interrelating the pars reticulata with the dopamine-containing pars compacta (Carpenter and Peter, 1972; Rinvik and Grofová, 1970). The output of the substantia nigra is directed not only to the striatum but also to the thalamus and other mesencephalic regions. It is consequently extremely difficult to specify the nature and route of the activity recorded in the striatum upon nigral stimulation. Second, the intricate synaptic organization within the striatum is compatible with a wide range of responses depending upon the momentary state of activity in small populations of caudate neurons (Hull *et al.*, 1973; Feltz and De Champlain, 1972*b*; Herz *et al.*, 1970).

Another approach has been to record from caudate neurons after depletion of striatal dopamine. Such studies have shown an enhanced sensitivity of caudate neurons to intophoretically applied dopamine, possibly a type of denervation hypersensitivity, but also a continued inhibition following electrical nigral stimulation (Feltz and De Champlain, 1972*b*). The effects of dopamine depletion on spontaneous striatal unit activity are similarly contradictory. The spontaneous activity of neurons in the putamen was increased following dopamine depletion (Ohye *et al.*, 1970), but no significant change in ipsilateral caudate unit activity could be observed by Buchwald *et al.*, (1972) who noted a concomitant significant decrease in activity in the contralateral caudate nucleus. The existence of striatal effects contralateral to the site of intervention has been observed in other studies as well (Chandu-Lall *et al.*, 1970; Krauthamer and Albe-Fessard, 1965).

6. CONCLUSION

Given the contradictory or, at best, equivocal nature of those studies which have attempted a neurophysiological or behavioral assessment of the role of dopamine in the activity of the neostriatum it seems premature to claim an immediate relationship between striatal dopamine and extrapyramidal motor functions predicated on an inhibitory action of dopamine; other possible dopaminergic actions remain to be explored.

At this point it is reasonably certain that dopamine is a crucial component in the intrastriatal modulation of neuronal activity. Because of its ubiquitous distribution throughout the entire extent of the neostriatum it probably participates in the "shaping" of the striatal activity prior to its emergence from the striatum. Given the ultrastructural organization of the neostriatum, a dopaminergic action exclusively on the large neurons with striatofugal axons appears most improbable; more likely it exerts its major effect on striatal interneurons. Given, in addition, the topographic precision of the striato–nigro–striatal projection system, an anatomical substratum is available for modulating selectively circumscribed zones of the neostriatum at any given moment in time. Its influence would extend to brain systems whose links with extrapyramidal motor functions, as traditionally defined, are extremely tenuous and highly state-dependent. Dopamine could thus serve as a powerful agent in assuring the functional plasticity of behaviorally adaptive sensorisensory and sensorimotor integration.

7. REFERENCES

Adinolfi, A. M., 1969, Degenerative changes in the entopeduncular nucleus following lesions of the caudate nucleus: An electron microscopic study, *Exptl. Neurol.* **25**:246.

Akert, K., and Andersson, B., 1951, Experimenteller Beitrag zur Physiologie des Nucleus caudatus, *Acta Physiol. Scand.* **9**:316.

Albe-Fessard, D., 1967, Organization of somatic central projections, in: *Contributions to Sensory Physiology Vol. 2,* (W. D. Neff, ed.), pp. 101–168, Academic Press, New York.

Albe-Fessard, D., and Fessard, A., 1963, Thalamic integrations and their consequences at the telencephalic level, in: *Progress in Brain Research, Vol. 1,* (G. Moruzzi, A. Fessard, and H. H. Jasper, eds.), pp. 115–148, Elsevier, Amsterdam.

Albe-Fessard, D., Levante, A., and Rokyta, R., 1971, Cortical projection of cat medial thalamic cells, *Intern. J. Neurosci.* **1**:327.

Albe-Fessard, D., Raieva, S., and Santiago, W., 1967, Sur les relations entre substance noire et noyau caudé, *J. Physiol. (Paris)* **59**:324.

Albe-Fessard, D., Massion, J., Hall, J., and Rosenblith, W., 1964, Modifications au cours de la veille ou du sommeil des valeurs moyennes des réponses centrales induites par des stimulations somatiques chez le chat libre, *C. R. Acad. Sci.* **258**:353.

Albe-Fessard, D., Oswaldo-Cruz, E., and Rocha-Miranda, C., 1960a, Activités évoquées dans le noyau caudé du chat en réponse à des types divers d'afférences. I. Etude macrophysiologique, *Electroencephalog. Clin. Neurophysiol.* **12**:405.

Albe-Fessard, D., Rocha-Miranda, C., and Oswaldo-Cruz, E., 1960b, Activités evoquées dans le noyau caudé du chat en réponse à des types divers d'afférences. II. Etude microphysiologique, *Electroencephalog. Clin. Neurophysiol.* **12**:649.

Allen, J. D., and Davison, C. S., 1973, Effects of caudate lesions on signaled and nonsignaled Sidman avoidance in the rat, *Behav. Biol.* **8**:239.

Andén, N. E., Carlsson, A., Dahlström, A., Fuxe, K., Hillarp, N. A., and Larsson, K., 1964, Demonstration and mapping out of nigro-neostriatal dopamine neurons, *Life Sci.* **3**:523.

Bartholini, G., and Pletscher, A., 1972, Drugs affecting monoamines in the basal ganglia, in: *Advances in Biochemical Psychopharmacology, Vol. 6,* (E. Costa, L. L. Iversen, and R. Paoletti, eds.), pp. 135–148, Raven Press, New York.

Bak, I. J., Hassler, R., Kim, J. S., and Kataoka, K., 1972, Amantadine actions on acetylcholine and GABA in striatum and substantia nigra of rat in relation to behavioral changes, *J. Neural Transmission* **33**:45.

Barbeau, A., 1962, Pathogenesis of Parkinson's disease: A new hypothesis, *Can. Med. Assoc. J.* **87**:802.

Battista, A. F., Goldstein, M., Nakatani, S., and Anagnoste, B., 1969, Ventrolateral thalamic lesions, *Arch. Neurol.* **21**:611.

Bédard, P., Larochelle, L., Parent, A., and Poirier, L. J., 1969*a*, The nigrostriatal pathway: a correlative study based on neuroanatomical and neurochemical criteria in the cat and the monkey, *Exptl. Neurol.* **25**:365.

Bédard, P., Larochelle, L., Parent, A., and Poirier, L. J., 1969*b*, Dopamine and serotonin in the striatum of the cat: effect of lesions in the intralaminar nuclei, *Arch. Neurol.* **20**:239.

Bell, C., Sierra, G., Buendia, N., and Segundo, J. P., 1964, Sensory properties of neurons in the mesencephalic reticular formation. *J. Neurophysiol.* **27**:961.

Benita, M., and Condé, H., 1971, Etude des afférences du noyau centre médian du thalamus du chat vers le cortex et les structures striopallidales, *Exp. Brain Res.* **12**:204.

Benita, M., and Krauthamer, G., 1966, Blocage par le froid de l'action inhibitrice des corps striés, *J. Physiol. (Paris)* **58**:205.

Bental, E., and Bihari, B., 1963, Evoked activity of single neurons in sensory association cortex of the cat, *J. Neurophysiol.* **26**:207.

Bloom, F. E., and Giarman, N. J., 1968, Physiologic and pharmacologic considerations of biogenic amines in the nervous system, *Ann. Rev. Pharmacol.* **8**:229.

Bloom, F. E., Costa, E., and Salmoiraghi, G. C., 1965, Anesthesia and the responsiveness of individual neurons of the caudate nucleus to acetylcholine, norepinephrine and dopamine administered by microelectrophoresis, *J. Pharmacol. Exptl. Therap.* **150**:244.

Boivie, J., 1971, The termination of the spinothalamic tract in the cat. An experimental study with silver impregnation methods, *Exp. Brain Res.* **12**:331.

Bolme, P., Fuxe, K., and Lidbrink, P., 1972, On the function of central catecholamine neurons—their role in cardiovascular and arousal mechanisms. *Res. Commun. Chem. Pathol. Pharmacol.* **4**:657.

Bowen, F. P., 1969, Visuomotor deficits produced by cryogenic lesions of the caudate, *Neuropsychologia* **7**:59.

Bowsher, D., 1965, The anatomophysiological basis of somatosensory discrimination, *Intern. Rev. Neurobiol.* **8**:35.

Bowsher, D., 1966, Some afferent and efferent connections of the parafascicular-center median complex, in: *The Thalamus* (D. P. Purpura and M. Yahr, eds.), pp. 99–127, Columbia University Press, New York.

Bowsher, D., Mallart, A., Petit, D., and Albe-Fessard, D., 1968, A bulbar relay to the centre median, *J. Neurophysiol.* **31**:288.

Brimblecombe, R. W., and Pinder, R. M., 1972, *Tremors and Tremorogenic Agents*, Scientechnica, Bristol.

Buchwald, N. A., Horvath, F. E., Soltysik, S., and Romero-Sierra, C., 1964, Inhibitory responses to basal ganglia stimulation, *Bol. Inst. Estud. Med. Biol. Mex.* **22**:363.

Buchwald, N. A., Levine, M. S., Hull, C. D., and Heller, A., 1972, Dopamine depletion and striatal unit firing, *Soc. Neurosci., 2nd Ann. Meeting,* (abstr.) p. 136.

Buchwald, N. A., Price, D. D., Vernon, L., and Hull, C. D., 1973, Caudate intracellular response to thalamic and cortical inputs, *Exptl. Neurol.* **38**:311.

Buser, P., and Bignall, K. E., 1967, Nonprimary sensory projections on the cat neocortex, *Intern. Rev. Neurobiol.* **10**:111.

Buser, P., Rougeul, A., and Perret, C., 1964, Caudate and thalamic influences on conditioned motor responses in the cat, *Bol. Inst. Estud. Med. Biol. Mex.* **22**:293.

Carpenter, M. B., and Peter, P., 1972, Nigrothalamic and nigrostriatal fibers in the Rhesus monkey, *J. Comp. Neurol.* **144**:93.

Carpenter, M. B., and Strominger, N. L., 1967, Efferent fibers of the subthalamic nucleus in the monkey—a comparison of the efferent projections of the subthalamic nucleus, substantia nigra and globus pallidus, *Am. J. Anat.* **121**:41.

Carpenter, M. B., Fraser, R. A. R., and Shriver, J. E., 1968, The organization of pallido-subthalamic fibers in the monkey, *Brain Res.* **11**:522.

Celesia, G., and Barr, A. N., 1970, Psychosis and other psychiatric manifestations of levodopa therapy, *Arch. Neurol.* **23**:193.

Chandu-Lall, J. A., Haase, G. R., Zivanovic, D., and Szekely, E. G., 1970, Dopamine interdependence between the caudate nuclei, *Exptl. Neurol.* **29**:101.

Chow, K. L., 1954, Lack of behavioral effects following destruction of some thalamic association nuclei in monkeys. *Arch. Neurol. Psychiat.* **71**:762.

Cianci, S. N., 1965, Effects of cortical and subcortical stimulation on delayed response in monkeys, *Exptl. Neurol.* **11**:104.

Cole, M., Nauta, W. J. H., and Mehler, W. R., 1964, The ascending efferent projections of the substantia nigra. *Trans. Am. Neurol. Assoc.* **89**:74.

Collins, R. J., and Simonton, V. R., 1967, Inhibition of evoked potentials by caudate stimulation and its antagonism by centrally acting drugs, *Intern. J. Neuropharmacol.* **6**:349.

Connor, J. D., 1970, Caudate nucleus neurones: Correlation of the effects of substantia nigra stimulation with iontophoretic dopamine. *J. Physiol.* **208**:691.

Cools, A. R., 1972, Athetoid and choreiform hyperkinesias produced by caudate application of dopamine in cats, *Psychopharmacologia* **25**:229.

Cools, A. R., 1973, Chemical and electrical stimulation of the caudate nucleus in freely moving cats: The role of dopamine, *Brain Res.* **58**:437.

Cooper, B. R., Breese, G. R., Grant, L. D., and Howard, J. L., 1973, Effects of 6-hydroxydopamine treatments on active avoidance responding: evidence for involvement of brain dopamine, *J. Pharmacol. Exptl. Therap.* **185**:358.

Costall, B., Naylor, R. J., and Olley, J. E., 1972, Catalepsy and circling behavior after intracerebral injections of neuroleptic, cholinergic and anticholinergic agents into the caudate-putamen, globus pallidus and substantia nigra of rat brain, *Neuropharmacologia* **11**:645.

Cowan, W. M., and Powell, T. P. S., 1966, Strio-pallidal projection in the monkey, *J. Neurol. Neurosurg. Psychiat.* **29**:426.

Crane, G. E., and Gardner, R., Jr. (eds.), 1968, *Psychotropic Drugs and Dysfunctions of the Basal Ganglia. A multidisciplinary workshop,* Public Health Service Publ. No. 1938, U.S. Govt. Printing Office, Washington, D.C.

Dahlström, A., and Fuxe, K., 1964, Evidence for the existence of monoamine-containing neurons in the central nervous system. I. demonstration of monoamines in the cell bodies of brain stem neurons, *Acta Physiol. Scand. Suppl.* **232**:25.

Deadwyler, S. A., Montgomery, D., and Wyers, E. J., 1971, Passive avoidance and carbachol excitation of the caudate nucleus, *Physiol. Behav.* **8**:631.

Dean, W. H., and Davis, G. D., 1959, Behavior changes following caudate lesions in Rhesus monkey, *J. Neurophysiol.* **22**:524.

Delacour, J., 1971, Effects of medial thalamic lesions in the rat: a review and an interpretation, *Neuropsychologia* **9**:157.

Demetrescu, M., Demetrescu, M. A. and Iosif, G., 1965, The tonic control of cortical responsiveness by inhibitory and facilitatory diffuse influences, *Electroencephalog. Clin. Neurophysiol.* **18**:1.

Desiraju, T., and Purpura, D. P., 1969, Synpatic convergence of cerebellar and lenticular projection to thalamus, *Brain Res.* **15**:544.

80 George M. Krauthamer

Dieckmann, G., and Hassler, R., 1967, Reizexperimente zur Funktion des Putamen der Katze, *J. Hirnforsch.* **10**:188.
Dieckmann, G., and Sasaki, K., 1970, Recruiting responses in the cerebral cortex produced by putamen and pallidum stimulation, *Exp. Brain Res.* **10**:236.
Divac, I., 1968a, Functions of the caudate nucleus, *Acta Biol. Exptl. Polish Acad. Sci.* **28**:107.
Divac, I., 1968b, Effects of prefrontal and caudate lesions on delayed response in cats, *Acta Biol. Exptl. Polish Acad. Sci.* **28**:149.
Divac, I., Rosvold, H. E., and Szwarcbart, M. K., 1967, Behavioral effects of selective ablation of the caudate nucleus, *J. Comp. Physiol. Psychol.* **63**:184.
Ermolaeva, V. Y., and Ermolenko, S. F., 1972, Reciprocal connections between the first and second somatosensory cortical areas and the caudate nucleus, *Arkh. Anat. Gistol. Embriol.* **63**:20 [translated in *Neurosci. Behav. Physiol.* **6**:325].
Ermolenko, S. F., 1971, Cortical projections of the caudal part of the head and body of the caudate nucleus in cats, *Arkh. Anat. Gistol. Embroil.* **61**:24, [translated in *Neurosci. Behav. Physiol.* **5**:364].
Faull, R. L. M., and Laverty, R., 1969, Changes in dopamine levels in the corpus striatum following lesions in the substantia nigra, *Exptl. Neurol.* **23**:332.
Feltz, P., and Albe-Fessard, A., 1972, A study of an ascending nigro-caudate pathway, *Electroencephalog. Clin. Neurophysiol.* **33**:179.
Feltz, P., and De Champlain, J., 1972a, Persistence of caudate unitary responses to nigral stimulation after destruction and functional impairment of the striatal dopaminergic terminals. *Brain Res.* **43**:595.
Feltz, P., and De Champlain, J., 1972b, Enhanced sensitivity of caudate neurones to microiontophoretic injections of dopamine in 6-hydroxydopamine treated cats, *Brain Res.* **43**:601.
Feltz, P., Krauthamer, G., and Albe-Fessard, D., 1967, Neurons of the medial diencephalon, I. somatosensory responses and caudate inhibition, *J. Neurophysiol.* **30**:55.
Fibiger, H. C., Zis, A. P., and McGeer, E. G., 1973, Feeding and drinking deficits after 6-hydroxydopamine administration in the rat: similarities to the lateral hypothalamic syndrome, *Brain Res.* **55**:135.
Fox, S. S., Kimble, D. P., and Lickey, M. E., 1964, Comparison of caudate nucleus and septal-area lesions on two types of avoidance behavior, *J. Comp. Physiol. Psychol.* **58**:380.
Frigyesi, T., and Machek, J., 1970, Basal ganglia-diencephalon synaptic relations in the cat. I. An intracellular study of dorsal thalamic neurons during capsular and basal ganglia stimulation, *Brain Res.* **20**:201.
Frigyesi, T. L., and Machek, J., 1971, Basal ganglia-diencephalon synaptic relations in the cat. II. Intracellular recordings from dorsal thalamic neurons during low frequency stimulation of the caudato-thalamic projection systems and the nigrothalamic pathway, *Brain Res.* **27**:59.
Frigyesi, T. L., and Purpura, D. P., 1967, Electrophysiological analysis of reciprocal caudato-nigral relations, *Brain Res.* **6**:440.
Frigyesi, T. L., and Rabin, A., 1971, Basal ganglia-diencephalon synaptic relations in the cat. III. An intracellular study of ansa lenticularis, lenticular fasciculus and pallidosubthalamic projection activities, *Brain Res.* **35**:67.
Frigyesi, T. L., Ige, A., Iulo, A., and Schwartz, R., 1971, Denigration and sensorimotor disability induced by ventral tegmental injection of 6-hydroxydopamine in the cat, *Exptl. Neurol.* **33**:78.
Fuxe, K., and Hanson, L. C. F., 1967, Central catecholamine neurons and conditioned avoidance behavior, *Psychopharmacologia* **11**:439.
Gold, P. E., and King, R. A., 1972, Caudate stimulation and retrograde amnesia: Amnesia threshold and gradient, *Behav. Biol.* **7**:709.

Goldman, P. S., and Rosvold, E., 1972, The effects of selective caudate lesions in infant and juvenile Rhesus monkeys, *Brain Res.* **43**:53.

Goldstein, M., Anagnoste, B., Owen, W. S., and Battista, A. F., 1967, The effects of ventromedial tegmental lesions on the disposition of dopamine in the caudate nucleus of the monkey, *Brain Res.* **4**:298.

Goldstein, M., Anagnoste, B., Battista, A. F., Owen, W. S., and Nakatani, S., 1969, Studies of amines in the striatum in monkeys with nigral lesions. The disposition, biosynthesis and metabolites of (^{3}H) dopamine and (^{14}C) serotonin in the striatum, *J. Neurochem.* **16**:645.

Green, R. H., Beatty, W. W., and Schartzbaum, J. S., 1967, Comparative effects of septo-hippocampal and caudate lesions on avoidance behavior in rats, *J. Comp. Physiol. Psychol.* **64**:444.

Gross, C. G., and Weiskrantz, L., 1964, Some changes in behavior produced by lateral frontal lesions in the macaque, in: *The Frontal Granular Cortex and Behavior* (J. M. Warren and K. Akert, eds.), pp. 74–101, McGraw-Hill, New York.

Gross, C. G., Chorover, S. L., and Cohen, S. M., 1965, Caudate, cortical, hippocampal and dorsal thalamic lesions in rats: Alternation and Hebb-Williams maze performance, *Neuropsychologia* **3**:53.

Gybels, J., Meulders, M., Callens, M. and Colle, J., 1967, Disturbances of visuomotor integration in cats with small lesions of the caudate nucleus, *Arch. Intern. Physiol. Biochim.* **75**:283.

Harman, P. J., Tankard, M., Hovde, C., and Mettler, F. A., 1954, An experimental anatomical analysis of the topography and polarity of the caudate-neocortex relationship in the primate, *Anat. Record* **118**:307.

Hopf, A., 1954, Orientierende Untersuchung zur Frage patho-anatomischer Veränderungen in Pallidum and Striatum bei Schizophrenie, *J. Hirnforsch.* **1**:96.

Hassler, R., and Bak, I. J., 1969, Unbalanced ratios of striatal dopamine and serotonin after experimental interruption of strionigral connection in rat, in: *Third Symposium on Parkinson's Disease* (F. J. Gillingham and I. M. L. Donaldson, eds.), pp. 29–38, Livingstone, Edinburgh.

Hassler, R., and Dieckmann, G., 1967, Arrest reaction, delayed inhibition and unusual gaze behavior from stimulation of the putamen in awake, unrestrained cats, *Brain Res.* **5**:504.

Hattori, T., Fibiger, H. C., McGeer, P. H., and Maler, L., 1973, Analysis of the fine structure of the dopaminergic nigrostriatal projection by electron microscopic autoradiography, *Exptl. Neurol.* **41**:599.

Haycock, J. W., Deadwyler, S. A., Sideroff, S. I., and McGaugh, J. I., 1973, Retrograde amnesia and cholinergic systems in the caudate-putamen complex and dorsal hippocampus of the rat, *Exptl. Neurol.* **41**:201.

Hedreen, J. C., 1971, Separate demonstration of dopaminergic and nondopaminergic projections of substantia nigra in the rat, *Anat. Record* **169**:338.

Herz, A., and Zieglgänsberger, W., 1968, The influence of microelectro-phoretically applied biogenic amines, cholinomimetics and procain on synaptic excitation in the corpus striatum, *Intern. J. Neuropharmacol.* **7**:221.

Herz, A., Zieglgänsberger, W., and von Freytag-Loringhoven, H., 1970, Development of fields of focal potentials in the caudate nucleus following microiontophoretic application of glutamic acid and GABA, *Electroencephalog. Clin. Neurophysiol.* **28**:247.

Hornykiewicz, O., 1972a, Neurochemistry of Parkinsonism, in: *Handbook of Neurochemistry, Vol. 7,* (A. Lajtha, ed.), pp. 465–501, Plenum Press, New York.

Hornykiewicz, O., 1972b, Dopamine and extrapyramidal motor function and dysfunction, *Res. Publ. Assoc. Res. Nervous Mental Disease* **50**:390.

Hull, C. D., Buchwald, N. A., and Ling, G., 1967, Effects of direct cholinergic stimulation of forebrain structures, *Brain Res.* **6**:22.

82 George M. Krauthamer

Hull, C. D., Bernardi, G. and Buchwald, N. A., 1970, Intracellular responses of caudate neurons to brain stem stimulation, Brain Res. 22:163.

Hull, C. D., Bernardi, G., Price, D. D., and Buchwald, N. A., 1973, Intracellular responses of caudate neurons to temporally and spatially combined stimuli, Exptl. Neurol. 38:324.

Johnson, T. N., 1961, Fiber connections between dorsal thalamus and corpus striatum in the cat, Exptl. Neurol. 3:556.

Johnson, T. N., Rosvold, H. E., and Mishkin, M., 1968, Projections from behaviorally defined sectors of the prefrontal cortex to the basal ganglia, septum, and diencephalon of the monkey, Exptl. Neurol. 21:20.

Jung, R., and Hassler, R., 1960, The extrapyramidal motor system, in: Handbook of Physiology. Sect. I., Vol. II (J. Field, H. W. Magoun, and V. E. Hall, eds.), pp. 863–927, Amer. Physiol. Soc., Washington, D.C.

Kaelber, W. W., 1967, Observations on striatal connections following total destruction of the nucleus medialis dorsalis in the cat, Proc. Soc. Exptl. Biol. 125:386.

Keller, H. H., Bartholini, G., and Pletscher, A., 1973, Drug-induced changes of striatal cholinergic and dopaminergic functions in rats with spreading depression, J. Pharm. Pharmacol. 25:433.

Kemp, J. M., and Powell, T. P. S., 1970, The cortico-striate projection in the monkey, Brain 93:525.

Kemp, J. M., and Powell, T. P. S., 1971a, The structure of the caudate nucleus of the cat: Light and electron microscopy, Phil. Trans. Roy. Soc. Lond. Ser. B 262:383.

Kemp, J. M., and Powell, T. P. S., 1971b, The synaptic organization of the caudate nucleus, Phil. Trans. Roy. Soc. London Ser. B 262:403.

Kemp, J. M., and Powell, T. P. S., 1971c, The site of termination of afferent fibres in the caudate nucleus, Phil. Trans. Roy. Soc. London Ser. B, 262:413.

Kemp, J. M., and Powell, T. P. S., 1971d, The termination of fibres from the cerebral cortex and thalamus upon dendritic spines in the caudate nucleus: A study with the Golgi method, Phil. Trans. Roy. Soc. London Ser. B 262:429.

Kemp, J. M., and Powell, T. P. S., 1971e, The connexions of the striatum and globus pallidus: synthesis and speculation, Phil. Trans. Roy. Soc. London Ser. B 262:441.

Kety, S. S., 1959, Biochemical theories of schizophrenia, Science 129:1528.

Khalifeh, R. R., Kaelber, W. W., and Ingram, W. R., 1965, Some efferent connections of the nucleus medialis dorsalis, Am. J. Anat. 116:341.

Kirkby, R. J. and Kimble, D. P., 1968, Avoidance and escape behavior following striatal lesions in the rat, Exptl. Neurol. 20:215.

Kitsikis, A., 1968, The suppression of arm movements in monkeys: threshold variations of caudate nucleus stimulation, Brain Res. 10:460.

Kitsikis, A., and Roberge, A., 1973, Behavioral and biochemical effects of α-methyltyrosine in cats, Psychopharmacologia 31:143.

Kitsikis, A., Roberge, A. G., and Frenette, G., 1972, Effect of L-dopa on delayed response and visual discrimination in cats and its relation to brain chemistry, Exptl. Brain Res. 15:305.

Klawans, H. L., Goetz, C., and Westheimer, R., 1972, Pathophysiology of schizophrenia and the striatum, Diseases Nervous Systems 33:711.

Kline, N. S., and Mettler, F. A., 1961, The extrapyramidal system and schizophrenia, in: Extrapyramidal System and Neuroleptics, (J. M. Bordeleau, ed.), pp. 487–491, Presses Universitares, Montreal.

Krauthamer, G., 1963, Inhibition of evoked potentials by striatal stimulation and its blockage by strychnine, Science 142:1175.

Krauthamer, G., and Bagshaw, M., 1963, Recherche des niveaux où les impulsions provenant des corps striés inhibent certaines afférences somatiques, J. Physiol. (Paris) 55:274.

Krauthamer, G., and Dalsass, M., 1972, Inhibition of polysensory responses by striatonigral stimulation, *Soc. Neurosci. 2nd Ann. Meeting* (abstr.) p. 138.

Krauthamer, G., and Yamaguchi, Y., 1964, Supression par la strychnine de l'action inhibitrice des corps striés, *J. Physiol. (Paris)* **56**:586.

Krauthamer, G., and Albe-Fessard, D., 1961, Inhibitions d'activités evoquées corticales et souscorticales par la stimulation des noyaux de la base et des régions limitrophes de la capsule interne, *C. R. Soc. Biol.* **155**:144.

Krauthamer, G., and Albe-Fessard, D., 1964, Electrophysiologic studies of the basal ganglia and striopallidal inhibition of nonspecific afferent activity, *Neuropsychologia* **2**:73.

Krauthamer, G., and Albe-Fessard, D., 1965, Inhibition of nonspecific sensory activities following striopallidal and capsular stimulation, *J. Neurophysiol.* **28**:100.

Krauthamer, G., Feltz, P., and Albe-Fessard, D., 1967a, Neurons of the medial diencephalon. II. Excitation of central origin, *J. Neurophysiol.* **30**:81.

Krauthamer, G., Liebeskind, J., and Salmon-Legagneur, A., 1967b, Reversible deficit on a delayed alternation task during subcortical cooling, *J. Physiol.* **190**:18p.

Kruger, L., and Albe-Fessard, D., 1960, Distribution of responses of somatic afferent stimuli in the diencephalon of the cat under chloralose anesthesia, *Exptl. Neurol.* **2**:442.

Kuo, J. S. and Carpenter, M. B., 1973, Organization of pallidothalamic projections in the Rhesus monkey, *J. Comp. Neurol.* **151**:201.

Lalley, P. M., Rossi, G. V., and Baker, W. W., 1970, Analysis of local cholinergic tremor mechanisms following selective neurochemical lesions, *Exptl. Neurol.* **27**:258.

Lamarche, M., and Buser, P., 1968, Suppression de la réaction de sursaut du chat sous chloralose par stimulation du noyau caudé, *Experientia* **24**:355.

Lewin, R. H., Dillard, G. V., and Porter, R. W., 1967, Extrapyramidal inhibition of the urinary bladder, *Brain Res.* **4**:301.

Li, C. L., 1966, Evidence of afferent fibers in the motor cortex from subcortical basal ganglia, *J. Neurosurg., Suppl. 2nd Symp. Parkinson's Dis., Pt. II* 222–226.

Liebman, J. M., and Butcher, L. L., 1973, Effects on self-stimulation behavior of drugs influencing dopaminergic neurotransmission mechanisms, *Naunyn-Schmiedebergs Arch. Exptl. Pathol. Pharmakol.* **277**:305.

Liles, S. L., and Davis, G. D., 1969a, Interrelation of caudate nucleus and thalamus in alteration of cortically induced movement. *J. Neurophysiol.* **32**:564.

Liles, S. L., and Davis, G. D., 1969b, Electrocortical effects of caudate stimulations which alter cortically induced movement, *J. Neurophysiol.* **32**:574.

Lindsley, D. F., Ranf, S. K., Sherwood, M. J., and Preston, W. G., 1973, Habituation and modification of reticular formation neuron responses to peripheral stimulation in cats, *Exptl. Neurol.* **41**:174.

McGeer, P. L., McGeer, E. G., Fibiger, H. C., and Wickson, V., 1971, Neostriatal choline acetylase and cholinesterase following selective brain lesions, *Brain Res.* **35**:308.

McLennan, H., and York, D. H., 1967, The action of dopamine on neurons of the caudate nucleus, *J. Physiol.* **189**:393.

MacLean, P. D., 1972, Cerebral evolution and emotional processes: New findings on the striatal complex, *Ann. N.Y. Acad. Sci.* **193**:137.

Mahut, M., 1964, Effects of subcortical electrical stimulation on discrimination learning in cats, *J. Comp. Physiol. Psychol.* **58**:390.

Maler, L., Fibiger, H. C., and McGeer, P. H., 1973, Demonstration of the nigrostriatal projection by silver staining after nigral injections of 6-hydroxydopamine, *Exptl. Neurol.* **40**:505.

Malitz, S., (ed.), 1972, L-*dopa and Behavior,* Raven Press, New York.

Malliani, A., and Purpura, D. P., 1967, Intracellular studies of the corpus striatum. II. Patterns of synaptic activities in lenticular and entopeduncular neurons, *Brain Res.* **6**:341.

Marco, L. A., Copack, P., Edelson, A. M. and Gilman, S., 1973a, Intrinsic connections of caudate neurons. I. Locally evoked field potentials and extracellular unitary activity, *Brain Res.* 53:291.

Marco, L. A., Copack, P., and Edelson, A. M., 1973b, Intrinsic connections of caudate neurons. Locally evoked intracellular responses, *Exptl. Neurol.* 40:683.

Means, L. W., Huntley, D. H., Anderson, H. P., and Harrell, T. H., 1973, Deficient acquisition and retention of a visual-tactile discrimination task in rats with medial thalamic lesions, *Behav. Biol.* 9:435.

Mehler, W. R., 1966, Further notes on the center median nucleus of Luys, in: *The Thalamus* (D. P. Purpura and M. D. Yahr, eds.), pp. 109–122, Columbia University Press, New York.

Mehler, W. R., Vernier, V. G., and Nauta, W. J. H., 1958, Efferent projections from dentate and interpositus nuclei in primates, *Anat. Record* 130:430.

Mettler, F. A., 1955, The experimental anatomophysiologic approach to the study of diseases of the basal ganglia, *J. Neuropathol. Exptl. Neurol.* 14:115.

Mettler, F. A., 1970, Nigrofugal connections in the primate brain, *J. Comp. Neurol.* 138:291.

Mettler, F. A., and Crandall, A., 1959, Relation between Parkinsonism and psychiatric disorder, *J. Nervous Mental Disease* 129:551.

Mettler, F. A., Ades, H. W., Lipman, E., and Culler, E. A., 1939, The extrapyramidal system, *Arch. Neurol. Psychiat.* 41:984.

Murphy, D. L., Henry, G. M., and Weingartner, H., 1972, Catecholamines and memory: enhanced verbal learning during L-dopa administration, *Psychopharmacologia* 27:319.

Murphy, D. L., Goodwin, F. K., Brodie, K. H., and Bunney, W. E., 1973, L-Dopa, dopamine, and hypomania, *Am. J. Psychiat.* 130:79.

Murray, M., 1966, Degeneration of some intralaminar thalamic nuclei after cortical removals in the cat, *J. Comp. Neurol.* 127:341.

Nakamura, S., and Sutin, J., 1972, The pattern of termination of pallidal axons upon cells of the subthalamic nucleus, *Exptl. Neurol.* 35:254.

Nauta, W. J. H., and Kuypers, H. G. J. M., 1958, Some ascending pathways in the brain stem reticular formation, in: *Reticular Formation of the Brain,* (H. H. Jasper, L. D. Proctor, R. S. Knighton, W. C. Noshay, and R. T. Costello, eds.), pp. 3–30, Little, Brown, Boston.

Nauta, W. J. H., and Mehler, W. R., 1966, Projections of the lentiform nucleus in the monkey, *Brain Res.* 1:3.

Nauta, W. J. H., and Whitlock, P. C., 1954, An anatomical analysis of the nonspecific thalamic projection, in: *Brain Mechanisms and Consciousness* (E. D. Adrian, F. Bremer, H. H. Jasper, and J. F. Delafresnaye, eds.), pp. 81–116, Blackwell, Oxford.

Nelson, C. N. and Bignall, K. E., 1973, Interactions of sensory and nonspecific thalamic inputs to cortical polysensory units in the squirrel monkey, *Exptl. Neurol.* 40:189.

Niimi, K., Ikeda, T., Kawamura, S., and Inoshita, H., 1970, Efferent projections of the head of the caudate nucleus in the cat, *Brain Res.* 21:327.

Noda, H., Manohar, S., and Adey, W. R., 1968, Responses of cat pallidal neurons to cortical and subcortical stimuli, *Exptl. Neurol.* 20:585.

Ohye, C., Bouchard, M., Boucher, R., and Poirier, L. J., 1970, Spontaneous activity of the putamen after chronic interruption of the dopaminergic pathway: effect of L-dopa, *J. Pharmacol. Exptl. Therap.* 175:700.

Okady, Y., Nitsch-Hassler, C., Kim, J. S., Bak, I. J., and Hassler, R., 1971, Role of γ-aminobutyric acid (GABA) in the extrapyramidal motor system. I. Regional distribution of GABA in rabbit, rat, guinea pig, and baboon CNS, *Exptl. Brain Res.* 13:514.

Olivier, A., Parent, A., Sirnard, H., and Poirier, L. J., 1970, Cholinesterasic striatopallidal and striatonigral efferents in the cat and the monkey, *Brain Res.* 18:273.

Orem, J., Schlag-Rey, M., Schlag, J., 1973, Unilateral visual neglect and thalamic intra-laminar lesions in cat, *Exptl. Neurol.* **40**:784.

Peeke, H. V. S., and Herz, M. J., 1971, Caudate nucleus stimulation retroactively impairs complex maze learning in the rat, *Science* **173**:80.

Poirier, L. J., Singh, P., Sourkes, T. L., and Boucher, R., 1967*a*, Effect of amine precursors on the concentration of striatal dopamine and serotonin in cats with and without unilateral brain stem lesions, *Brain Res.* **6**:654.

Poirier, L. J., Singh, P., Boucher, R., Bouvier, G., Oliver, A., and Larochelle, P., 1967*b*, Effect of brain lesions on striatal monoamines in the cat, *Arch. Neurol.* **17**:601.

Poirier, L. J., McGeer, E. G., Larochelle, L., McGeer, P. L., Bédard, P., and Boucher, R., 1969, The effect of brain stem lesions on tyrosine and tryptophan hydroxylases in various structures of the telencephalon of the cat, *Brain Res.* **14**:147.

Portig, P. J., and Vogt, M., 1969, Release into the cerebral ventricles of substances with possible transmitter function in the caudate nucleus, *J. Physiol.* **204**:687.

Potegal, M., Copack, P., de Jong, J. M. B. V., Krauthamer, G., and Gilman, S., 1971, Vestibular input to the caudate nucleus, *Exptl. Neurol.* **32**:448.

Powell, T. P. S., and Cowan, W. M., 1956, A study of thalamo-striate relations in the monkey, *Brain* **79**:364.

Prado-Alcala, R. A., Grinberg-Zylberbaum, J., Alvarez-Leefmans, J., and Brust-Carmona, H., 1973, Suppression of motor conditioning by the injection of 3 M KCl in the caudate nucleus of cats, *Physiol. Behav.* **10**:59.

Precht, W., and Yoshida, M., 1971, Blockage of caudate-evoked inhibition of neurons in the substantia nigra by picrotoxin, *Brain Res.* **32**:229.

Purpura, D. P., 1970, Operations and processes in thalamic and synaptically related neural subsystems, in: *The Neurosciences. II.* (F. O. Schmitt, ed.), pp. 458–470, Rockefeller University Press, New York.

Purpura, D. P., and Malliani, A., 1967, Intracellular studies of the corpus striatum. I. Synaptic potentials and discharge characteristics of caudate neurons activated by thalamic stimulation, *Brain Res.* **6**:325.

Purpura, D. P., Housepian, E. M., and Grundfest. H., 1958, Analysis of caudate-cortical connections in neuraxially intact and télencéphale isolé cats, *Arch. Ital. Biol.* **96**:145.

Purpura, D. P., Frigyesi, T. L., and Malliani, A., 1967, Intrinsic synaptic organization and relations of the corpus striatum, in: *Neurophysiological Basis of Normal and Abnormal Motor Activities* (M. D. Yahr and D. P. Purpura, eds.), pp. 177–204, Raven Press, New York.

Rasminsky, M., Mauro, A. J., and Albe-Fessard, D., 1973, Projections of medial thalamic nuclei to putamen and cerebral frontal cortex in the rat, *Brain Res.* **61**:69.

Rinvik, E., and Grofová, I., 1970, Observations on the fine structure of the substantia nigra in the cat, *Exptl. Brain Res.* **11**:229.

Robertson, R. T., and Thompson, R. F., 1973, Effects of subcortical ablations on cortical association responses in the cat, *Physiol. Behav.* **10**:245.

Robertson, R. T., Lynch, G. S., and Thompson, R. F., 1973, Diencephalic distributions of ascending reticular systems, *Brain Res.* **55**:309.

Rocha-Miranda, C. E., 1965, Single unit analysis of cortex-caudate connections, *Electroencephalog. Clin. Neurophysiol.* **19**:237.

Rosvold, H. E., and Delgado, J. M. R., 1956, The effect on delayed-alternation test performance of stimulating or destroying electrically structures within the frontal lobes of the monkey's brain, *J. Comp. Physiol. Psychol.* **49**:365.

Rosvold, H. E., and Szwarcbart, M., 1964, Neural structures involved in delayed-response performance, in: *The Frontal Granular Cortex and Behavior* (J. M. Warren and K. Akert, eds.), pp. 1–15, McGraw-Hill, New York.

Rosvold, H. E., Mishkin, M., and Szwarcbart, M., 1958, Effects of subcortical lesions in monkeys on visual-discrimination and single-alternation performance, *J. Comp. Physiol. Psychol.* **51**:437.

Rougeul, A., Perret, C., and Buser, P., 1967, Effets comportementaux et électrographiques de stimulations électriques du thalamus chez le chat libre, *Electroencephalog. Clin. Neurophysiol.* **23**:410.

Rubinstein, E. H., and Delgado, J. M. R., 1963, Inhibition induced by forebrain stimulation in the monkey, *Am. J. Physiol.* **205**:941.

Scheibel, M. E., and Scheibel, A. B., 1970, Elementary processes in selected thalamic and cortical subsystems—the structural substrates, in *The Neurosciences, II.,* (F. O. Schmitt, ed.), pp. 443–457, Rockefeller University Press, New York.

Scheibel, M. E., and Scheibel, A. B., 1972, Input-output relations of the thalamic nonspecific system, *Brain Behav. Evol.* **6**:332.

Schildkraut, J. J., and Kety, S. S., 1967, Biogenic amines and emotion, *Science* **156**:21.

Schmaltz, L. W., and Isaacson, R. L., 1968, Effects of caudate and frontal lesions on retention and relearning of a DRL schedule, *J. Comp. Physiol. Psychol.* **65**:343.

Schoenfeld, R. I., and Seiden, L. S., 1969, Effect of α-methyltyrosine on operant behavior and brain catecholamine levels, *J. Pharmacol. Exptl. Therap.* **167**:319.

Schulman, S., 1964, Impaired delayed response from thalamic lesions, Studies in monkeys, *Arch. Neurol.* **11**:477.

Sedgwick, E. M., and Williams, T. D., 1967, The response of single units in the caudate nucleus to peripheral stimulation, *J. Physiol.* **189**:281.

Segundo, J. P., and Machne, X., 1956, Unitary responses to afferent volleys in lenticular nucleus and claustrum, *J. Neurophysiol.* **19**:325.

Shellenberger, M. K., 1971, Effects of α-methyltyrosine on spontaneous and caudate-induced electroencephalographic activity and regional catecholamine concentrations in the cat brain, *Neuropharmacology* **10**:347.

Shute, C. C. D., and Lewis, P. R., 1967, The ascending cholinergic reticular system: neocortical, olfactory and subcortical projections, *Brain* **90**:497.

Siegel, J., and Lineberry, C. G., 1968, Caudate-capsular induced modulation of single-unit activity and mesencephalic reticular formation, *Exptl. Neurol.* **22**:444.

Snyder, S. H., Taylor, K. M., Horn, A. S., and Coyle, J. T., 1972, Psychoactive drugs and neurotransmitters: Differentiating dopamine and norepinephrine neuronal functions with drugs, *Res. Publ. Assoc. Res. Nervous Mental Disease* **50**:359.

Spehlmann, R., Creutzfeldt, O. D., and Jung, R., 1960, Neuronale Hemmung im Motorischen Cortex nach elektrischer Reizung des Caudatum, *Arch. Psychiat. Nervenkr.* **201**:332.

Stevens, J. R., Kim, C., and MacLean, P. D., 1961, Stimulation of caudate nucleus, *Arch. Neurol.* **4**:47.

Strick, P. L., 1973, Light microscopic analysis of the cortical projection of the thalamic ventrolateral nucleus in the cat, *Brain Res.* **55**:1.

Szabo, J., 1962, Topical distribution of the striatal efferents in the monkey, *Exptl. Neurol.* **5**:21.

Szabo, J., 1967, The efferent projections of the putamen in the monkey, *Exptl. Neurol.* **19**:463.

Szabo, J., 1970, Projections from the body of the caudate nucleus in the Rhesus monkey, *Exptl. Neurol.* **27**:1.

Tennyson, V. M., and Marco, L. A., 1973, Intrinsic connections of caudate neurons. II. Fluorescence and electron microscopy following chronic isolation, *Brain Res.* **53**:307.

Teuber, H.-L., 1964, The riddle of the frontal lobe function in man, in: *The Frontal Granular*

Cortex and Behavior (J. M. Warren and K. Akert, eds.), pp. 410–441, McGraw-Hill, New York.

Teuber, H.-L., and Mishkin, M., 1954, Judgement of visual and postural vertical after brain injury, *J. Psychol.* **38**:161.

Teuber, H.-L., and Proctor, F., 1964, Some effects of basal ganglia lesions in subhuman primates and man, *Neuropsychologia* **2**:85.

Thompson, R. F., and Bettinger, L. A., 1970, Neural substrates of attention, in: *Attention: Contemporary Theory and Analysis* (D. Mostofsky, eds.), pp. 367–401, Appleton Century Crofts, New York.

Thompson, R. F., and Shaw, J. A., 1965, Behavioral correlates of evoked activity recorded from association areas of the cerebral cortex, *J. Comp. Physiol. Psychol.* **60**:329.

Thompson, R. F., Johnson, R. H., and Hoopes, J., 1963, Organization of auditory, somatic sensory, and visual projections to association fields of cerebral cortex in the cat, *J. Neurophysiol.* **26**:343.

Ungerstedt, U., 1971, Adipsia and aphagia after 6-hydroxydopamine induced degeneration of the nigro-striatal dopamine system, *Acta Physiol. Scand. Suppl.* **367**:95.

Ungerstedt, U., Butcher, L. L., Butcher, S. G., Andén, N. E., and Fuxe, K., 1969, Direct chemical stimulation of dopaminergic mechanisms in the neostriatum of the rat, *Brain Res.* **14**:461.

Van Rossum, J. M., 1970, Mode of action of psychomotor stimulating drugs, *Intern. Rev. Neurobiol.* **12**:307.

Voneida, T. J., 1960, An experimental study of the course and destination of fibers arising in the head of the caudate nucleus in the cat and monkey, *J. Comp. Neurol.* **115**:75.

Wang, G. H., and Akert, K., 1962, Behavior and reflexes of chronic striatal cats, *Arch. Ital. Biol.* **100**:48.

Warburton, J. W., 1967, Memory disturbance and the Parkinson syndrome. *Brit. J. Med. Psychol.* **40**:169.

Webster, K. E., 1965, The cortico-striatal projection in the cat, *J. Anat.* **99**:329.

Weiss, T., and Fifkova, E., 1963, The effect of neocortical and caudatal spreading depression on "circling movements" induced from the caudate nucleus, *Physiol. Bohemoslov.* **12**:332.

Wyers, E. J., Peeke, H. V. S., Williston, J. S., and Herz, M. J., 1968, Retroactive impairment of passive avoidance learning by stimulation of the caudate nucleus, *Exptl. Neurol.* **22**:350.

Chapter 4

Catecholamines in Activation, Stereotypy, and Level of Mood

A. Randrup, I. Munkvad, R. Fog, and I. H. Ayhan

Sct. Hans Hospital
The Research Laboratory, Department E
Roskilde, Denmark

1. INTRODUCTION

Studies of the effects of psychoactive drugs have contributed much to the present knowledge of the role of catecholamines in behavioral physiology. Since drugs are never completely specific, i.e., no drug acts on only one system in the brain, the knowledge derived from pharmacological experiments is beset with a corresponding uncertainty. Evidence from several experiments, preferably carried out using very different methods, is therefore necessary for conclusions about association between a specific system in the brain and a certain behavior. In the following we shall try to expound such evidence about the association of catecholaminergic systems in the brain with behavioral activation and stereotypy, and we shall explore the possible relations of animal experiments with clinical observations comprising also mental phenomena such as thinking and mood.

2. BEHAVIORAL ACTIVATION AND STEREOTYPY INDUCED BY AMPHETAMINES IN ANIMALS

The activating effect of amphetamines (including apomorphine and dopa) even in small doses is not a general one affecting all kinds of behavior, but it is selective: certain items of behavior ·are quantitatively increased while others are concurrently decreased or abolished. 0.25–1 mg/kg of *d*-amphetamine given subcutaneously to rats thus produces selective activation of sniffing, locomotion, and rearing while there is little grooming activity (Fog, 1970; Ayhan and Randrup, 1973*a*,*b*). Gradual increase of the amphetamine dose in the interval 1–10 mg/kg leads first to further decrease and eventually to disappearance of grooming activity; then, locomotion and rearing are also decreased and finally disappear, so that only sniffing remains. At 10 mg/kg the maximal stereotypy is reached. Sniffing, often accompanied by licking and biting, is performed continuously and usually covers only a small area at or near the bottom of the cage; sometimes backward locomotion is seen (Randrup *et al.*, 1963; Arnfred and Randrup, 1968; Munkvad and Randrup, 1966; Fog, 1970; Scheel-Kruger, 1972).

With the higher doses of amphetamine the stereotyped behavior does not appear immediately after a subcutaneous dose, but develops gradually through a prephase with selective stimulation comparable to that seen with the smaller doses; after the period of maximal stereotypy there is again a postphase with similar selective stimulation (Randrup *et al.*, 1963; Schiørring. 1971).

Other examples of selectivity of the amphetamine stimulation and inhibition come from experiments with vervet monkeys (Kjellberg and Randrup, 1971, 1972*a*) and with cats (Muller-Calgan and Hotovy, 1961; Norton, 1967). Many forms of behavior may be selectively stimulated by amphetamines or turned into a continuously performed stereotypy. The quality of the behavior resulting from an amphetamine injection seems to depend on animal species, dose of amphetamine, time after injection, environmental conditions, and previous learning procedures.

Extreme stereotypy has been described in many mammalian species, including rodents, such as the mouse, rat, and guinea pig (sniffing, licking, biting), cats (looking from side to side, sniffing, or certain grooming activities), dogs (circling or running back and forth along a fixed route, etc.), monkeys (grooming, staring, seizing bars, repertoires of body and limb movements) (Randrup and Munkvad, 1967, 1968, 1974, 1975; Randrup *et al.* 1973; Ellinwood and Duarte-Escalante, 1972), and humans (see below). In monkeys, simple movements such as chewing (as distinct from biting) protrusion of the tongue, prolonged writhing motions, repetitious myoclonic jerks of neck and shoulders, etc., have also been observed (Ellinwood and Duarte-Escalante, 1972; Kjellberg and Randrup, 1972*a*).

It now seems to be generally agreed that the stereotyped behavior produced by amphetamines is mediated by the action of these drugs on brain dopamine. This contention is based on a comprehensive body of evidence referring mostly to the extreme, maximal stereotypy of rats mentioned above. This evidence has been reviewed several times recently (Randrup and Munkvad, 1968, 1970, 1975; Randrup et al., 1974; Sayers, 1972; Ernst, 1971, 1972). Pertinent parts of the evidence is the specific antagonism of the stereotypy by neuroleptics (Randrup and Munkvad, 1965, 1968, 1975; Randrup et al., 1973), which are blockers of dopamine (for references see Randrup et al., 1973; Cools, 1973; Kety and Matthysse, 1974; Soudijn and Wijngaarden, 1972; York, 1972) and the inhibition or elicitation of the stereotypy by lesions of microinjections of amphetamines or dopamine in the dopamine-rich areas (mainly corpus striatum) of the forebrain (Fog, 1972; Sayers, 1972; Costall and Naylor, 1974; Randrup et al., 1973). Also electrical stimulation of the dopaminergic nigrostriatal pathway has led to stereotyped behavior (Anlezark et al., 1971; Crow, 1972). Some experiments with other species e.g., mice (Pedersen and Christensen, 1972) and cats (Cools, 1971, 1973) support the main body of evidence from the rat experiments.

If we accept that the amphetamine-induced stereotyped behavior is due to overactivity of dopaminergic brain systems, then the study of this behavior will help us to understand the physiological role of brain dopamine. This would imply that the dopaminergic systems in the brain influence many, probably all, types of behavior in mammals. Other evidence supporting this contention is available. In a recent paper we reviewed such evidence concerning locomotion, aggression, and other social activities in rats, mice, and monkeys, eating and drinking (Randrup et al., 1973). The restoration by neuroleptics of grooming suppressed by amphetamines in rats was reported some years ago (Randrup and Munkvad, 1965) and was recently confirmed in experiments with the specific dopamine blocker spiramide (Kjellberg and Randrup, unpublished). Each of these behavioral items is, however, also influenced by other mechanisms in the brain, e.g., locomotion by noradrenergic mechanisms, and eating by noradrenergic and serotonergic mechanisms. Probably each behavioral item is influenced by a mosaic of systems, dopaminergic systems being components of this mosaic (Randrup et al., 1974).

Stereotypy was described above as the extreme result of selective stimulation of one or a few items of behavior with concurrent inhibition of others. This implies that stereotypy is a feature of the whole pattern of behavior. Stereotypy can, however, also be a feature of the performance of each item of behavior. Thus, Figure 1 shows stereotyped features in the locomotion of an amphetaminized rat. This observation was made in the prephase before the whole pattern of behavior has reached maximal stereotypy (Schiørring, 1971, and in prep.). Other examples of stereotyped routes of locomotion followed by amphetaminized rats were given by Lat

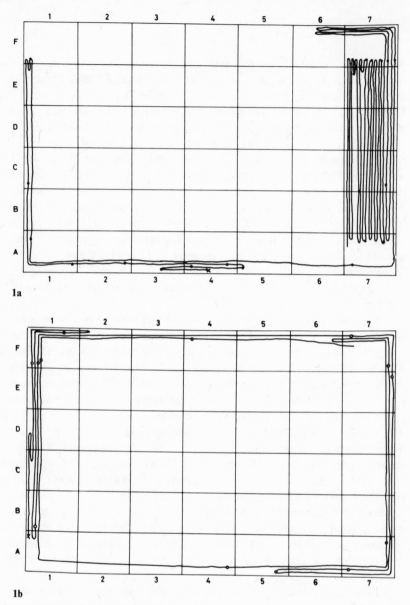

Figure 1a. Route of an amphetaminized rat in a 3 × 3.5 m² cage. There is a period with apparently normal exploration (left in the figure) and a period with repetitive running forth and back (right). The floor of the cage was divided in squares numbered after the chess board principle as indicated in the figure. The observer followed the rat through a one-way screen and recorded its route of locomotion by speaking into a tape recorder.

Figure 1b. Route of a control rat. The figures are representative examples from experiments by Schirring (1971) comprising 13 rats given 5 mg/kg *d*-amphetamine sulfate and ten placebo rats. The locomotion of the amphetamine rat was recorded in the prephase, before the drug took maximal effect. All the locomotion shown in the figure was along the walls of the cage.

(1965), and similar observations have been made with dogs (Willner *et al.*, 1970; Nymark, 1972; Randrup and Munkvad, 1968), monkeys (Randrup and Munkvad, 1967; Kjellberg and Randrup, 1972*a*) and man (Rylander, 1972; Connell, 1956, see case IV in Appendix B).

In monkeys, amphetamine often elicits stereotyped self-grooming; this is restricted to a certain part of the body in contrast to normal grooming which covers the whole body (Kjellberg and Randrup, 1972*a*; Ellinwood, 1971; Ellinwood and Duarte-Escalante, 1972). It often seems that amphetamines selectively stimulate a fraction of an item of normal behavior rather than the whole item (see also Ellinwood *et al.*, 1973; Ellinwood and Duarte-Escalante, 1972).

As may be expected the stereotyped behavior is incompatible with the performance of normal functions. We do not, however, regard stereotypy as the cause of functional impairment, but rather consider that selective stimulation and inhibition, stereotypy, and functional impairment are features of the same process. An example of functional impairment developing concurrently with the emergence of stereotypy is given in Figure 2, which illustrates the effects of amphetamine on operant behavior, showing lever-pressing by a rat in a Skinner box for avoidance of electrical shocks to the feet. The drug takes effect gradually. Immediately after injection the rat works rather normally following the rate of lever-pressing required by the

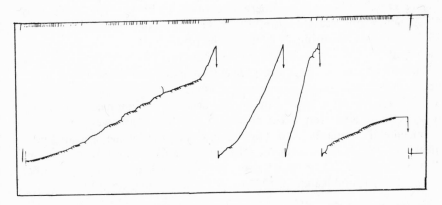

Figure 2. Effects of amphetamine on lever-presses of a rat working to avoid electric shocks to the feet. *d*-Amphetamine sulfate, 10 mg/kg, was given subcutaneously just before the start of the session. Schedule: the first lever-press given, when the electric shock was on, delivered a 15 sec shock-free period (escape) while succeeding presses during the shock-free period delayed the next shock onset for 25 sec (avoidance). The curve shows cumulative recording of lever-presses and covers 104 min beginning at the start of the session; the pen resets after 500 responses; the short oblique lines designate escape responses. On top a record by an event marker: lower position = shock on, upper position = shock off (Lyon and Randrup, 1972; Randrup and Munkvad, 1971).

schedule. The rate then increases out of proportion to the schedule and the rat goes into a stereotyped phase with very quick continuous lever-pressing; in this phase it also performs continuous sniffing, licking, or biting at or off the lever (Randrup and Munkvad, 1970; Lyon and Randrup, 1972). Then follows a phase in which the rat responds only when receiving the shock, and finally, the operant behavior breaks down completely. The rat then sits sniffing and licking the bars of the cage floor, although these give shock continuously.

This process may also be seen as a gradual decrease of adaptability or of influence of environmental factors (shocks and schedule of avoidance) on the behavior. In the last phase the behavior is shaped only by the amphetamine effect, the rat performs the same stereotyped behavior as it does in its home cage. This might perhaps be regarded as "autistic" behavior. In terms of motivation it may be considered that under amphetamine, the performance of stereotyped behavior could become a reward in itself. Robinson and Daley (1967) found that restrained rats upon receiving apomorphine would actually "work" to obtain a gnawable object. However, more experiments are necessary (and strongly indicated) to elucidate the changes in motivation associated with stereotyped behavior elicited by amphetamine and apomorphine. Other examples of functional impairment under amphetamine come from experiments on exploratory activity (Robbins and Iversen, 1973; Dyne and Hughes, 1970; Hughes, 1972; see also Figure 1), social activity (Kjellberg and Randrup, 1971, 1972b; Schiørring, 1972; Schiørring and Randrup, 1971), and drinking (Nielsen and Lyon, 1973). The functional impairments can be partially but not completely antagonized by neuroleptics (Kjellberg and Randrup, 1971; Nielsen and Lyon, 1973; Randrup *et al.*, unpublished data from experiments on avoidance behavior of rats and social behavior of monkeys).

In certain experiments with operant behavior the animals may appear to work more effectively under amphetamine. This can however be due to an incidental compatibility of the response required by the special experiment with the items of behavior selectively stimulated by the dose of amphetamine given. This is revealed by control experiments requiring another response (Lyon and Randrup, 1972; Randrup and Munkvad, 1971).

3. POSSIBLE ROLE OF NORADRENALINE IN BEHAVIORAL ACTIVATION AND STEREOTYPY INDUCED BY MORPHINE

In rats, doses of 5–100 mg/kg of morphine cause mainly sedation and catalepsy, but when the rats become tolerant, this effect is replaced by activation. With 100–125 mg/kg of morphine the activity of the rats is stereotyped and somewhat similar to amphetamine stereotypy. With morphine, however, licking or biting of paws is more predominant, and the stereotyped activity is now and then interrupted by spells of very quick running or rearing, lasting 2–5 sec (Fog, 1970; Ayhan and Randrup, 1972).

Pharmacologically there are also differences between the stereotypy induced by chronic morphine and the amphetamine stereotypy, particularly with respect to drugs antagonizing noradrenaline such as the α-blockers, phenoxybenzamine and aceperone, and the inhibitor of noradrenaline synthesis, FLA-63. These drugs all inhibit the morphine stereotypy in doses which barely affect the amphetamine stereotypy. In comparison the neuroleptic spiramide (blocker of dopamine) inhibits the two types of stereotypy to about the same extent. This indicates a role of noradrenaline in morphine stereotypy, an indication, which is further supported by an experiment, that morphine stereotypy inhibited by FLA-63 can be restored by intraventricular injection of noradrenaline (Ayhan and Randrup, 1972).

Small single doses of morphine (1–2 mg/kg) produce excitation in rats, and this excitation is also sensitive to drugs inhibiting noradrenaline (Ayhan and Randrup, 1973a). Behaviorally, this excitation differs from that produced by small doses of amphetamine by being less selective. While amphetamine selectively stimulates certain items of behavior (e.g., locomotion, rearing) and concurrently inhibits others (e.g., grooming, particularly grooming with the hind leg) the morphine-stimulated rats are more varied, comprising many items of behavior: locomotion and rearing *as well as* grooming, in particular, much grooming with the hind leg, eating, drinking (Fog, 1970; Ayhan and Randrup, 1973a), and various forms of social behavior, e.g., sniffing of the anal–genital region and a form of play (also seen in untreated rats) in which two rats are touching each other with the forepaws and the one is alternatively over and under the other (unpublished observations).

In mice, morphine produces stimulation in the dose range 5–100 mg/kg. With 5–10 mg/kg the activity is varied (as with the smaller doses of morphine in rats). With increasing dose, however, the behavioral repertoire becomes gradually more restricted, first grooming is diminished and finally disappears, then rearing, and with 100 mg/kg the activity is very stereotyped, consisting of locomotion only, the locomotion being accompanied by very little sniffing. This stereotypy can be clearly distinguished from the amphetamine stereotypy, which in mice consists predominantly of continuous sniffing, licking, or biting with some, but not much, locomotion. The experiments with mice in our laboratory (Ayhan, unpublished) also indicate a role of noradrenaline in the stimulation of mice by morphine, and this is supported by other recently published experiments (Kuschinsky and Hornykiewicz, 1973; Carroll and Sharp, 1972a).

In our experiments, the morphine stimulation was completely antagonized by small doses of noradrenaline blockers, such as phenoxybenzamine and aceperone, and the mice became cataleptic. Application of the noradrenaline blockers alone did not produce catalepsy. This indicates to us that in mice morphine blocks dopamine as it does in rats (producing catalepsy), but in mice the concurrent stimulation of noradrenaline is so strong that it overcomes the cataleptic effect of the dopamine blockade. The contention that morphine also blocks the dopamine system in mice is supported by biochemical experiments on mouse brain, showing that morphine affects dopamine metabolites and turnover in a way similar to a neuroleptic but different from amphetamine (Fukui and Takagi, 1972; Fukui *et al.*, 1972; cf. Roffler-Tarlov *et al.*, 1971, and the discussion in Ayhan and Randrup, 1973*a*).

Association of increased noradrenergic activity in the brain with behavioral activation is also supported by other experimental results, i.e., the behavioral activation after intraventricular injection of small doses of noradrenaline (Benkert, 1969; Herman, 1970; Segal and Mandell, 1970; Geyer and Segal, 1973; Geyer, 1973) and the sedative effect of noradrenaline inhibitors (Janssen *et al.*, 1965, 1967; Rolinski and Scheel-Krüger, 1973).

The behavioral activation induced by morphine seems to be inhibited also by all changes in dopaminergic activity in the brain, both increase in this activity by apomorphine, amphetamine, or dopa (Ayhan and Randrup, 1973*b*; Kuschinsky and Hornykiewicz, 1973) and decrease by neuroleptics or lesions in the striata (Carroll and Sharp, 1972*a*; Ayhan and Randrup, 1972, 1973*a*, unpublished; Kuschinsky and Hornykiewicz, 1973). According to the interpretation above, this would mean that noradrenaline activation can cause stimulation of behavior only when the dopaminergic system is functioning within limits near the normal.

Excitatory effects of morphine are reported in many mammalian species, e.g., cat, horse, sheep, pig, bear, and hedgehog (Guinard, 1890; Krueger, 1941) and have also been observed in certain human individuals (Krueger *et al.*, 1941; Isbell, 1971, Carroll and Sharp, 1972*b*). It remains to be seen if these excitatory effects are pharmacologically analogous to those in rats and mice, particularly with respect to noradrenaline.

4. EFFECTS OF AMPHETAMINES AND NEUROLEPTICS ON ACTIVATION, STEREOTYPY, AND MOOD IN HUMANS

Amphetamines elicit stereotyped behavior ("punding," Rylander, 1972) in humans as in other mammals (Randrup and Munkvad, 1967; Ellinwood *et al.*, 1973), and it seems reasonable to assume that in humans also the stereotyped behavior is mediated by brain dopamine. Many items of behavior can be selectively stimulated and become stereotyped in humans, e.g., bathing, cleaning of the house or a particular item, mechanical work on cars, radios, etc., combing the hair, repeating the same words or sentences for hours, walking the streets, etc. (Rylander, 1969, 1971, 1972; Ellinwood et al., 1973; further references in Randrup and Munkvad, 1967, 1970, 1971, 1974; Randrup et al., 1974).

As in the monkeys (see above), very simple "neurological" movements can be stimulated or elicited in man by amphetamines including dopa, e.g., movements of mouth and tongue, jerky movements of legs, screwing or twisting movements of the body, etc. (Rylander, 1971, 1972; Ashcroft et al., 1972; Calne, 1970; further references in Kjellberg and Randrup, 1972a; Randrup and Munkvad, 1974a; Randrup et al., in 1974). The items of behavior and movements that are actually stimulated seem to depend on individuality, dose of amphetamine, environmental factors, etc.

An interesting example of compatibility of the stereotyped behavior with topical requirements (compare the text on operant behavior in the section on animals above) is given by Rylander (1969):

"An odd phenomenon indicating the deepgoing effects of large doses of central stimulants is a sort of automatic and stereotype behavior which can go on for hours. The addict plucks at some object in a compulsive manner, for instance taking apart and putting together a watch or a telephone. Women sort out their handbags again and again or tidy up their flats whether it needs tidying or not. Some make use of this curious state. If the flat really needs tidying they take a strong so-called tidy-pump and then start the job. This is then done in a meticulous way and with pleasure, whether they in fact like tidying or not."

Ordinarily, the stereotyped behavior is associated with functional impairment as in the animals (Kalus et al., 1942; Kalus, 1950; Sjoqvist and Tottie, 1969; Ellinwood and Cohen, 1972; Randrup and Munkvad, 1971) and the abnormal states elicited by amphetamines in humans often appear similar to schizophrenia, so much that misdiagnoses are made (Randrup and Munkvad, 1972).

Neuroleptics antagonize (but do not completely eliminate) the symptoms of schizophrenia and the "amphetamine psychosis" and seem to antagonize most or perhaps all "fundamental" as well as "accessory" symptoms (Cole and Davis, 1968; Angrist, 1974) including stereotyped activities (Munkvad et al., 1971). Since blockade of dopamine seems to be the only common and characteristic property of neuroleptics (Randrup et al., 1973; Cools, 1973; Soudijn and Wijngaarden, 1972; Carlsson et al., 1972; Kety and Matthysse, 1974), this indicates an association of brain dopamine with most all the symptoms of schizophrenia. Based on the effect of amphetamines and neuroleptics the hypothesis has been advanced that absolute or relative overactivity of dopaminergic systems in the brain is an important feature in the pathogenesis of schizophrenia (Munkvad and Randrup, 1970; Randrup and Munkvad, 1970, 1972, 1974).

As pointed out previously (Randrup and Munkvad, 1974) it cannot be ruled out, however, that abnormalities in other areas of the brain could elicit schizophrenic symptoms, and that these, although elicited by another system, could be antagonized by reduction of the activity of dopaminergic systems by neuroleptic treatment. In any case, some association between brain dopamine and the symptoms of schizophrenia, fundamental as well as accessory, seems highly probable.

We are now trying to find out to what extent the various symptoms of schizophrenia and amphetamine psychosis (described in traditional clinical terms) can be seen as directly related to the stereotypy and the selective stimulation and inhibition observed in the amphetaminized animals and humans, and described in purely behavioral terms. Stereotyped behavior, of course, forms an important link here, since this has often been observed and described in behavioral terms in schizophrenic patients (Bleuler, 1972; Munkvad *et al.*, 1971) as well as in amphetaminized humans and animals. Mannerism and automatism appear to be quite closely associated with stereotypy. Autism has at least the relation to stereotypy that both terms designate behavior that is determined exclusively from within and not influenced by the environment (see the text associated with Figure 2). Rylander (1972) states that during the stereotyped activity ("punding") of amphetamine addicts, all sorts of social interaction is excluded: "Eighty-four percent keep quite silent and 95% say that they do not listen if they are spoken to. 'I am living in my own world quite secluded,' one of the addicts said. They are not at all interested in what others are doing and they never try to get into contact with others. The same sort of autistic behavior Randrup has observed in animals."

Other human symptoms, such as changes in affective behavior (aggression, blunted affect) and social withdrawal appear to be directly parallel to the similar phenomena observed in amphetaminized animals (see above and Randrup *et al.*, 1973) in which these phenomena are seen as examples of selective stimulation and inhibition. In still other cases, the relation of clinically described symptoms to observations in amphetaminized animals is not so clear and direct, but it seems that here is an area where further clarification is possible. As an example we shall discuss stereotypy and activation of thinking.

Munkvad *et al.* (1971), who made a clinical trial with the neuroleptic pimozide (probably the most specific dopamine blocker), noted this antagonized stereotyped thinking as well as stereotyped behavior in schizophrenic patients. Stereotyped thinking has also been reported in amphetamine addicts (Kalus, 1950; Scher, 1966; Ellinwood, 1967, 1972; Ellinwood et al., 1973).

Such observations in humans give rise to epistemological problems, since thinking and behavior are not immediately comparable; the relations of these entities, with the observations they are based on, are different. A more thorough treatment of these problems will be attempted by one of us (Randrup, in prep.) but here it may suffice to note, that both behavior and thoughts are supposed to be associated with certain processes in the brain, and these processes are directly comparable. Further, the brain processes associated with behavior and thinking may well be related. Thus, the psychologist and epistemologist Piaget (1964) thinks that thoughts originate from internalized actions, and Ellinwood et al. (1973), writing on amphetamine intoxication, state "that a common attitudinal–postural mechanism may subserve both the motor stereotypies and the constricted perceptual and cognitive patterns."

On this clinical and epistemological basis it seems reasonable to assume that hyperactivity of brain dopamine is associated with stereotyped thinking. An association of brain dopamine with activated or accelerated thinking ("Ideenflucht," Bleuler, 1972) as observed in manic patients (see further below) and amphetamine addicts (Angrist et al., 1969) also appears likely.

An interesting example of connections between paranoid thinking, hallucinations, and steroeotyped behavior (in both man and animals) is provided by the following observations:

Ellinwood (1969, 1971, 1972) describes amphetamine-induced grooming stereotypies (incessant examining, rubbing, and picking of certain areas of the skin) in rhesus monkeys (see also Kjellberg and Randrup, 1972a) and humans. Many of the humans, Ellinwood states, developed stereotyped delusions of parasitosis and spent many hours examining their skin and digging out imagined encysted parasites. Similar cases are described in the other German literature about methamphetamine abuse (Staehelin, 1941, Daube, 1942; see also Rylander, 1971) and have also been observed among schizophrenic patients (Ellinwood, 1969, 1972; Munkvad, personal observations).

While many cases of amphetamine psychosis show resemblance to schizophrenia, some authors have reported cases which appear to be reminiscent of manic-depressive psychosis or have mixed manic-depressive and schizophrenic symptomatology (Tatetsu, 1960; Sano and Nagasaka, 1956; O'Flanagen and Taylor, 1950; Rylander, 1969; Kellner, 1960; Harder, 1947; Angrist et al., 1969). In this connection it should be noted that stereotyped behavior can be an important component of the clinical picture of mania, and "neurological" dyskinesias similar to those seen in amphetamine addicts have been observed in patients with bipolar affective illness, apparently unrelated to drug treatment (Ashcroft *et al.*, 1972).

This raises the question of possible relations of brain catecholamines (and particularly dopamine) to manic-depressive psychosis and to mood. It may at first glance be considered improbable that brain dopamine should be associated with both schizophrenia and manic-depressive psychosis, but this would be in keeping with the results of the animal experiments which indicate that brain dopamine is associated with many behavioral features. The net result (the clinical picture) of, e.g., dopamine overactivity, would then depend on the state of the rest of the brain (individuality, other abnormalities) environmental factors, subdivisions within the dopamine area in the forebrain (see below), etc.

The idea that brain dopamine is associated with mania and depression actually receives support from an important body of pharmacological and biochemical evidence.

In our opinion the antimanic effect of neuroleptics is an important item of this body of evidence. This effect is generally recognized, and some neuroleptics, which are regarded as very specific dopamine blockers have particularly strong antimanic effect, e.g., haloperidol. Recent data indicate that certain neuroleptics (e.g., benperidol and clotiapine) have mainly antimanic effect, and others (e.g., sulpiride) have mainly antiautistic and antidelusional effects, while still others (e.g., haloperidol) exert all three effects (Bobon *et al.*, 1972, 1972a). However, all these neuroleptics give Parkinsonian side effects (Bobon *et al.*, 1972), indicating their dopamine-blocking action. It seems possible that these observations open new possibilities for investigating differences between the actions of various neuroleptics upon brain dopamine. There may be differences in the action on the single synapse and functional subdivisions within the dopamine-rich area in the forebrain which can also be considered; one neuroleptic may act most strongly on one certain subdivision and another neuroleptic mainly on other subdivisions. That such subdivisions exist appears very likely on anatomical grounds, particularly in the higher mammals, such as monkey and man, where the putamen and the caudate nucleus (the two areas which contain the bulk of the dopamine in the brain) are clearly separated anatomically (see also McKenzie, 1972; Costall and Naylor, 1974).

Another piece of evidence, which specifically indicates an association of brain dopamine with affective psychoses, is the finding of abnormal values of the dopamine metabolite homovanillic acid in cerebrospinal fluid from depressed and manic patients (van Praag and Korf, 1971; Papeschi and McClure, 1971; Ashcroft *et al.*, 1972; Roos and Sjöström, 1969; Nordin *et al.*, 1971; Sjöström, 1972; Mendels *et al.*, 1972; Bowers, 1973; Goodwin *et al.*, 1973; Post *et al.*, 1973). Coexistence and other connections between

Parkinson's disease and depression (Patrick and Levy, 1922, Mandell *et al.*, 1962; Warburton, 1967; Mindham, 1970; Müller-Fahlbusch, 1972) also indicate an association with dopamine.

In agreement with the antimanic effect of neuroleptics, depression (also states similar to the endogenous depression) appears as a not uncommon side effect of this type of drugs, also of specific dopamine blockers such as fluphenazine and haloperidol (Alarcon and Carney, 1969; Forrest, 1969; Segal and Ropschitz, 1969; Helmchen and Hippius, 1969; Simonson, 1964; Bohaček, 1965; Boardman and Fullerton, 1960; Delay *et al.*, 1963).

Several drugs which influence mania, hypomania, and depression, such as monoamine oxidase inhibitors, reserpine, α-methyl-p-tyrosine, dopa, have effect on brain dopamine, but since these drugs also affect other substances in the brain, e.g., noradrenaline and serotonin, the evidence derived from them is less specific than that derived from the specific dopamine blockers among the neuroleptics. The same is true for electroconvulsive therapy (Papeschi *et al.*, 1974a, 1974b).

The most direct experiments on the relations of catecholamines with mood are probably those of Gunne *et al.* (1970, 1972). They elicited "euphoria," assessed by patients' self-rating, by intravenous injections of amphetamine and found that this could be inhibited by the inhibitor of catecholamine synthesis, α-methyltyrosine. They also found that the euphoria was reduced by pretreatment with the specific dopamine-blocker pimozide, while α- and β-blockers of noradrenaline were without effect (see also Jonsson *et al.*, 1971; Änggård *et al.*, 1971).

Like thoughts, mood would be assumed to be associated with certain brain processes, but mood has no clear relations to observations in animals, and our discussion of this topic has therefore been based on observations of humans only.

5. REFERENCES

Alarcon, R. de, and Carney, M. W. P., 1969, Severe depressive mood changes following slow-release intramuscular fluphenazine injection, *Brit. Med. J.* 3:564.
Änggård, E., Jönsson, L. E., and Gunne, L.-M., 1971, Pharmacological blockade of amphetamine effects in subjects dependent on central stimulants, *Acta Pharmacol. Toxicol. Suppl.* 4:2.
Angrist, B., 1974, Amphetamine Psychosis, in: *Catecholamines and Their Enzymes in the Neuropathology of Schizophrenia* (S. Kety and S. Matthysse, eds.), *J. Psychiat. Res.* 11:1.
Angrist, B., Schweitzer, J., Friedhoff, A. J., Gershon, S., Hekimian, L. J., and Floyd, A., 1969, The clinical symptomatology of amphetamine psychosis and its relationship to amphetamine levels in urine, *Int. Pharmacopsychiatry* 2:125.

Anlezark, G. M., Arbuthnott, G. W., Christie, J. E., and Crow, T. J., 1971, Role of cerebral dopamine in action of psychotropic drugs, *Brit. J. Pharmacol.* **41**:406.

Arnfred, T., and Randrup, A., 1968, Cholinergic mechanism in brain inhibiting amphetamine-induced stereotyped behavior, *Acta Pharmacol. Toxicol.* **26**:384.

Ashcroft, G. W., *et al.*, 1972, Modified amine hypothesis for the etiology of affective illness, *Lancet* 1972:573.

Ayhan, I. H., and Randrup, A., 1972, Role of brain noradrenaline in morphine-induced stereotyped behavior, *Psychopharmacologia* **27**:203.

Ayhan, I. H., and Randrup, A., 1973a, Behavioral and pharmacological studies on morphine-induced excitation of rats. Possible relation to brain catecholamines, *Psychopharmacologia* **29**:317.

Ayhan, I. H., and Randrup, A., 1973b, Inhibitory effects of amphetamine, L-dopa and apomorphine on morphine-induced behavioral excitation of rats, *Arch. Intern. Pharmacodyn.* **204**:283.

Benkert, O., 1969, Measurement of hyperactivity in rats in a dose-response curve after intrahypothalamic norepinephrine injection, *Life Sci.* **8**:943.

Bleuler, M., 1972, *Lehrbuch der Psychiatrie,* Springer-Verlag, Berlin, Heidelberg, New York.

Boardman, R. H., and Fullerton, A. G., 1960, Iatrogenic parkinsonism, *J. Mental Sci.* **106**:1468.

Bobon, J., Pinchard, A., Collard, J., and Bobon, D. P., 1972, Clinical classification of neuroleptics, with special reference to their antimanic, antiautistic, and ataraxic properties. *Comprehensive Psychiat.* **13**:123.

Bobon, J., Bobon, D. P., Pinchard, A., Collard, J., Ban, T. A., Buck, R. de, Hippius, H., Lambert, P. A., and Vinar, O., 1972a, A new comparative physiognomy of neuroleptics: a collaborative clinical report. *Acta Psychiat. Belgica* **72**:542.

Bohaček, N., 1965, Discussion working group 4, in: *Neuro-Psychopharmacology,* (D. Bente and P. B. Bradley, eds.), pp. 175–178, Elsevier Publishing Company, Amsterdam.

Bowers, M. B., Jr., 1973, 5-Hydroxyindoleacetic acid (5HIAA) and homovanillic acid (HVA) following probenecid in acute psychotic patients treated with phenothiazines, *Psychopharmacologia* **28**:309.

Calne, D. B., 1970, L-Dopa in the treatment of parkinsonism, *Clin. Pharmacol. Therap.* **11**:6.

Carlsson, A., Persson, T., Roos, B. E., and Wålinder, J., 1972, Potentiation of phenothiazines by α-methyltyrosine in treatment of chronic schizophrenia, *J. Neural Transmission* **33**:83.

Carroll, B. J., and Sharp, P. T., 1972a, Monoamine mediation of the morphine-induced activation of mice, *Brit. J. Pharmacol.* **46**:124.

Carroll, B. J., and Sharp, P. T., 1972b, An animal model of mania, *Psychopharmacologia* **26** (Suppl. 1972):10.

Cole, J. O., and Davis, J. M., 1968, Clinical efficacy of the phenothiazines as antipsychotic drugs, in: *Psychopharmacology,* (D. H. Efron, ed.), pp. 1057–1063, Public Health Service Publ. No. 1836, U.S. Government, Printing Office, Washington, D.C.

Connell, P. H., 1956, Amphetamine psychosis, Thesis, Maudsley Hospital, University of London.

Cools, A. R., 1971, The function of dopamine and its antagonism in the caudate nucleus of cats in relation to the stereotyped behaviour, *Arch. Intern. Pharmacodyn.* **194**:259.

Cools, A. R., 1973, The Caudate Nucleus and Neurochemical Control of Behavior, Thesis, Universitet Nijmegen, Holland.

Costall, B. and Naylor, R. J., 1974, Extrapyramidal and mesolimbic involvement with the stereotypic activity of *d*- and *l*-amphetamine, *European J. Pharmacol.* **25**:121.

Crow, T. J., 1972, A map of the rat mesencephalon for electrical self-stimulation, *Brain Res.* **36**:265.

Daube, H., 1942, Pervitinpsychosen, *Nervenarzt* **15**:20.

Delay, J., Pichot, P., Lemperiere, T., and Bailly, R., 1963, L'emploi des butyrophenones en psychiatrie etude statistique et psychometrique, in: *Symposium Internazionale Sull'Haloperidol E Triperidol,* pp. 305–319, Istituto Luso Farmaco D'Italia, Milano.

Dyne, L. J., and Hughes, R. N., 1970, Effects of methylphenidate on activity and reactions to novelty in rats, Psychonomic Sci. **19**(5):267.

Ellinwood, E. H., 1967, Amphetamine psychosis: I. Description of the individuals and process, *J. Nervous Mental Disease* **144**:273.

Ellinwood, E. H., 1969, Amphetamine psychosis: A multi-dimensional process, *Seminars Psychiatry* **1**:208.

Ellinwood, E. H., 1971, Comparative methamphetamine intoxication in experimental animals, *Pharmakopsychiat. Neuropsychopharmakol.* **4**:357.

Ellinwood, E. H., 1972, Amphetamine psychosis: individuals, setting, and sequences, in: *Current Concepts of Amphetamine Abuse,* (E. H. Ellinwood, and S. Cohen, eds.), pp. 143–157, U.S. Government Printing Office, Washington, D.C.

Ellinwood, E. H., and Cohen, S. (eds.), 1972, *Current Concepts of Amphetamine Abuse,* U.S. Government Printing Office, Washington, D.C.

Ellinwood, E. H., and Duarte-Escalante, O., 1972, Chronic methamphetamine intoxication in three species of experimental animals, in: *Current Concepts of Amphetamine Abuse,* (E. H. Ellinwood and S. Cohen, eds.), pp. 59–68, U.S. Government Printing Office, Washington, D.C.

Ellinwood, E. H., Sudilovsky, and Nelson, L. M., 1973, Evolving behavior in the clinical and experimental amphetamine (model) psychosis, *Am. J. Psychiat.* **730**(10):1088.

Ernst, A. M., 1971, Chemical stimulation of central dopaminergic receptors in the striatal body of rats, in: *The Correlation of Adverse Effects in Man with Observation in Animals* (S. B. de Baker, ed.), pp. 18–23, Excerpta Med. Intern. Congr. Series 220, Amsterdam.

Ernst, A. M., 1972, Relationship of the central effect of dopamine on gnawing compulsion syndrome in rats and the release of serotonin, *Arch. Intern. Pharmacodyn.* **199**:219.

Fog, R., 1970, Behavioral effects in rats of morphine and amphetamine and of a combination of the two drugs, *Psychopharmacologia* **16**:305.

Fog, R., 1972, On stereotype and catalepsy: studies on the effect of amphetamines and neuroleptics in rats, *Acta Neurol. Scand. Suppl.* **48**:50 (Thesis).

Forrest, A., 1969, Depressive changes after fluphenazine treatment, *Brit. Med. J.* October:69.

Fukui, K., and Tagaki, H., 1972, Effect of morphine on the cerebral contents of metabolites of dopamine in normal and tolerant mice: its possible relation to analgesic action, *Brit. J. Pharmacol.* **44**:45.

Fukui, K., Shiomi, H., and Tagaki, H., 1972, Effect of morphine on tyrosine hydroxylase activity in mouse brain, *European J. Pharmacol.* **19**:123.

Geyer, M., 1973, Dissociation of some behavioral effects of intraventricular dopamine and norepinephrine, *Dissertation Abst.* **33**(11):5539.

Geyer, M. A., and Segal, D. S., 1973, Differential effects of reserpine and α-methyl-p-tyrosine on norepinephrine and dopamine induced behavioral activity, *Psychopharmacologia* **29**:131.

Goodwin, F. K., Post, R. M., Dunner, D. L., and Gordon, E. K., 1973, Cerebrospinal fluid amine metabolites in affective illness: the probenecid technique, *Am. J. Psychiat.* **130**(1):73.

Guinard, L., 1890, Action physiologique de la morphine chez le chat, *C. R. Acad, Sci. (Paris)* **111**:981.

Gunne, L. M., Änggård, E., and Jönsson, L. E., 1970, Blockade of amphetamine effects in human subjects, in: *International Institute on the Prevention and Treatment of Drug De-*

pendence, I.C.A.A. (A. Tongue and E. Tongue, eds.), pp. 249–255, Lausanne, Switzerland.

Gunne, L. M., Änggård, E., and Jönsson, L. E., 1972, Clinical trials with amphetamine-blocking drugs. *Psychiat. Neurol. Neurochir.* 75:225.

Harder, A., 1947, Uber Weckamin-Psychosen, *Schweiz. Med. Wochschr.* 37/38:982.

Helmchen, H., and Hippius, H., 1967, Depressive Syndrome im Verlauf neuroleptischer Therapie, *Nervenarzt* 38(10):455.

Herman, Z. S., 1970, The effects of noradrenaline on rat's behaviour, *Psychopharmacologia* 16:369.

Hughes, R. N., 1972, Methylphenidate-induced inhibition of exploratory behaviour in rats, *Life Sci.* 11:161.

Isbell, H., 1971, Clinical aspects of the various forms of nonmedical use of drugs, *Anesthesia Analgesia Current Res.* 50:886.

Janssen, P. A. J., Niemegeers, C. J. E., and Schellekens, K. H. L., 1965, Is it possible to predict the clinical effects of neuroleptic drugs (major tranquilizers) from animal data? I. *Arzneimittel-Forsch.* 15:104.

Janssen, P. A. J., Niemegeers, C. J. E., Schellekens, K. H. L., and Lenaerts, F. M., 1967, Is it possible to predict the clinical effects of neuroleptic drugs (major tranquilizers) from animal data? IV, *Arzneimittel-Forsch.* 17:841.

Jönsson, L. E., Änggård, E., and Gunne, L.-M., 1971, Blockade of intravenous amphetamine euphoria in man, *Clin. Pharmacol. Therap.* 12:889.

Kalus, F., 1950, Über die psychotischen Bilder bei chronischem Pervitinmissbrauch (II), *Psychiat. Neurol. Med. Psychol.* 2:138:

Kalus, F., Kucher, I., and Zutt, J., 1942, Über Psychosen bei chronisher Pervitinmissbrauch, *Nervenarzt* 15:8.

Kellner, E., 1960, Preludinsucht und Preludinpsychose, *Ther. Ggw.* 11:524.

Kety, S., and Matthysse, S. (eds.), 1974, Catecholamines and their enzymes in the Neuropathology of Schizophrenia, *J. Psychiatric Res.* 11:1.

Kjellberg, B., and Randrup, A., 1971, The effects of amphetamine and pimozide, a neuroleptic, on the social behavior of vervet monkeys (ceropithecus sp), in: *Advances in Neuro-Psychopharmacology,* (O. Vinař, Z. Votava, and P. B. Bradley, eds.), pp. 305–310, North-Holland Publishing Company, Amsterdam. Avicenum, Czechoslovak Medical Press, Prague.

Kjellberg, B., and Randrup, A., 1972a, Stereotypy with selective stimulation of certain items of behavior observed in amphetamine-treated monkeys (cercopithecus), *Pharmakopsychiatr. Neuropsychopharmakol.* 5:1.

Kjellberg, B., and Randrup, A., 1972b, Changes in social behaviour in pairs of vervet monkeys (cercopithecus) produced by single, low doses of amphetamine, *Psychopharmacologia Suppl.* 26:117.

Krueger, H., Eddy, N. B., and Sumwalt, M., 1941, *The Pharmacology of the Opium Alkaloids, Part 1,* Supplement 165, Public Health Reports, U.S. Government Printing Office, Washington, D.C.

Kuschinsky, K., and Hornykiewicz, O., 1973, Morphine-induced locomotor activity in mice: involvement of central dopaminergic and noradrenergic neurons, in: *IV Congress of the Polish Pharmacological Society* (M. R. Mazur, ed.), p. 27, Lodz.

Lát, J., 1965, The spontaneous exploratory reactions as a tool for psychopharmacological studies. A contribution towards a theory of contradictory results, in: *Pharmacology of Conditioning, Learning and Retension* (M. Ya. Mikhel'son, V. G. Longo, and Z. Votava, eds.), pp. 47–66, Pergamon Press, Czechoslovak Medical Press, Prague.

Lyon, M., and Randrup, A., 1972, The dose-response effect of amphetamine upon avoidance behavior in the rat seen as a function of increasing stereotype, *Psychopharmacologia* **23**:334.

Mandell, A. J., Markham, C. H., Tallman, F. F., and Mandell, M. P., 1962, Motivation and ability to move, *Am. J. Psychiat.* **119**:554.

McKenzie, G. M., 1972, Role of the tuberculum olfactorium in stereotyped behavior induced by apomorphine in the rat, *Psychopharmacologia* **23**:212.

Mendels, J., Frazer, A., Fitzgerald, R. G., Ramsey, T. A., and Stokes, J. W., 1972, Biogenic amine metabolites in cerebrospinal fluid of depressed and manic patients, *Science* **175**:1380.

Mindham, R. H. S., 1970, Psychiatric symptoms in Parkinsonism, *J. Neurol. Neurosurg. Psychiat.* **33**:188.

Müller-Calgan, H., and Hotovy, R., 1961, Verhaltensänderungen der Katze durch verschiedene zentralerregand wirkende Pharmaka, *Arzneimittel-Forsch.* **11**:642.

Müller-Fahlbusch, H., 1972, *Klinische und Katamnestische Untersuchungen zum Parkinsonismus*, Georg Thieme Verlag, Stuttgart.

Munkvad, I., and Randrup, A., 1966, The persistence of amphetamine stereotypies of rats in spite of strong sedation, *Acta Psychiat. Scand. Suppl.* **191**:178.

Munkvad, I., and Randrup, A., 1970, Evidence indicating the role of brain dopamine in the psychopharmacology of schizophrenic psychoses, in: *Psihofarmakologija 2* (N. Bohacek, ed.), pp. 45–47, Medicinska Naklada, Zagreb.

Munkvad, I., Hein, G., and Herskin, B., 1971, The treatment of chronic schizophrenics with pimozide (Orap), *Clin. Trials J.* **8**(Suppl. II):67.

Nielsen, E. B., and Lyon, M., 1973, Drinking behavior and brain dopamine: Antagonistic effect of a neuroleptic drug (Pimozide) upon amphetamine- or apomorphine-induced hypodipsia, *Psychopharmacologia* **33**:299.

Nordin, G., Ottosson, J.-O., and Ross, B.-E., 1971, Influence of convulsive therapy on 5-hydroxyindoleacetic acid and homovanillic acid in cerebrospinal fluid in endogeneous depression, *Psychopharmacologia* **20**:315.

Norton, S., 1967, An analysis of cat behaviour using chlorpromazine and amphetamine, *Intern J. Neuropharmacol.* **6**:307.

Nymark, M., 1972, Apomorphine provoked stereotypy in the dog, *Psychopharmacologia* **26**:361.

O'Flanagan, P. M., and Taylor, R. B., 1950, A case of recurrent psychosis associated with amphetamine addiction, *J. Mental Sci.* **96**:1033.

Papeschi, R., and McClure, D., 1971, Homovanillic and 5-hydroxyindoleacetic acid in cerebrospinal fluid of depressed patients. *Arch. Gen. Psychiat.* **25**:352.

Papeschi, R., Randrup, A., and Lal, S., 1974*a*, Effect of ECT on dopaminergic and noradrenergic mechanisms. I. Effect on the behavioral changes induced by reserpine, α-methyl-*p*-tyrosine or amphetamie, *Psychopharmacologia* **35**:149.

Papeschi, R., Randrup, A., and Munkvad, I., 1974*b*, Effect of ECT on dopaminergic and noradrenergic mechanisms. II. Effect on dopamine and noradrenaline concentrations and turnovers, *Psychopharmacologia* **35**:159.

Patrick, H. T., and and Levy, D. M., 1922, Parkinson's disease, *Arch. Neurol. Psychiat.* **7**:711.

Pedersen, V., and Christensen, A. V., 1972, Antagonism of methyl-phenidate-induced stereotyped gnawing in mice, *Acta Pharmacol. Toxicol.* **31**:488.

Piaget, J., 1964, *Six Etudes de Psychologie*, Gonthier, Paris.

Post, R. M., Kotin, J., Goodwin, F. K., and Gordon, E. K., 1973, Psychomotor activity and cerebrospinal fluid amine metabolites in affective illness, *Am. J. Psychiat.* **130**(1):67.

Randrup, A., and Munkvad, I., 1965, Special antagonism of amphetamine-induced abnormal behaviour, *Psychopharmacologia* **7**:416.

Randrup, A., and Munkvad, I., 1967, Stereotyped activities produced by amphetamine in several animal species and man, *Psychopharmacologia* **11**:300.

Randrup, A., and Munkvad, I., 1968, Behavioural stereotypies induced by pharmacological agents, *Pharmakopsychiat. Neuropsychopharmakol.* **1**:18.

Randrup, A., and Munkvad, I., 1970, Biochemical, anatomical and psychological investigations of stereotyped behavior induced by amphetamine, in: *Amphetamines and Related Compounds* (E. Costa and S. Garattini, eds.), pp. 695–713, Raven Press, New York.

Randrup, A., and Munkvad, I., 1971, Behavioural toxicity of amphetamine studied in animal experiments, in: *The Correlation of Adverse Effects in Man with Observations in Animals* (S. B. de Baker, ed.), pp. 6–16, Excerpta Med. Congr. Series No. 220, Amsterdam.

Randrup, A., and Munkvad, I., 1972, Evidence indicating an association between schizophrenia and dopaminergic hyperactivity in the brain, *Orthomol. Psychiat.* **1**(1):2.

Randrup, A., and Munkvad, I., 1975, Stereotyped behavior, in: *Section 25, International Encyclopedia of Pharmacology and Therapeutics* (O. Hornykiewicz, ed.), Pergamon Press, Toronto (in press).

Randrup, A., and Munkvad, I., 1974, Pharmacology and physiology of stereotyped behavior, in: *Catecholamines and Their Enzymes in the Neuropathology of Schizophrenia* (S. Kety and S. Matthysse, eds.) *J. Psychiatric Res.* **11**:1.

Randrup, A., Munkvad, I., and Udsen, P., 1963, Adrenergic mechanisms and amphetamine-induced abnormal behaviour, *Acta Pharmacol. Toxicol.* **20**:145.

Randrup, A., Munkvad, I., and Scheel-Krüger, J., 1973, Mechanisms by which amphetamines produce stereotypy, aggression and other behavioural effects, in: *Psychopharmacology, Sexual Disorders and Drug Abuse* (T. Bau *et al.*, eds.), North Holland, Amsterdam, and Avicenum, Prague.

Robbins, T., and Iversen, S. D., 1973, A dissociation of the effects of *d*-amphetamine on locomotor activity and exploration in rats, *Psychopharmacologia* **28**:155.

Robinson, P., and Daley, M., 1967, Apomorphine-induced reinforcement, *Psychonomic Sci.* **7**:117.

Roffler-Tarlov, S., Sharman, D. F., and Tegerdine, P., 1971, 3,4-Dihydroxyphenylacetic acid and 4-hydroxy-3-methoxyphenylacetic acid in the mouse striatum: a reflection of intra- and extra-neuronal metabolism of dopamine?, *Brit. J. Pharmacol.* **42**:343.

Rolinski, Z., and Scheel-Krüger, J., 1973, The effect of dopamine and noradrenaline antagonists on amphetamine induced locomotor activity in mice and rats, *Acta Pharmacol. Toxicol.* **33**:385.

Roos, B. E., and Sjöström, R., 1969, 5-hydroxyindoleacetic acid (and homovanillic acid) levels in the cerebrospinal fluid after probenecid application in patients with manic-depressive psychosis, *Pharmacol. Clin.* **1**:153.

Rylander, G., 1969, Clinical and medico-criminological aspects of addition to central stimulating drugs, in: *Abuse of Central Stimulants* (F. Sjoquist and M. Tottie, eds.), pp. 251–273, Almqvist and Wiksell, Stockholm.

Rylander, G., 1971, Stereotypy in man following amphetamine abuse, in: *The Correlation of Adverse Effects in Man with Observations in Animals* (S. B. de Baker, ed.), pp. 28–31, Excerpta Med. Internl. Congr. Series No. 220, Amsterdam.

Rylander, G., 1972, Psychoses and the punding and choreiform syndromes in addiction to central stimulant drugs, *Psychiat. Neurol. Neurochir.* **75**:203.

Sano, I., and Nagasaka, 1956, Uber chronische Weckaminsucht in Japan, *Fortschr. Neurol. Psychiat.* **24**:391.

Sayers, A. C., 1972, An investigation into hyperkinesia and akinesia induced by certain stimulant drugs, Thesis, University of Aston in Birmingham.

Scheel-Krüger, J., 1972, Behavioural and biochemical comparison of amphetamine derivatives cocaine, benztropine and tricyclic antidepressant drugs, *European J. Pharmacol.* 18:63.

Scher, J., 1966, Patterns and profiles of addiction and drug abuse, *Arch. Gen. Psychiat.* 15:539.

Schiørring, E., 1971, Amphetamine-induced selective stimulation of certain behaviour items with concurrent inhibition of others in an open-field test with rats, *Behaviour* 34:1.

Schiørring, E., 1972, Social isolation and other behavioural changes in a group of three vervet monkeys (cercopithecus) produced by single, low doses of amphetamine, *Psychopharmacologia Suppl.* 26:117.

Schiørring, E., An open-field study on spontaneous locomotion with amphetamine-treated rats, In preparation.

Schiørring, E., and Randrup, A., 1971, Social isolation and changes in the formation of groups induced by amphetamine in an open-field test with rats, *Pharmakopsychiatr. Neuropsychopharmakol.* 4:2.

Segal, D. S., and Mandell, A. J., 1970, Behavioral activation of rats during intraventricular infusion of norepinephrine, *Proc. Natl. Acad. Sci. (U.S.)* 66:289.

Segal, M., and Ropschitz, D., 1969, Depressive changes after fluphenazine treatment, *Brit. Med. J.* 3:169.

Simonson, M., 1964, Phenothiazine depressive reaction, *J. Neuropsychiat.* 5:259.

Sjöqvist, F., and Tottie, M., (eds.), 1969, *Abuse of Central Stimulants,* Almqvist and Wiksell, Stockholm.

Sjöström, R., 1972, Studier av mano-depressiv psykos, *Forskning och Praktik* (Sandoz) 4:102.

Soudijn, W., and Wijngaarden, I. van, 1972, Localization of [³H]pimozide in the rat brain in relation to its anti-amphetamine potency, *J. Pharm. Pharmacol.* 24:773.

Staehelin, J. E., 1941, Pervitin-Psychose, *Z. Ges. Neurol. Psychiat.* 173:589.

Tatetsu, S., 1960, Pervitin-psychosen, *Folia Psychiat. Neurol. Japon. Suppl.* 6:25.

Van, Praag, H. M., and Korf, J., 1971, Retarded depression and the dopamine metabolism, *Psychopharmacologia* 19:199.

Warburton, J. W., 1967, Depressive symptoms in Parkinson patients referred for thalamotomy, *J. Neurol. Neurosurg. Psychiat.* 30:368.

Willner, J. H., Samach, M., Angrist, B. M., Wallach, M. B., and Gershon, S., 1970, Drug-induced stereotyped behavior and its antagonism in dogs, *Commun. Behav. Biol.* 5:135.

York, D. H., 1972, Dopamine receptor blockage—A central action of chlorpromazine on striatal neurones, *Brain Res.* 37:91.

Chapter 5

Functional Interrelationships of Principal Catecholaminergic Centers in the Brain

N. P. Bechtereva, D. K. Kambarova, and
V. K. Pozdeev

Institute of Experimental Medicine
Leningrad, USSR

1. THE ROLE OF BIOGENIC AMINES IN THE MEDIATION OF CERTAIN CENTRAL NERVOUS SYSTEM FUNCTIONS

The central nervous system is truly remarkable in its ability to maintain stable normal function amidst myriad environmental factors which tend to disrupt its equilibrium. It maintains its functional balance by means of adaptive mechanisms. During the normal course of existence external forces act on the organism, altering its internal environment so that important elements fall outside their range of optimal functioning. Exceeding the optimal range activates specialized adaptive mechanisms which tend to restore the internal environment to the optimal state. Thus, the initial change acts as a stimulus to processes which tend to reverse that change. This regulatory pattern of action and reaction is ineffective only when the initial change is so extreme as to be irreversible or when the mechanisms to counter the initial change are either weakened or absent.

The symptoms of Parkinsonism (rigidity, tremor, salivation, hypersebaceous secretion, etc.) are known to be hyperreactions resulting from the deficiency or absence of inhibitory influences. Much data have already been obtained on the disturbances in the central mediation system in Parkinsonian patients. A number of studies (Barbeau *et al.*, 1961, 1966; Bertler, 1964; Carlsson, 1959; 1972; Ehringer and Hornykiewicz, 1960; Friedhoff *et al.*, 1963, 1964; Hornykiewicz, 1964, 1966) have convincingly shown the connection between disturbances in dopaminergic mediation in the extrapyramidal system and the motor disorders in Parkinsonian patients. Moreover, the pathognomic character of these disturbances has been demonstrated. Neurophysiological studies (Connor, 1970; Feltz, 1970; Hull *et al.*, 1970) showed that the dopaminergic systems exert a predominantly inhibitory effect on the nigrostriatum. Therefore, the Parkinsonian syndrome may be regarded as a condition in which essential variables have exceeded their normal functional limits because of a deficiency in certain inhibitory adaptive mechanisms of dopaminergic and probably serotonergic mediation.

Pathological signs similar to the symptoms of "authentic" Parkinsonism can be seen in patients who have undergone prolonged treatment with reserpine or chlorpromazine. These drugs are known to suppress the activity of adrenergic and serotonergic systems, and reserpine depletes the stores of catecholamines and serotonin in brain tissue.

The importance of the brain mediatory mechanisms is obvious from experiments with LSD-25 and mescaline, drugs which cause healthy subjects to develop psychopathological symptoms similar to those observed in acute schizophrenia (disociation of mental processes, inadequacy of affect, elements of catatonia, etc.). The action of these drugs is followed by displays which suggest the participation of systems of adrenergic mediation. While mescaline is structurally similar to adrenaline and an adrenomimetic substance, LSD-25 is a structural analog and competitive antagonist of serotonin. Thus, although these drugs have a relatively isolated influence upon different biochemical systems, they produce similar clinical effects. This finding should be considered in any attempt to understand the causes of hyperreactions and to identify the cerebral systems involved

The fact that similar psychopathological states can be induced through action on a different biochemical substrate, and that Parkinsonism, a disease due to a deficit of dopamine, noradrenaline and serotonin, can be treated with cholinolytics suggests that syndrome character is determined not only by disturbances in a single biochemical neuromediatory system, but also by disturbances in the interrelationships between biochemical systems.

Paradoxical as it seems, pathological reactions (disease symptoms) are determined less by the inactive or partially active systems than by the brain systems which are functionally dominant due to the dysfunction of the former. It is probable that in some, and perhaps in the majority of cases, the intrinsic cause or "precondition" of chronic brain disturbances lies in the interaction between genetically defective brain structures and the environment. Disturbed environment–brain system interaction may produce changes in certain brain systems which cause the systems to lose their proper initial stability. If the organism survives this loss of stability, the initial changes may lead to secondary changes which result in the organism's arriving at a new balance, a stable pathological condition resulting from the previous pathological and compensatory alterations. Although the new balance is qualitatively different from the healthy state, it may often be just as stable because the function's control "scheme" becomes fixed in long-term memory.

In medical research, success in identifying disease processes and developing modes of treatment hinges on the proper choice of methodological approach to studying the disease. We feel that viewing CNS disease as a disturbance in homeostasis makes it possible to develop better methods of treatment and to open new perspectives on the pathogenic control of disease.

If one adopts this view of CNS disorders, it is clear that there are two principal possibilities for controlling disease: to compensate for deficient or damaged mechanisms (the pathogenic approach) or to restore CNS balance at another functional level by suppressing the activity of the "healthy" systems (the symptomatic approach). The latter method is the more common form of treatment, but whether the two methods are equally successful in achieving therapeutic effect is open to question.

Just as in a closed ecological system, a population explosion (of hares, for example) may occur only when there is a decrease in limiting factors (of foxes or wolves, for instance), so in CNS chronic disease, the symptoms of disease (of hyperreaction) may arise when there is damage or deficit in the hyperreaction-limiting mechanisms. This conclusion is significant because efforts to control disease by suppressing the function of a biochemical substratum have the effect of restoring the balance in the biochemical systems at a lower-than-normal functional level. In such treatment, as a rule, no attempt is made to increase the deficient system's adaptability, i.e., to restore its ability to restrict hyperreactions.

The pathogenic approach to disease treatment is any method which attempts to restore the initial level of neurochemical balance. The rationale behind the pathogenic approach is that if a restoration of the biochemical substratum's lost functions can be initiated, then previous compensatory changes may be reversed, and a "normal" balance may ultimately be attained. Achievement of a "normal" level of function is impossible with symptomatic therapy because the method tends to suppress the activity of the relatively healthy systems.

A number of objections may be raised about the efficacy of pathogenic therapy. It may reasonably be asked why pathogenic therapy has not been able to cure Parkinsonism even though its pathogenic mechanism is more or less known and there are means available to compensate for the pertinent neuromediatory deficiency. There may be a number of reasons for the failure of pathogenic treatment in Parkinsonism: (i) there may be a difficulty in overcoming the stable pathological condition if it has already been fixed in long-term memory; (ii) the secondary compensatory changes may be particularly resistant to reversal; and finally, (iii) our knowledge of the biochemical transformations in pathologically altered systems may be incomplete, and thus, treatment based on this knowledge may be ineffective.

In the clinic it is possible to study biochemical substances in the biological fluids (blood, spinal fluid, urine). The composition of these biological fluids reflects to a certain extent the biochemical processes in the organism. However. analysis of these fluids can provide only limited information about the fine dynamic biochemical processes in the CNS. Additional data will become obtainable with new developments in chemistry and pharmacology.

A great number of studies have demonstrated that pharmacological analysis of CNS neurochemistry can be a useful method of studying the biochemical organization of the brain. The experimental use of drugs with adrenergic or cholinergic action made it possible to suggest the role of disturbances in the higher vegetative centers of the diencephalic portions of the brain and in unspecific structures in the brain stem in the generation of pathology stemming from hyperfunction of adrenergic mediation. In other studies of similar design (Bechtereva *et al.,* 1963, 1965) data were obtained about disorders in the system of serotonergic mediation. In pathology resulting from hyperfunction it was found clinically valuable to suppress the functional activity of the serotonergic systems along with that of the adrenergic systems (Kambarova, 1967).

In the USSR, an approach which combined neuropharmacological, behavioral, and EEG studies was already in use ten years ago in the study of patients with paroxysmal disorders of nonepileptic type (Raynaud's disease). Based on the principle of the "black box," this kind of study provides an opportunity to compare pharmacological results with data obtained from EEG and clinical studies and suggests general answers to the questions posed earlier about the structures and mechanisms involved in disease. The EEG and clinical data alone did not provide adequate answers about the fine cerebral mechanisms involved in disease processes.

Unique possibilities for studying the human brain were provided with the introduction into clinical practice of implanted electrodes for diagnosis and treatment of CNS diseases. Long-term contact with various cerebral areas made it possible to develop and use a complex method involving the observation of clinical, biochemical, and neurophysiological parameters. Thus, clinicians were able as never before to study the dynamics of disease symptoms and pathogenesis. Direct contact with the brain allowed researchers to control neurophysiological activity at the fine neuronal–glial level and to relate electrical activity patterns with concomitant changes in biochemical and clinical parameters. These relationships provided a new perspective on the organization of different kinds of cerebral activity and on possible pharmacological and electrical treatments for brain dysfunctions.

In the present study comparative clinical, neurophysiological, and biochemical examinations were performed on Parkinsonian and epileptic patients. Different experimental procedures were used with the two types of patients because in Parkinsonism the biochemistry of the pathological process is relatively well known, while in epilepsy, despite a great number of studies, the biochemical mechanisms remain poorly understood. Accordingly, for each disease the biochemical, clinical, and neurophysiological parameters chosen for study were those considered most representative of the peculiarities of that disease.

In both Parkinsonian and epileptic patients the biochemical parameters studied were circadian urinary excretion rhythms and 24-hr excretion levels of 3,4-dihydroxyphenylalanine (D), catecholamines [3,4-dihydroxyphenethylamine (DA), noradrenaline (NA), and adrenaline (A)], and 5-hydroxyindolacetic acid (5-HIAA).

Estimation of catecholamine and dihydroxyphenylalanine content of urine was performed by the fluorometric trihydroxyindole method modified by Matlina and Menshikov (1967). Estimation of the 5-HIAA content was performed by the spectrophotometric method of Udenfriend *et al.* (1965). The urine samples were taken six times during a 24-hr period, and each sample was studied separately. Estimates of 24-hr excretion levels were statistically processed [the mean value (M) and the mean error (m)]. A coefficient was calculated to estimate the difference between the mean statistical values. The reliability of the difference was calculated for n-1 number of observations (Kaminsky, 1959; 1964).

In both Parkinsonian and epileptic patients neurophysiological studies were performed with intracerebral electrodes implanted, according to clinical indications, into deep brain structure (thalamic nuclei, caudate nucleus, basal ganglia, and midbrain tegmentum) and limbic structures (amygdala, uncus, and hippocampus). The dynamics of slow electric processes (SEP), neuronal impulse activity (IA), muscle tone, and speed of movements (in Parkinsonism) and electroencephalogram and electrosubcorticogram (ESCoG) (in epilepsy) were studied under ordinary conditions and after the administration of adren-, seroton-, and cholinergic drugs.

In Parkinsonian patients, the neurotropic drugs tested were L-dopa (600–3000 mg), in some cases L-dopa combined with the monoaminoxidase inhibitor iprazid (25–50 mg), dezeril* (0.1%, 1–3 ml iv), the central N-cholinolytic, pediphen (2.5%, 1–2 ml im), and the central m-cholinolytic, metamyzil (0.25%, 1–2 ml im). Observations of muscle tone, movement speed, and changes of SEP and IA were made at rest, and during motor tests (flexing of extremities) and psychological tests (of short-term verbal memory) given prior to and after the administration of neurotropic drugs. SEP and IA measurements were made by the method of Bechtereva *et al.* (1970) and Iliukhina (1972).

In the epileptic patient group the drugs administered were L-dopa (1000–2000 mg orally), dezeril (3 mg orally or 0.1%–3.0 ml iv), and corazol (10%, 5–8 ml iv). Biochemical and clinical parameters were studied concurrently with the diagnostic and therapeutic effects produced by the implanted electrodes. All studies were made not earlier than 3–5 days after the termination of ordinary treatment.

In all, 10 Parkinsonian and 16 epileptic patients between the ages of 18 and 40 were examined. During examination and treatment the patients were hospitalized and had an ordinary diet. To provide a control, healthy subjects were maintained on the same regimen and examined by the same method.

Certain difficulties in the clinical–biochemical and clinical–psychological studies account for incomplete identification of the examination spectra in different patients. However, even under these conditions the data obtained were sufficient to allow the formulation of certain preliminary but clinically and theoretically significant conclusions.

2. RESULTS OF THE STUDIES

2.1. Biochemical Examinations of Healthy Subjects

Nine healthy adults, six men and three women, ages 26 to 37, were examined under ordinary life conditions (Table I). Figure 1 shows the 24-hr patterns of catecholamine and D excretion in five subjects (2 men and 3 women) and the patterns of 5-HIAA excretion in three subjects (2 men and 1 woman). For these substances, high levels of excretion during wakefulness (10 AM to 12 PM) are characteristic. During night sleep, excretion is minimal as a rule. Peaks of maximum excretion occur at different moments during wakefulness. The specific character of the catecholamines D, and 5-HIAA excretion rate curves varies between patients and in the same patient. In healthy subjects, the excretion rates of the studied substances fell within the

---

* Methysergide bimaleinate.

following ranges: A, from 0.008 to 0.85 μg/hr; NA, from 0.4 to 3.8 μg/hr; DA, from 4.0 to 33.0 μg/hr; D, from 0.5 to 7.5 μg/hr; 5-HIAA, from 0.15 to 0.9 mg/hr.

The character of the excretion curves from each substance during one examination was different (Figure 2-I). The closest resemblance is observed between the D and DA curves. The NA/5-HIAA and A curves are distinct and, as a rule, have no resemblance to the curves for other substances, although occasionally NA excretion peaks coincided with those of DA excretion.

2.2. Examination of Parkinsonian Patients

Ten patients with grave bilateral rigidity-tremor form of Parkinsonism were examined. Ordinarily the electrodes were implanted into the hemisphere contralateral to the side of more obvious signs.

2.2.1. Background Biochemical Data for Seven Men and Three Women Measured after Three Treatment-Free Days

The 24-hr excretion of D, DA, and NA in Parkinsonian patients is lower than in normals (Table I). We have observed normal and Parkinsonian values respectively as follows: D, 49.70 $\pm$ 5.06 and 27.40 $\pm$ 4.11 μg/24 hr (t-3,4); DA, 350.30 $\pm$ 36.50 and 275.80 $\pm$ 43.36 μg/24 hr (t-1.31); NA, 42.90 $\pm$ 4.48 and 20.30 $\pm$ 4.03 μg/24 hr (t-3.75).

Excretion of A in Parkinsonism remains within normal limits: 6.48 $\pm$ 1.15 μg/24 hr as compared with the normal 7.60 $\pm$ 0.77 μg/24 hr; the difference between these values is insignificant (t- -0.81).

Excretion of 5-HIAA in urine in Parkinsonism is definitely reduced: 3.40 $\pm$ 0.25 mg/24 hr as compared with 6.60 $\pm$ 0.46 mg/24 hr in normal, (t-6.1).

The excretion of these substances varies widely: A, from 0.12 to 2.0 μg/hr; NA, from 0.25 to 6.6 μg/hr; D, from 0.2 to 6.0 μg/hr; DA, from 4.0 to 55.0 μg/hr; 5-HIAA, from 0.03 to 0.44 mg/hr (Figures 3; 4-III).

As in normals, the greatest excretion rates are observed during wakefulness from 10 AM to 12 PM. During night-sleep, excretion is minimal. Excretion peaks occur at different moments during wakefulness, and the time of peaking varies between subjects and in the same subject (Figures 5; 4-II). Also, as in normals, the character of the excretion curves during a single examination is different for each substance (Figure 2-II). In some cases, A excretion peaks coincide with NA, DA, and D peaks.

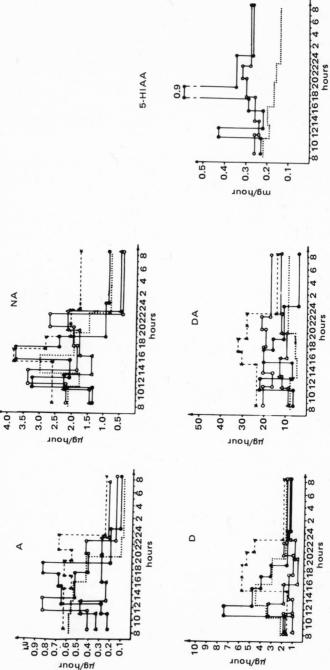

Figure 1. Catecholamines, D, and 5-HIAA 24-hr excretion levels in normal. Five practically healthy adult subjects were examined: two men (designated with dotted line and black circles) and three women.

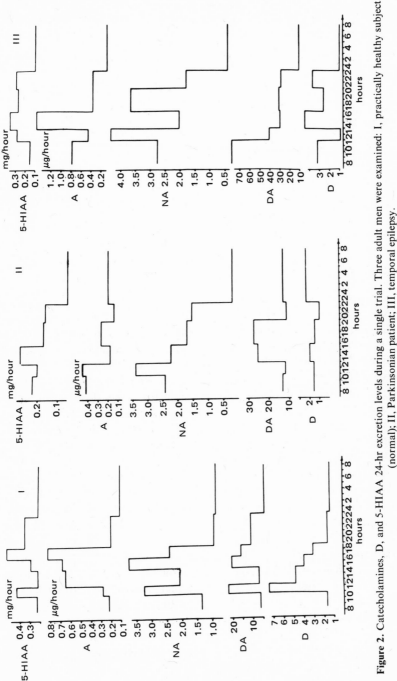

Figure 2. Catecholamines, D, and 5-HIAA 24-hr excretion levels during a single trial. Three adult men were examined: I, practically healthy subject (normal); II, Parkinsonian patient; III, temporal epilepsy.

Table I. Mean Values of the 24 hr Excretion of Catecholamines, D, and 5-

The subjects	The number of subjects	D (µg/24 hr)		DA (µg/24 hr)	
		$M \pm m$	t	$M \pm m$	t
Healthy subjects	9	49.70 ± 5.06		350.30 ± 36.50	
Parkinsonian patients after 3-day discontinuation of the drug treatment (background)	10	27.40 ± 4.11	3.4[a]	275.80 ± 43.36	1.31
Parkinsonian patients after per os administration of 1,0–3,0 g L-dopa	8	447.80 ± 44.85	8.82[a]	13011.70 ± 2111.67	6.0[a]
The difference of the mean statistical values: Parkinsonian patients baseline and after L-dopa administration			9.3[a]		6.03[a]

[a] The difference is positive.

2.2.2. Background Neurophysiological Examinations

Changes of SEP in response to motor and psychological tests may be characterized as: (i) Reproducible patterns which occur during either psychological or motor tests; (ii) reproducible patterns which occur during both types of test (Figures 6; 7). The constant component is the important parameter of "level of relatively stable functioning" (LRSF) of neuronal–glial populations within different subcortical structures (the thalamic ventrolateral nucleus and center median, the globus pallidus and the caudate nucleus). In similar experimental conditions, the LRSF was found to differ not only in different subcortical structures, but also in different areas of the same subcortical structure and within the same neuronal–glial population on different days.

Analysis of the LRSF dynamics and responses to tests revealed a correlation between LRSF and SEP reproducible patterns. For each neuronal–glial population, individual levels of LRSF were determined which correlated with SEP reproducible changes during certain kinds of activity (Iliukhina, 1972) (Figure 8).

Comparative studies of SEP changes in the ventrolateral thalamic nucleus, globus pallidus, and caudate nucleus measured at rest and in response to motor and psychological tests revealed that the ventrolateral nucleus had the highest level of activity (Figure 9). Out of the nine neuronal–glial populations studied in the ventrolateral nucleus, seven participated in motor or mental activity, while in the globus pallidus only two of the nine areas studied participated in such activity. No area studied in the caudate nucleus displayed any reproducible changes during the tests.

HIAA in Parkinsonism and the Estimation of Their Difference from Normal

NA (μg/24 hr)		A (μg/24 hr)		5-HIAA (mg/24 hr)	
$M \pm m$	t	$M \pm m$	t	$M \pm m$	t
42.90 ± 4.48		7.60 ± 0.77		6.60 ± 0.46	
20.30 ± 4.03	3.75[a]	6.48 ± 1.15	0.81	3.40 ± 0.25	6.1[a]
52.07 ± 9.28	0.88	4.50 ± 0.54	3.3[a]	2.60 ± 0.23	7.78[a]
	3.14[a]		1.55		2.33

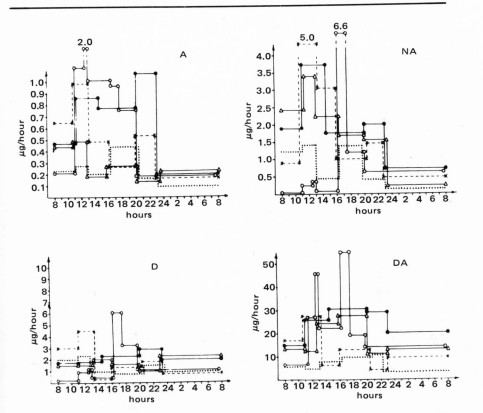

Figure 3. Catecholamines and D 24-hr excretion levels in five Parkinsonian patients measured 3 days after the discontinuation of drug treatment. Two men (designated with black balls and triangles) and three women.

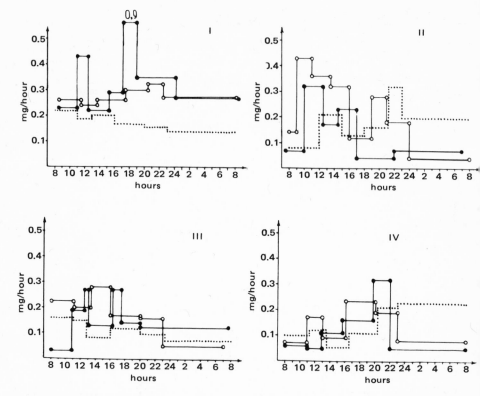

Figure 4. 5-HIAA 24-hr excretion levels in normals (I) and in Parkinsonian patients measured 3 days after the discontinuation of drug treatment (II and III), and after a single per os administration of 1.0 g L-dopa at noon–2 PM (IV). I, two adult practically healthy men and one woman (designated by light circles); II, three examinations of a Parkinsonian patient (woman) with a month interval between examinations; III, Parkinsonian patients: one man (light balls) and two women; IV, the same patients after L-dopa administration (designations the same as in part III of the figure).

Background studies of neural activity and changes in firing rates during tests revealed that certain areas within the globus pallidus, putamen, and certain thalamic structures (ventrolateral nucleus, anterior-medial group of nuclei, and center median) exhibited characteristic reproducible patterns during motor and psychological tests.

Study of the functional characteristics of the above structures showed that the neuronal populations of the brain subcortical structures are usually polyfunctional, i.e., a single neuronal population participates in responses to both motor and psychological tests (Figure 10). Obvious fractionality of functional features of the structures united into certain nuclear units according to a morphological property was revealed. Thus, within a single nucleus, there were areas which responded to neither psychological nor motor activity as well as areas which responded to both types of activity. Furthermore, increase in the firing rate within a single nucleus could occur in different phases of the psychological test (presentation, retention, verbal response), in response to only the contra- or the ipsilateral extremities (Figure 10). (The side is defined in relation to the hemisphere operated upon.) The last type of response was characteristic mainly of populations within the ventrolateral and central thalamic nuclei.

2.2.3. Biochemical Data during Pharmacological Tests

L-*Dopa.* Biochemical examination after L-dopa administration showed that the excretion rates for D, DA, and NA increased sharply 3–6 hr after

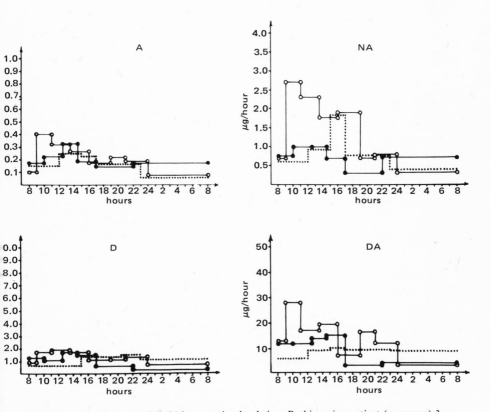

Figure 5. Catecholamines and D 24-hr excretion levels in a Parkinsonian patient (a woman) 3 days after the discontinuation of drug treatment. The patient was examined three times with a month interval between examinations.

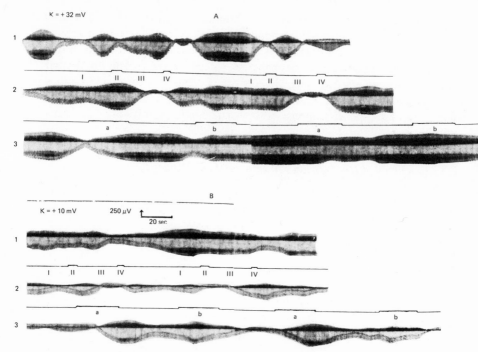

Figure 6. The SEP pattern in one globus pallidus area: (1) during wakefulness at rest; (2) during psychological tests; (3) during motor tests; (A) before and (B) 30 min after dezeril administration. 2. The Roman numerals mark the phases of the psychological tests: I, before test presentation; II, test presentation; III, retention in memory phase; IV, verbal response phase. 3. a, the time of contralateral limb movement; b, the time of ipsilateral limb movement. The side is defined in relation to the side of area of the SEP recording.

K, the compensation of the SEP constant component (mv) characterizes the level of relatively stable functioning (LRSF) of the neuronal–glial population. A, SEP reproducible pattern is observed only during the psychological test (III). The neuronal–glial population did not respond to the motor tests. B, After the dezeril administration, the SEP reproducible pattern for the psychological test disappears (2), and the reproducible response appears only during movements of the contralateral limb.

ingestion. The respective rates increased to 60–70 µg/hr, 1700–2900 µg/hr, and 3.0–15.6 µg/hr (Figure 11). These rates then decreased slightly but remained higher than background levels for 24 hr. After L-dopa, A excretion remained essentially the same. Mean values and statistics are shown in Table I. The 24-hr D excretion rate rises from 27.40 ± 4.11 µg/24 hr before treatment to 447.80 ± 44.85 µg/24 hr after L-dopa. Similarly, the DA rate increases from 275.80 ± 43.36 to 13011.70 ± 2111.67 µg/24 hr, and the NA rate rises as well (from 20.30 ± 4.03 to 52.07 ± 9.28 µg/24 hr), although not as much as the D and DA rates. After treatment, NA excretion attains the level observed in healthy subjects (t-0.88; the difference between these values is insignificant). The A 24-hr excretion decreases slightly after L-dopa administration (from 6.48 ± 1.15 to $4.50 \pm 0.54\,\mu g/24$ hr), but the decrease is statistically insignificant (t-1.55).

Interestingly, the already depressed 5-HIAA excretion rate in Parkinsonian patients decreases even further after L-dopa administration (from

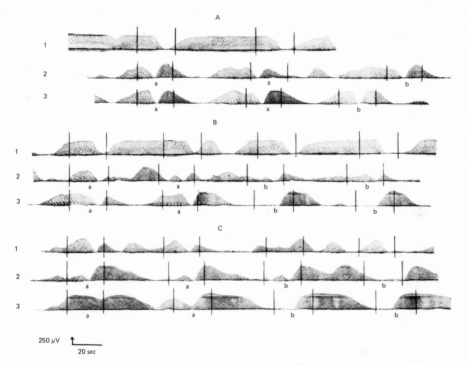

Figure 7. The SEP pattern in one area of the ventrolateral thalamic nucleus during psychological (1) and motor tests of the upper (2) and lower (3) limbs before the administration of L-dopa and iprazid (A), and in 30–40 min (B), and 2 or 2.5 hr (C) after administration. The time of completion of the test is shown by vertical lines. a, The active flexing of the upper and lower ipsilateral limb; b, the active flexing of the upper and lower contralateral limb. The side is defined in relation to the side of the area of the SEP recording. The area under study is polyfunctional because the SEP reproducible pattern appears in response to both mental and motor tests. B, the SEP reproducible pattern is maintained during the psychological test (1); the SEP reproducible pattern disappears during the motor test for the upper limbs (2); a peculiar reproducible pattern of the SEP occurs during movement of the ipsi-(3a) and contralateral (3b) limbs. C, The SEP reproducible pattern only occurs during first two tests and then disappears (1); the SEP reproducible pattern occurs only during movement of the ipsilateral arm (2) the SEP reproducible pattern occurs only during movement of the contralateral leg.

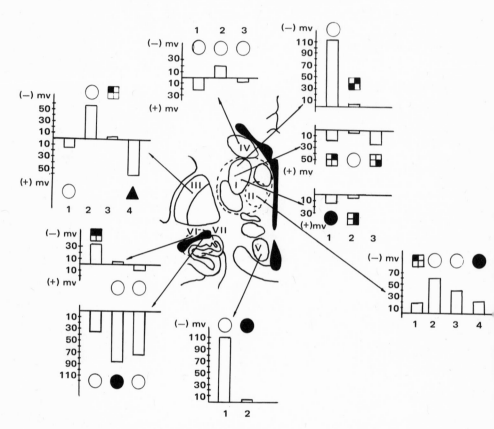

Figure 8. The dependence of occurrence of the SEP reproducible pattern during tests on the level of the relative stable functioning (LRSF, its value in mV is marked on the ordinate with arabic numerals) in the neuronal–glial populations of the n. ventrolateralis (I), n. centromedialis thalami (II), globus pallidus (III), n. caudatus (IV), n. ruber (V), n. amygdala (VI), hippocampus (VII). The arabic numerals on abscissa mark the days of examination. The white circle: the SEP reproducible pattern during test is absent. The black circle: the SEP reproducible changes are observed during psychological and motor tests (a polyfunctional population). In the square divided into four parts the SEP pattern during motor tests is shown. The upper part of the square shows the SEP pattern during flexing of the upper limbs: in the right, ipsi-, and in the left, contralateral sides with regard to the side of the SEP recording. The lower part of the square: the same for the lower limbs. The black part represents the reproducible pattern of SEP.

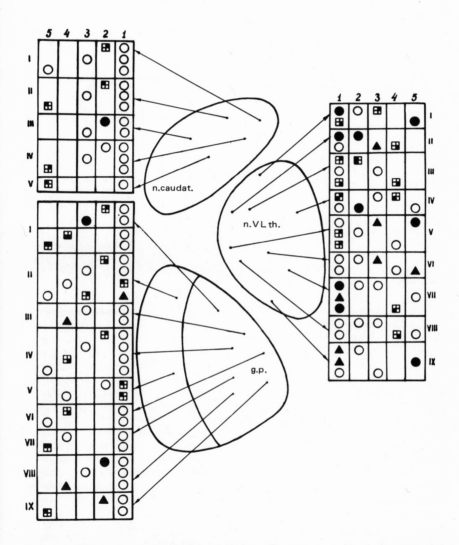

Figure 9. SEP in the neuronal–glial populations (Roman numerals) of the n.VL thal. (n. ventrolateralis thalami), G.P. (globus pallidus), and n. caudatus during psychological and motor tests before (1) and after administration of L-dopa with iprazid (2), dezeril (3), met-amyzil (4), and pediphen (5). Other marks the same as in Figure 8.

126 N. P. Bechtereva et al.

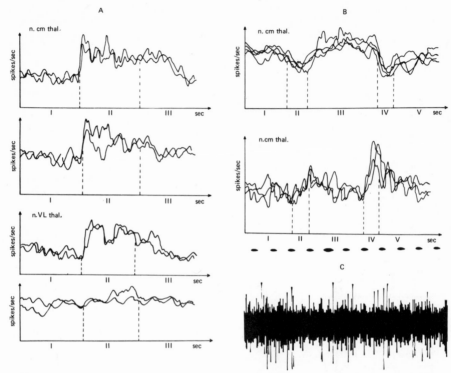

Figure 10. A variant of the neuronal populations' responses to different tests. The integral recording of the impulse activity superimposition. Dynamics of the neuronal populations' impulse activity: left (A), during voluntary movement of the limb; right (B), during a psychological test; (C), the analogue representation of the neural activity. Abscissa: time in sec; Roman numerals: background and the test's phases. Left: I, the initial background; IIa movement of the contralateral limb, IIb ipsilateral limb (with regard to the area of recording); III, the background after the test performance; Right: I, the initial background; II, presentation of the test; III, the retention in memory phase; IV, the verbal response; V, the background after the test performance. The disrupted vertical lines limit a motor test, presentation of a psychological test, and the verbal response. Ordinate: the relative amount of the impulse discharges. Abbreviations: n.cm.thal., n. centrum medianum thalami; n.VL thal., n. ventrolateralis thalami. 1, Obvious increase in the firing rate on movement of both limbs. 2, Increase in the IA on movement of the contralateral limb. 3, Decrease in the IA during the II and IV, and increase during the III phase of the test. 4, Increase in the IA during the presentation and the response phases.

3.40 ± 0.25 to 2.60 ± 0.23 mg/24 hr; *t*-2.33). Figure 4 (III and IV) shows the 24-hr 5-HIAA excretion rates in the same patients both before therapy (III) and after L-dopa administration (IV). The curves indicate a reversal in excretion pattern. Before therapy the excretion rate decreases during the day. However, after L-dopa administration, excretion is low during the day (from noon to 6 PM, the period when patients were given L-dopa), and then, when most of the L-dopa has been metabolized and excreted, 5-HIAA excretion rises, and in some cases, remains high during the night.

2.2.4. Clinical Data during Pharmacological Tests

Clinical signs were observed after the administration of L-dopa, dezeril, L-dopa plus iprazid, pediphen, and metamyzil. Changes in muscle tone and speed of hand movements after drug administration are shown in Figure 12 (Smirnov, 1967; Bechtereva et al., 1969).

Some decrease in muscle tone was common after the administration of practically all the drugs. However, the degree of tone-change depended on both the particular drug tested and the patient's condition at the moment of examination. The greatest decreases in tone were observed when there was a high initial level of tone. This pattern was typical regardless of the day of

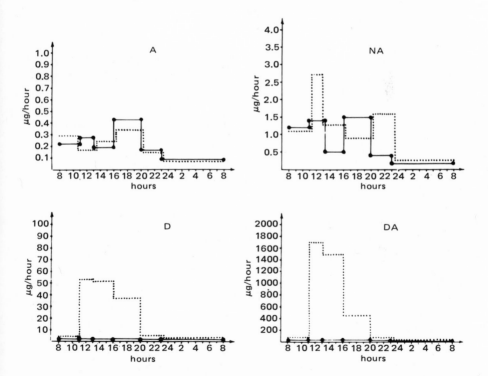

Figure 11. The intensity of the catecholamines and D 24-hr excretion in a Parkinsonian patient (a woman) three days after discontinuation of the drug treatment (the background, solid line), and after oral administration of 1.0 g L-dopa in the afternoon.

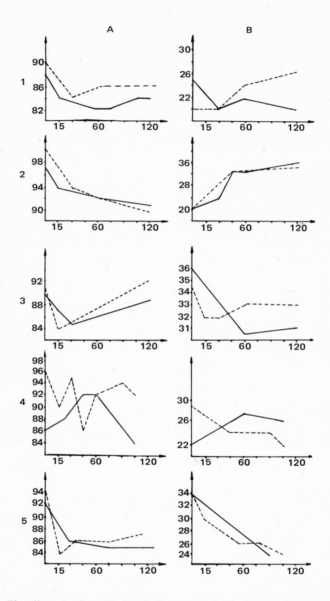

Figure 12. The effect of L-dopa (1), dezeril (2), metamyzil (3), pediphen (4), L-dopa combined with iprazid (5) on muscle tone (A) and the speed of arm movement (B), contralateral in regard to the hemisphere operated upon. The solid and dotted lines mark the above parameters during different days. See the text. A: ordinate, myotones (the relative units of the muscle tone); abscissa, the time in minutes after drug administration. B: ordinate, the time necessary for performance of a standard motor act (in seconds); abscissa, the time in minutes after drug administration.

examination, and was seen even in patients with high tone on one side. In such cases the amplitude of the first shift (from background level to first minimum) was greater on the side where the tone had been higher.

Differences were observed in the time of onset of muscle tone shifts and in the muscle tone patterns related to a particular drug. After the administration of L-dopa, dezeril, or L-dopa plus iprazid, muscle tone decreased almost linearly during the first 15–30 min and then remained at a virtually constant level for the following 2.0–2.5 hr. Administration of cholinolytics was followed by complex fluctuating changes in muscle tone. The phase of decrease in tone was considerably shorter after the administration of cholinolytics than after the administration of L-dopa or dezeril.

Obvious changes in the speed of hand movements [assessed by the method of Bayevsky and Smirnov (Smirnov, 1967)] after drug administration were recorded. The comparative analysis of these data revealed that adren-, seroton-, and cholinergic drugs had distinctly different effects on the speed of hand movements. After L-dopa administration, an increase of movement speed was sometimes observed. Maximal increase occurred after the administration of L-dopa plus iprazid. After dezeril administration there was an increase in movement speed coupled with a decrease in muscle tone. After the administration of cholinolytics, there was usually a dissociation between changes in movement speed and muscle tone: in some cases an initial decrease in tone was followed by a slowing of movement, while in other cases an initial increase in tone was followed by a slowing of movement, and in other cases an initial increase in tone was accompanied by an acceleration of movement. In a very few cases a decrease in tone with an acceleration of movement was observed.

2.2.5. Neurophysiological Data During Pharmacological Tests

The studies of SEP were made using L-dopa, dezeril, metamyzil, and pediphen. Increases in adrenergic activity induced by administration of L-dopa led to a basic reordering of SEP patterns in the subcortical structures. Changes in LRSF and SEP reproducibility were observed during various tests.

L-*Dopa Plus Iprazid.* After L-dopa plus iprazid administration distinct and varied patterns of LRSF occurred in different areas of the ventrolateral thalamic nucleus, globus pallidus, and the caudate nucleus. The greatest changes in LRSF were noted in a number of neuronal–glial populations in the globus pallidus (from 3 to 59 mV). Lesser changes were noted in the ventrolateral thalamic nucleus (from 2 to 30 mV), and the smallest changes were observed in the caudate nucleus (from 4 to 11 mV).

The principal drug-induced readjustments in the systems controlling mental and motor activity were the emergence of reproducible responses to mental and motor tests in the caudate nucleus and the pallidum. Prior to drug administration these structures had reacted to neither mental nor motor activity (Figure 9). Changes in SEP after drug administration were also seen in the ventrolateral thalamic nucleus (VTN). In background studies, the VNT responded with a singular reproducible pattern of SEP to all kinds of activity. However, L-dopa plus iprazid induced a variety of changes in the reproducible pattern depending on the kind of test (Figure 7).

Figure 9-1 shows that an increase in dopamine and serotonin concentrations in the brain affects the participation of brain structures in different kinds of activity. In structures where prior to drug administration there had been a maximal number of SEP reproducible changes (the VTN), after treatment there was a sharp drop in the number of observed changes. Conversely, in structures which in background studies had scarcely participated in any kind of activity (the globus pallidus and caudate nucleus), there was an increase in the number of neuronal–glial populations responding to tests with reproducible changes.

Dezeril. As a result of dezeril treatment, the LRSF level shifted. As with L-dopa plus iprazid, maximal shifts were observed in areas of the globus pallidus (24–30 mV), and minimal ones were seen in the caudate nucleus and the VTN (not more than 9 mV). Dezeril treatment produced no significant decreases in the number of reproducible responses to tests in the VTN: only one response disappeared after drug administration (Figure 9-2). However, dezeril did not alter the "specialization" of certain neuronal–glial populations. It tended to "switch on" hitherto inactive populations, particularly during mental activity.

In the globus pallidus, dezeril administration produced SEP response changes in only certain areas. One monofunctional neuronal–glial population switched from participation in mental activity to participation in movements of the contralateral hand (Figure 6). Another area of the same structure, initially unresponsive to any test, became polyfunctional (active in both mental and motor activity) after drug treatment. The functional condition of the caudate nucleus was unaffected by drug treatment modifying serotonergic mediation (Figure 9-3).

Metamyzil. Cholinergic drugs, and metamyzil in particular, had far less effect on LRSF levels than L-dopa or dezeril. In background studies of the VTN, a characteristic pattern of SEP was observed in response to the various tests. After metamyzil administration this pattern was absent in all tests except for motor tests of the legs. In the globus pallidus, after metamyzil treatment, reproducible changes of SEP occurred during both motor and mental tests (Figure 9-4).

Pediphen. After pediphen administration the changes in LRSF were fairly similar in all structures tested. Within each structure considerable oscillation in LRSF was observed (1–5 mV and 10–40 mV). In the VTN pe-diphen's effect on SEP dynamics differed from that of metamyzil in that the areas initially responding to only one kind of test became chiefly polyfunc-tional. On the other hand, in structures of the striopallidar system (the globus pallidus and caudate nucleus), pediphen treatment limited neuronal–glial involvement to motor activity alone (Figure 9-5).

2.2.6. Data on Impulse Activity Changes during Pharmacological Tests

L-*Dopa*. The effect of L-dopa administration on central neurons impulse activity (IA) was to alter the typical pattern of activity of neuronal populations. The character of the IA changes varied not only in different structures, but also in different areas of the same nucleus. After L-dopa administration there was considerable suppression of IA in the thalamic nuclei and particularly in the center median, while in the VLT the change in the mean firing rate was less obvious. In certain areas within the nuclei of the extrapyramidal system (the globus pallidus, red nucleus, and substantia nigra) L-dopa treatment was generally followed by a rather considerable increase in spontaneous rhythmic neural activity (Figure 13-I). We limit our

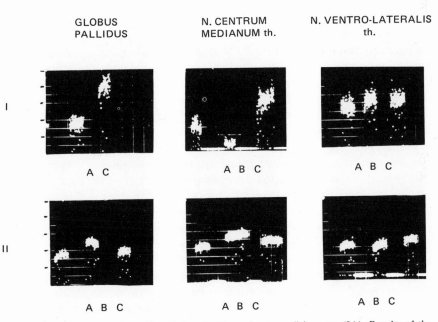

Figure 13. Effects of L-dopa (I) and dezeril (II) on the mean firing rate (IA). Results of the Dudac-4000 analyzer processing of IA data. Ordinates: the relative firing rate; Abscissa: the IA pattern in time.

discussion to "certain areas" because the extent of the increase differed according to the placement of the electrodes. The drug's effect disappeared in 5-7 hr. The changes in activity depended to a certain extent on the elapsed time after drug administration, and correlated with background activity changes.

The drug-induced changes in the activity patterns of neuronal populations were sometimes quite marked. In various areas of the VLT, for example, there was a diminishing (or disappearance) of the characteristic pattern of evoked responses to motor tests observed in background studies. Figure 14 shows a pretreatment neuronal response to movements of contra- and ipsilateral limbs recorded in the VLT. It is quite evident that the neuronal–glial population responds equally to limb movements on either side of the body. Within 30-60 min after L-dopa administration, there was a reduction of the neuronal response for the contralateral limb, and a disappearance of the response to the ipsilateral limb (Figure 14). L-dopa administration also produced significant changes in the IA pattern of another area of the VLT. Within 1.5 hr the background pattern of responses to contra- and ipsilateral limb movements became reversed (Figure 14).

Activity pattern changes similar to those observed in the VLT were seen in the center median, but in the latter area the changes lasted longer (more than 2-3 hr after drug administration).

In the globus pallidus two kinds of responses to motor tests were typical after L-dopa administration: the appearance of reproducible neuronal responses to movement on both sides where before treatment there were no responses; and the loss of response to movement on one side (more often the ipsilateral) where before treatment there were responses to movements on both sides.

In short-term verbal memory tests following L-dopa treatment, IA pattern changes were variable both in different brain structures and in the same anatomical unit. In some areas of the center median the reaction to treatment was simply a reduced firing rate during verbal response (Figure 15), while in other areas of the same structure the IA pattern underwent a more complicated transformation. For the first 30 min after drug administration there was an increase in firing rate only during the presentation phase, but later (in 1.5 hr) the firing rate increased during the verbal response phase as well (Figure 15). Thereupon, in this case too, the transformation of the neuronal populations' functional features was revealed.

In memory tests in the VLT, all IA changes after L-dopa administration occurred during the presentation and verbal response phase. Drug treatment deactivated many areas of this structure (Figure 15). In contrast to the thalamic nuclei, the globus pallidus demonstrated a drug-induced increase in firing rate often accompanied by marked responses during presentation and verbal response phases (Figure 15).

Dezeril. Dezeril, as a rule, was found to facilitate neuronal activity. Firing rates increased within 15 min of administration, and the rates remained fast for an hour or more depending on the dosage. This pattern of neuron spike activity was particularly clear in populations in the center median and the globus pallidus. In the VLT the drug reaction was slower: firing rates increased 15–30 min after administration and remained high for 1–2 hr (Figure 13).

Dezeril administration was followed by changes in the functional activities of midbrain neuronal populations. As noted earlier, an increase in firing rate during movement of both upper limbs was observed more frequently in the VLT than in the nuclei of the extrapyramidal system. This pattern was not significantly altered by dezeril treatment, but the drug produced considerable increases in background firing rates. In the nucleus and the substantia nigra, dezeril also increased firing rates. In the thalamic center median, dezeril initially had an effect similar to L-dopa. This similarity lasted about an hour, and then a dezeril-specific pattern emerged. Thus, before drug treatment, one area of the center median responded to limb movement on both sides but exhibited a stronger reaction to contralateral movement. Within 15–30 min after dezeril administration the area's response to ipsilateral limb movement became as strong as its contralateral response. After 2 hr the background response patterns were reestablished (Figure 16). In the globus pallidus, which typically exhibits no response to limb movement, dezeril treatment induced an obvious bilateral response (increase in firing rate) (Figure 16).

According to the IA data, dezeril had an effect on the portion of the brain involved in short-term memory. In memory tests the clearest changes were observed in the globus pallidus and the thalamic center median. In these structures dezeril produced an increase in the background firing rate often accompanied by changes in the reproducible pattern during the three phases of the memory test. In the globus pallidus the firing rate was increased during the presentation and verbal response phases (Figure 16), while in center median IA was reduced during the verbal response phase but significantly increased during the presentation and retention phases (Figure 16).

2.3. Examination of Epileptic Patients

Patients with so-called temporal epilepsy were studied. From the symptomatological standpoint, the disease was characterized by psychosensory fits and psychomotor seizures, disorders of the affective-mnestic type (constant mood disturbances, frequently of a depressive

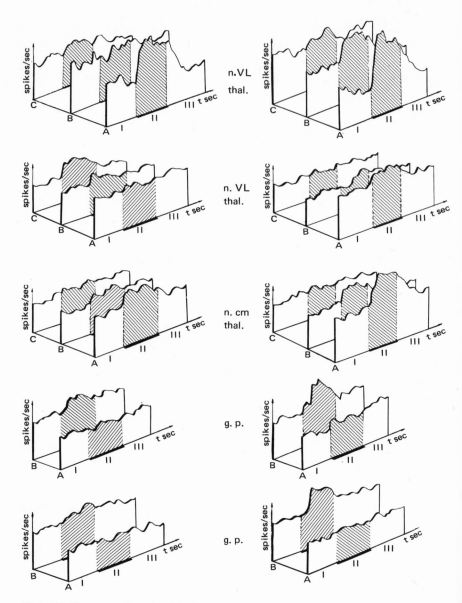

Figure 14. The averaged graphs of the impulse activity firing rate during voluntary movements of the ipsilateral (left) and contralateral (right) limbs. A, the IA before L-dopa administration; B, the IA 30 min after L-dopa administration; C, the IA 1.5–3 hr after L-dopa administration. The phase of the motor test performance is shown as crosshatched. n.VL thal. (the upper part), equal increase in the IA during movement of one or another limb; after L-dopa administration the response to movement of the ipsilateral limb disappears, and that to movement of the contralateral limb decreases. n.VL thal. (the lower part), absence of the neuronal response to movement of the ipsilateral limb, and appearance of the reproducible neuronal response to

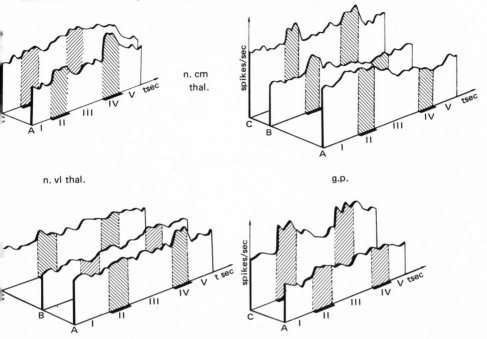

Figure 15. The averaged graphs of the IA firing rate during psychological tests after L-dopa administration. A, B, C, see Figure 14. The phases of the test presentation and of the verbal response are crosshatched. n.cm thal.: Left, in 1.5 hr after L-dopa administration (C), the peculiar pattern of the IA dynamics during the verbal response phase disappears (IV). Right, in another area of the same nucleus, in 30 min after L-dopa administration (B), a neuronal response appears at the test presentation phase (II), and in 1.5 hr at the verbal response phase, too (IV). n.VL thal., In 30 min after L-dopa administration (B), the peculiar IA pattern disappears during the verbal response (IV), and in 1.5 hr (C) the IA increase during the test presentation phase (II). g.p., After L-dopa administration (C), obvious responses of the neuronal population occurred during the test presentation phase (II) and the verbal response phase (IV).

character; emotional paroxysms—dysphoria, fears, anxiety, sadness, and paroxysmal disorder, recall of memories from the remote past).

2.3.1. Background Biochemical Data for Epileptic Patients

The 24-hr DA excretion rate (269.90 ± 67.29 μg/24 hr) tends to be decreased (t-1.05), and the NA rate (27.50 ± 5.32 μg/24 hr) is clearly

---

movement of the contralateral limb. After L-dopa administration the responses become opposite to the initial ones. n.cm. thal. (n.centrum medianum thalami), In 1.5–2 hr after L-dopa administration, the reproducible response of the neuronal population to movements of both limbs disappears. g.p., In 30 min after L-dopa administration, the increase in the IA occurs during movements of both limbs, this effect being more obvious during movement of the contralateral limb.

Table II. Mean Statistical Values of the 24-hr Excretion of Catecholamines, D,
The effect of neuropharmacological tests on excretion of these substances in epileptic patients
were compared with regard to each

The subjects	Number of subjects	D (μg/24 hr) M ± m	t	DA (μg/24 hr) M ± m	t
Healthy subjects	9	49.70 ± 5.06		350.30 ± 36.50	
Epileptic patients 3 days after discontinuation of the drug treatment	16	54.40 ± 9.08	0.45	269.90 ± 67.29	1.05
Baseline after iv administration of 2 ml of 10% corasol solution	7	64.50 ± 12.20 / 101.50 ± 49.15	0.73	172.10 ± 47.42 / 258.20 ± 32.51	1.50
Baseline after per os administration of 0,5–1.0 g L-dopa	16	54.40 ± 9.08 / 4182.90 ± 1696.99	2.43[a]	269.90 ± 67.29 / 12275.70 ± 1701.34	7.05[a]
Baseline after per os administration of 3 mg dezeril	10	63.00 ± 9.52 / 87.80 ± 31.16	0.76	251.30 ± 78.32 / 256.80 ± 69.30	0.05

[a] The difference is positive.

decreased (*t*-2.21) as compared with normal rates (Table II). On the contrary, A excretion (8.10 ± 1.05 μg/24 hr) tends to be greater than normal (*t*-1.31). The D rate (54.40 ± 9.08 μg/24 hr) does not noticeably differ from the normal (*t*-0.45), while the 5-HIAA rate (4.40 ± 0.71 μg/24 hr) is considerably decreased (*t*-2.59).

In epileptics DA and NA 24-hr excretion is not only reduced in total, but is also much more variable than normal. In general DA and NA excretion during wakefulness is greater than normal, whereas excretion during sleep is considerably reduced (Figures 17 and 1). The A excretion pattern shows a slight but similar increase in variability. D excretion sometimes drop to a very low level during night sleep. 5-HIAA excretion (Figure 17) also tends to decrease during night sleep. The excretion rates for these substances vary within the following limits: A, 0.02–1.5 μg/hr; NA, 0.25–5.5; DA, 2.0–106.2; D, 0.2–4 μg/hr; and 5-HIAA, 0.01–0.9 mg/hr.

Analysis of the excretion curves during a single study reveals that excretion rates for the different substances vary independently. Thus, if in normals some similarity exists between the D and DA curves, in epileptics this relationship is greatly disturbed.

2.3.2. Background Neurophysiological Data

Among the epileptic patients there were widely differing EEG patterns ranging from practically normal to grave diffuse changes with obvious poly-

and 5-HIAA in Epilepsy, and the Estimation of Their Difference from Normal
(baseline was established, then the neuropharmacological test was accomplished, the data obtained
neuropharmacological test separately).

NA (μg/24 hr)		A (μg/24 hr)		5-HIAA (mg/24 hr)	
$M \pm m$	t	$M \pm m$	t	$M \pm m$	t
42.90 ± 4.48		7.60 ± 0.77		6.60 ± 0.46	2.59[a]
27.50 ± 5.32	2.21[a]	8.10 ± 1.05	1.31	4.40 ± 0.71	
20.70 ± 3.06	0.45	9.50 ± 2.24	0.95	4.30 ± 0.88	1.33
18.30 ± 4.30		14.60 ± 4.86		2.60 ± 0.93	
27.50 ± 5.32	1.86	8.10 ± 1.05	0.17	4.40 ± 0.71	1.88
42.20 ± 5.81		7.80 ± 1.44		2.80 ± 0.47	
26.20 ± 4.44	0.14	9.50 ± 1.72	1.25	2.70 ± 1.06	1.52
27.40 ± 7.01		14.70 ± 3.78		4.70 ± 0.78	

morphism and a prevalence of slow and, in some cases, epileptiform (i.e., Spike complexes) waves in different portions of the hemispheres. For this group of patients, characteristically, there was an absence of permanently localized foci of pathological activity. On different days and during different tests severe bioelectrical changes were observed in different portions of one or both hemispheres.

The ESCoG changes were different from those of the EEG. Because of the direct contact with different brain areas, and particularly with the limbic system, the pathological changes showed up very clearly, and thus it was possible to identify the areas of gravest dysfunction. For example, in the case of patient Zh. who had suffered for nearly 20 years from temporal epilepsy, and ESCoG showed clear signs of epileptogenesis (rough delta and theta rhythms, spike-wave complexes, sharp-wave/slow wave complexes, spikes, etc.) in the left medial-basal structures, while EEGs recorded over a period of 3 years had shown obvious focal changes in the right hemisphere. The ESCoG made it possible to define the areas of greatest disorder, to estimate more accurately their degree of stability, and to view the dynamics of pathological changes during diagnostic and therapeutic procedures (Fig. 18).

2.3.3. The Dynamics of Clinical, Biochemical, and Electrophysiological Parameters During Neuropharmacological Tests

Corazol, a drug known to decrease seizure activity threshold, was used to locate the epileptogenic focus. As a rule, the dosage level used was the

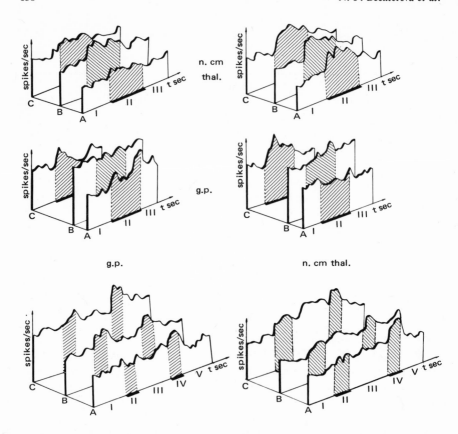

Figure 16. The averaged graphs of the IA firing rate during motor (upper part) and psychological (lower part) tests prior to (A) and after (B and C) dezeril administration. n.cm thal., A: a bilateral response with prevailing reaction to the movement of the contralateral limb; B, in 30 min after dezeril administration increase of the IA frequency during the movement of the ipsilateral limb; C, in 2 hr, the background IA returns. g.p., A: no response of the neuronal population to movements of any limb; C: in 1 hr after dezeril administration, an obvious increase in the IA frequency occurs during movements of both limbs. g.p., A: the increase in the IA frequency only occurs during the verbal response phase (IV); B and C: in 30 min and in 1 hr, an obvious increase in the IA frequency occurs during the test presentation phase (II), and then during the verbal response too (IV). n.cm thal., A: the increase in the IA frequency only occurs during the verbal response phase (IV); B and C: in 30 min or 1.5 hr, the increase in the IA frequency occurs during all three phases of the test (II, III, IV).

amount necessary to produce the first signs of increase in epileptiform (local or diffuse) changes. Administration of the drug was usually discontinued on the first subclinical bioelectrical signs to prevent the development of a seizure. In some cases, besides the EEG and ESCoG changes, other signs of

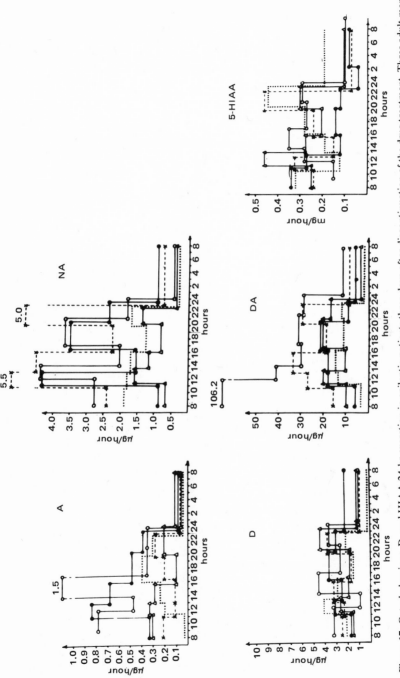

Figure 17. Catecholamines, D, and HIAA 24-hr excretion in epileptic patients three days after discontinuation of the drug treatment. Three adult men and two women (designated with, respectively, triangles and crosses).

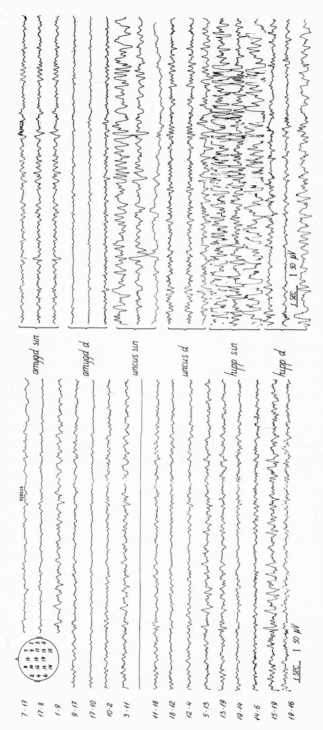

Figure 18. The EEG (left) and electrosubcorticogram (ESCoG) (right) of a patient with temporal epilepsy. In the EEG: the local epileptiform changes revealed over the right hemisphere; in the ESCoG: in the medio-basal structures of the left hemisphere.

disease or paroxysm could be detected (emotional disturbances, mainly of mood; different kinds of aura; and local motor disorders).

The aim of pharmacological tests with L-dopa and dezeril was to define, if possible, the role of the adren- and serotonergic systems in epileptogenesis and in the permanent mental disturbances which accompany the paroxysmal component of epilepsy. Dezeril and L-dopa were found to produce similar clinical effects. With a single exception, administration of these drugs intensified psychopathological symptoms to varying degrees. Typically, within 3–4 hr after drug administration, emotional tension and anxiety increased, mood became bad, and the patient would develop a feeling that disaster or a fit was imminent. In three cases patients had fits similar to spontaneous ones 3 hr after drug administration.

The effect of L-dopa and dezeril differed, in the L-dopa simply induced the above-described symptom intensification, while dezeril, as a rule, exerted a biphasic effect. It caused an initial period of behavioral suppression (indifference, drowsiness) which was followed within 30–60 min by symptom intensification.

EEG and ESCoG Data. EEG and ESCoG readings after dezeril and L-dopa administration revealed changes which indicated the close connection between clinical and electrical signs. The first phase of the dezeril effect (behavioral suppression) was characterized by the appearance of signs of increasing synchronization. There was an increase in the amplitude and period of the waves, and the appearance of rhythmic forms of activity. During the second phase in both the EEG and ESCoG obvious epileptiform signs appeared and/or increased. The signs included both local and diffuse effects (paroxysmal discharges consisting of complexes of spikes and slow waves, local pathological signs; Figures 19, 20).

L-Dopa administration tended to increase the signs of epileptogenesis in both the EEG and the ESCoG, but the signs appeared against the background of electrographical activation (decrease in the amplitude and period of waves). L-Dopa's effect was more obvious in the EEG (Figures 21, 22).

2.3.4. Biochemical Data during Pharmacological Studies

Biochemical studies explored the effects of corazol, L-Dopa, and dezeril on the excretion of catecholamines, D, and 5-HIAA in epileptic patients. The drugs were administered at 10 or 11 AM after the patient had been off all medication for three days.

Corazol. Corazol was administered in a dose of 10%, 2.0 or 6.0 ml iv. Corazol had no effect on the 24-hr excretion of D or A, but a tendency toward some increase was noted, and the dispersion of parameters

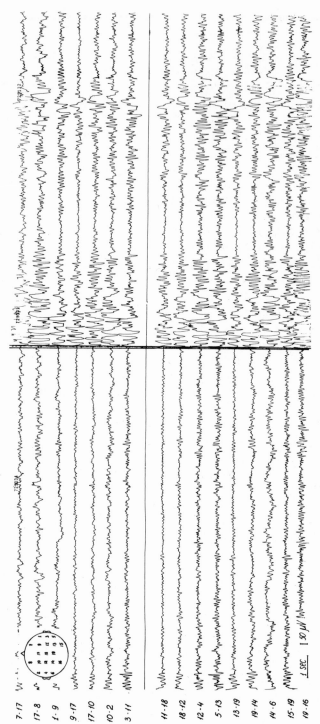

Figure 19. The EEG before (left) and after (right) dezeril administration. A significant enhancement of epileptiform activity is observed.

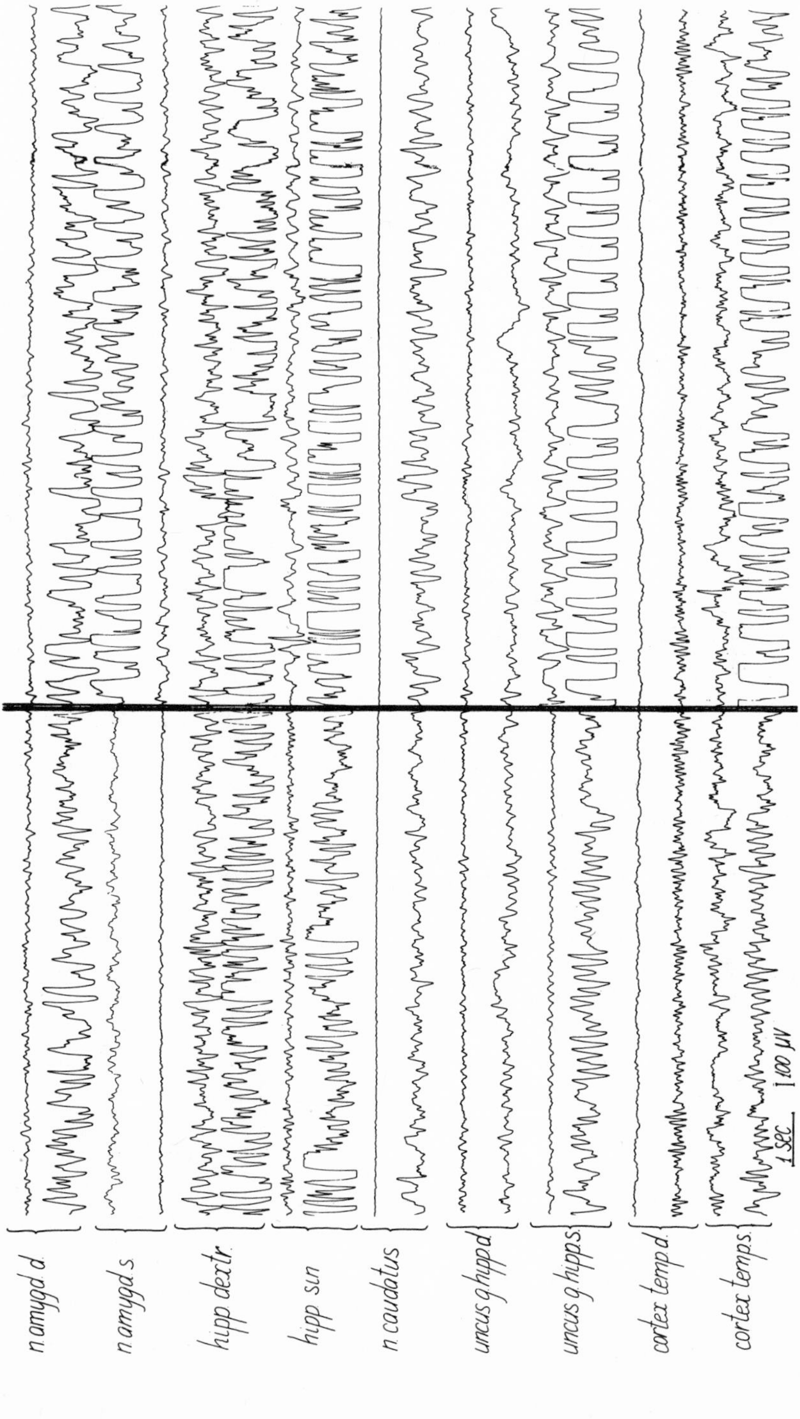

Figure 20. The ESCoG before (left) and after (right) dezeril administration. A significant enhancement of epileptiform activity is observed.

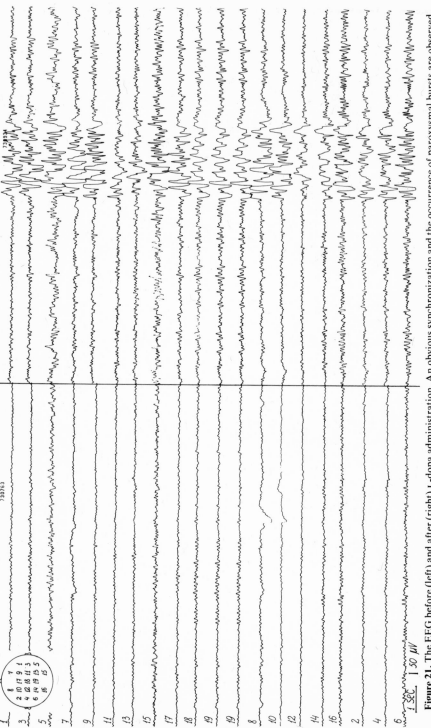

Figure 21. The EEG before (left) and after (right) L-dopa administration. An obvious synchronization and the occurrence of paroxysmal bursts are observed.

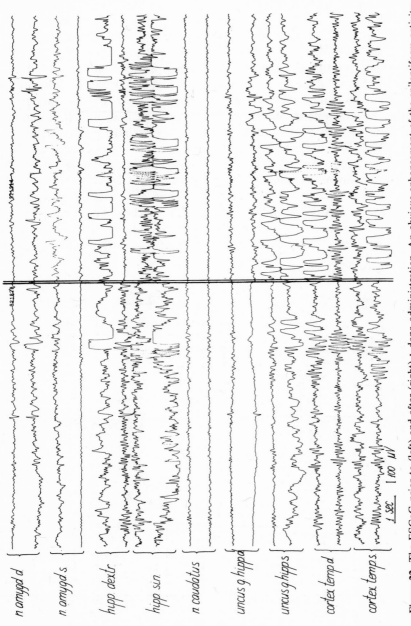

Figure 22. The ESCoG prior to (left) and after (right) L-dopa administration. An obvious enhancement of the epileptiform activity can be noted.

considerably increased (Table II). After corazol treatment, NA 24-hr excretion was similar to background values. DA excretion increased markedly from the background level of 172.10 ± 47.42 μg/24 hr to 258.20 ± 32.51 μg/24 hr (*t*-1.5). The 5-HIAA excretion tended to decrease (from the background level of 4.30 ± 0.88 mg/24 hr to 2.60 ± 0.93; *t*-1.33).

Analysis of the 24-hr excretion patterns provides more information about the effects of corazol administration (Figure 23). Within 3 hr after corazol administration there was a sharp drop in A, D, and NA excretion (From 1 PM to 4 PM). A and D excretion then increased, with D excretion attaining a peak 10 hr after administration and remaining high even during night sleep. By contrast, NA excretion continued to decrease, almost reached zero (0.02 μg/hr) 10 hr after corazol administration (8 PM to 11 PM), and then increased remaining high during night sleep. After corazol the DA excretion pattern was an inversion of the NA pattern: after drug administration DA excretion increased steadily, reaching a peak within 5 hr (from 4 PM to 8 PM). Then it gradually decreased, although it remained high during night sleep. Thus, corazol during the first 10 hr after administration,

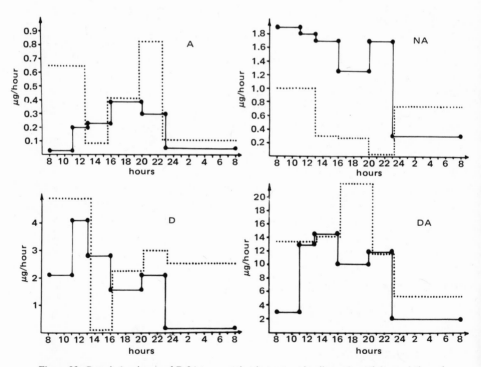

Figure 23. Catecholamines and D 24-hr excretion in temporal epilepsy (an adult man) three days after discontinuation of the drug-treatment (black circles), and after iv administration at 11 AM of 2 ml of 10% corazol solution.

disrupted the positive correlation between the biologically active catecholamines and produced an increase in DA and a decrease in NA.

L-*Dopa.* L-Dopa was administration in a dose of 1.0–3.0 g. After L-dopa, DA, and D excretion rates increased sharply, reaching levels of 2000.0 and 70 μg/hr, respectively. Both rates remained very high for 3–6 hr and then decreased, but neither dropped to its initial level during the 24 hr after drug administration. A and NA excretion rates remained essentially unchanged. 5-HIAA excretion decreased substantially within 3–6 hr after L-dopa administration, sometimes reaching zero values. Then, it gradually increased and remained relatively high during night sleep, i.e., an effect like that in Parkinsonism was observed (Figures 24, 25).

After L-dopa administration the 24-hr excretion levels were as follows: DA increased markedly from a background level of 269.90 $\pm$ 67.29 μg/24 hr to 12275.70 $\pm$ 1701.34 μg/24 hr; D excretion also increased substantially from 54.40 $\pm$ 9.08 to 4182.90 $\pm$ 1696.99 μg/24 hr; 5-HIAA levels also decreased (2.80 $\pm$ 0.47 after L-dopa as compared to a background level of 4.40 $\pm$ 0.71 mg/24 hr); A excretion remained at background levels (t-0.17); and NA excretion increased somewhat from 27.50 $\pm$ 5.32 to 42.20 $\pm$ 5.81 μg/24 hr, thus practically attaining the level in normals (42.90 $\pm$ 4.48 μg/24 hr) (Figure 25).

Dezeril. After dezeril administration excretion patterns did not change sharply (Figure 26). The excretion rates for the catecholamines and D were depressed for 8–10 hr after drug treatment (10–12 PM), and were elevated above background levels during night sleep. The 5-HIAA excretion rate remained somewhat higher than background levels for the entire 24-hr period after dezeril administration.

In most cases dezeril treatment did not substantially affect 24-hr excretion levels. The 24-hr excretion of the catecholamines remained essentially at background levels: DA excretion was 256.80 $\pm$ 69.30 μg/24 hr, with a background level of 251.30 $\pm$ 8.32 μg/24 hr (t-0.05); NA excretion was 27.40 $\pm$ 7.01 μg/24 hr with a background level of 26.20 $\pm$ 4.44 μg/24 hr (t-0.14); A excretion increased slightly from a background level of 9.50 $\pm$ 1.72 to 14.70 $\pm$ 3.78 μg/24 hr (t-1.25). D excretion increased insignificantly, but the difference from the background values was insignificant (Table II). Only the 5-HIAA excretion level showed a noticeable change, increasing from a background level of 2.70 $\pm$ 1.06 mg/24 hr to 4.70 $\pm$ 0.78 mg/24 hr (t-1.52).

2.3.5. Changes in Biochemical, Electrophysiological, and Clinical Parameters Produced by Electrical Effects Administered through Implanted Electrodes

As an illustration, we present the case of patient SH. For 17 years he has suffered from temporal epilepsy with psychosensory fits and obvious

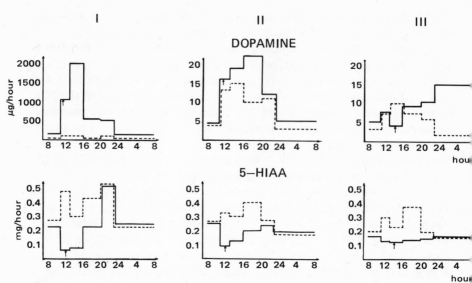

Figure 24. The neuropharmacological effects on DA and 5-HIAA excretion (I, 1.0 g L-dopa orally at 12 AM; II, 2 ml of 10% corazol solution iv at 12 AM) and the effect of polarization (III) of the right hippocampus at 2 PM in a patient (a woman) with temporal epilepsy. The dotted line shows the excretion of these substances three days after discontinuation of the drug treatment (the background).

emotional disturbance sufficiently severe to have required his hospitalization on several occasions. SH's EEG record from the last 4 years reveals weak and diffuse pathological changes in the form of some polymorphism with no distinct signs of focal pathology. The infrequent occurrence of slow waves (low and moderate amplitude theta waves) over the left temporal area suggests that the epileptic focus is localized on the left side. However, the patient's ESCoG, recorded with electrodes implanted in the medial-basal structures of both hemispheres and with electrical effects and neuropharmacological tests, revealed a distinct epileptogenic focus in the right limbic structures.

Table III presents the results of biochemical examinations performed after the patient had been subjected to electrical effects. The data are interesting because they show how electrical diagnostic stimulation of the brain can provide information about the mediator metabolism in the organism and, presumably, in the brain. Almost any electrical effect which activates epileptiform signs causes a considerable increase in the excretion of the biochemical substances under study. Particularly remarkable is the parallel between biochemical, clinical, and electrophysiological data.

The most serious epileptiform changes were revealed in the limbic structures of the right hemisphere (hippocampus, amygdala, and uncus of the hippocampal convolution) where the functionally significant epilepto-

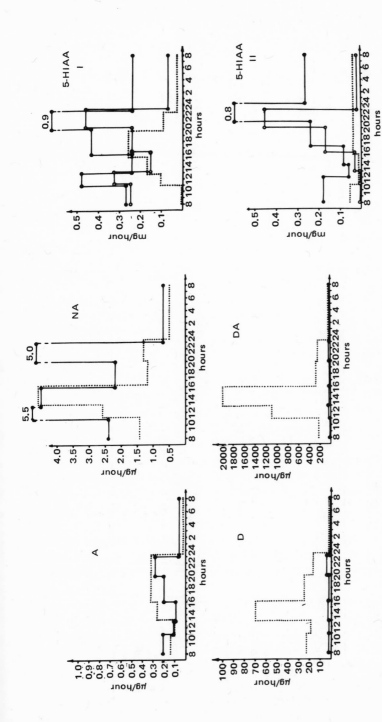

Figure 25. Catecholamines, D, and 5-HIAA 24-hr excretion three days after discontinuation of the drug treatment (the background) and after oral administration of 1.0 g L-dopa at 12 PM in epileptic patient C. The D, DA, NA, and A excretion was studied in an adult woman (black circles). The 5-HIAA excretion was studied in three women: I, background; II, after L-dopa administration. On the last figures, black circles show the excretion pattern in patient C.

Table III. Excretion of Catecholamines, D, and 5-HIAA without (Baseline) and during Electrical Effects on Brain of Patient SH (Diagnosis: Temporal Epilepsy)

Electrical effects Structures	II (μg/24 hr)		DA (μg/24 hr)		NA (μg/24 hr)		A (μg/24 hr)		5-HIAA (mg/24 hr)	
	Left	Right	Left	Right	Left	Right	Left	Right	Left	Right
Stimulations										
Baseline	65.05		48.76		22.74		8.33		4.4	
Hippocampus	196.27	70.17	104.17	271.10	28.61	14.76	26.99	27.38	5.5	5.3
Amygdala	261.60	257.62	177.85	177.38	68.77	40.17	22.87	26.99	8.7	8.1
Baseline	177.21		55.20		33.57		10.73		4.0	
Caudate nucleus	121.76	85.25	42.44	51.57	27.04	14.02	13.43	18.57	11.1	4.1
Baseline	163.80		115.92		31.00		22.56		4.5	
Polarizations										
Hippocampus	107.21	835.53	122.39	7000.99	29.48	201.04	20.66	81.45	2.06	0.94
Baseline	174.67		131.84		27.46		27.44		2.87	
Amygdala	46.38		79.11		22.06		15.52		2.6	
Baseline	75.68		96.82		33.89		14.85		1.84	

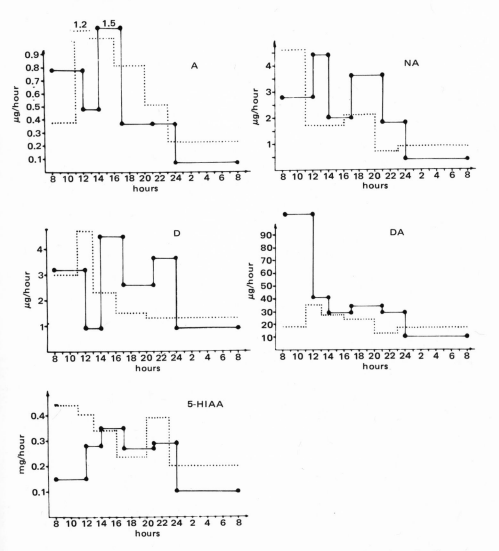

Figure 26. Catecholamines, D, and 5-HIAA excretion in temporal epilepsy three days after discontinuation of the drug treatment (the background is designated with black circles) and after oral administration of 3 mg dezeril at 11 AM. An adult man was examined.

genic focus was localized. Even weak stimulation of the right hippocampus (Figure 27), produced general subclinical ESCoG changes which were usually associated with visceral auras and mood changes, and sometimes accompanied by auditory hallucinations and rare clonic switches (the elements of psychosensory and psychomotor seizures). All these symptoms could occur separately; their occurrence depended on the quality of the stimulation.

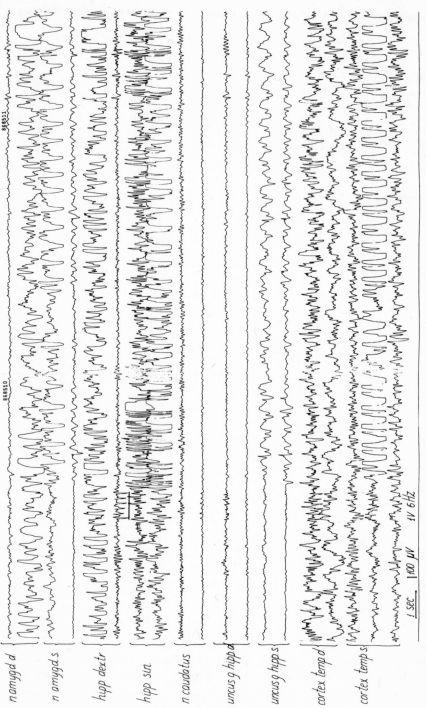

Figure 27. The electrosubcorticogram pattern during stimulation of the right hippocampus area, showing the absence of any considerable changes in the stimulation area, and obvious distant effects.

Stimulation of the left hippocampus (Figure 28) produced varied electrophysiological phenomena (reverberation, after-discharges, etc.) in that structure, while stronger stimulation produced paroxysmal changes primarily in the limbic structures of the left hemisphere. Subclinical seizures were not usually observed during stimulation of the left hippocampus. Analysis of catecholamine (CA) and 5-HIAA excretion revealed that stimulation of these structures tended to increase the excretion of D, DA, and A without affecting the excretion of the other substances.

Stimulation of the right and left amygdala produced clinical and bioelectrical displays which showed a worsening of the patient's condition. Excretion analyses indicated that the site of stimulation (right or left side) had no significant effect on excretion.

Of some interest are the results of stimulation of the caudate nucleus which apparently exerts an inhibitory influence on the epileptogenic structures. In the case of SH., the inhibitory effect of the caudate nucleus on epileptiform activity was negligible, being quite distinct after a single stimulus or at a stimulation frequency of 2/sec, and less obvious at a stimulation frequency of 10–30 sec. During the test the patient did not note any unusual sensations which might have been caused by the stimulation.

To study the effects of temporal suppression of various structures on patient condition and ESCoG epileptiform changes, electrical anodal polarizations (EP) of 1 mA at maximum were created around a pair of electrodes in various areas of the brain. EP of structures with a high threshold of seizure readiness produced the desired polarization effect. However, EP of an epileptogenic focus (of a structure with an extremely low threshold of seizure readiness) abruptly activated the epileptic process, producing clear clinical effects.

Table III shows the results of EP of the right hippocampus, an epileptogenic focus. EP caused a psychomotor fit (with no loss of consciousness) followed by an abrupt worsening of the patient's emotional state (dysphoria, malice, nagging, etc.). In the ESCoG during this period, generalized epileptiform waves were recorded, and excretion analysis showed an unprecedented increase in catecholamine excretion and a sharp drop in 5-HIAA excretion. Other changes occurred during the temporal suppression of the left hippocampus and the left amygdala. During EP of the latter structure there was a striking change in the patient's emotional state; he became responsive, kind, and satisfied with the therapeutic course. This positive effect lasted for the unusually long time of two days.

In the ESCoG a considerable decrease in the focal and general epileptiform changes was noted, and excretion analysis showed a considerable drop below background levels in the excretion of D, DA, and A. In this patient

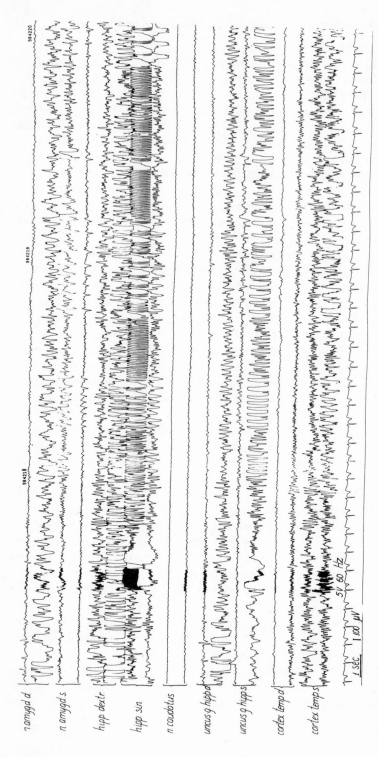

Figure 28. The electrocorticogram changes during stimulation of the right hippocampus area. Obvious local effects spreading over the mediobasal structures of the same hemisphere.

the pattern of excretion of DA and 5-HIAA following corazol, L-dopa, and dezeril shows a similarity to the pattern observed after electrically affecting the brain (Figure 24).

Table IV presents the baseline values of catecholamine and 5-HIAA excretion for patient Z, who has an epileptogenic focus in the left limbic structures and in the left amygdala. Z's most notable symptoms consist of emotional disturbances (dysphoria with great malice and aggressiveness). In Z, electrical stimulation of the right central thalamic nucleus produced clear sexual sensations which led to an improvement in mood (increase responsiveness and the disappearance of malice and aggressiveness). Repeated stimulation of this area once a week for a month showed that the observed effect was reproducible. Excretion analysis during these stimulations revealed a peculiar pattern: with repeated stimulation, DA, A, and 5-HIAA excretion dropped while NA excretion increased. This pattern was related to an improvement in emotional state, sleep, and other behavioral parameters, a fact which suggests that the observed biochemical shifts have a positive significance.

ES (60/sec, 5 V) and EP (1mA, 1–5 min) were also performed on the midbrain tegmentum of patient Z. These procedures were followed by a distinct worsening of the patient's condition (appearance of visceral aura, reduced psychosensory fit, depression, melancholy, and fear). ES and EP were found to alter excretion levels, producing a particularly noticeable increase in DA excretion.

The above examples show that there is a slight correlation between certain clinical, electrophysiological, and biochemical parameters.

Table IV. Excretion of Catecholamines, D, and 5-HIAA without (Baseline) and during Electrical Stimulations of the Right Thalamic Central Nucleus, and during Electrical Polarization of the Midbrain Tegmentum of Patient Z (Diagnosis: Temporal Epilepsy)

Electrical effects	D (μg/24 hr)	DA (μg/24 hr)	NA (μg/24 hr)	A (μg/24 hr)	5-HIAA (mg/24 hr)
Baseline	123.53	104.31	32.60	20.42	4.6
Stimulations	55.05	245.91	13.47	26.84	7.4
	33.57	156.37	21.55	24.29	4.4
	86.30	128.61	24.26	23.08	5.6
	39.08	106.40	31.90	14.81	2.7
	129.30	81.55	85.10	15.16	2.2
Polarization	135.41	222.09	39.95	16.01	3.1
	165.40	200.40	25.60	23.30	3.0

3. DISCUSSION

This study employed a combination of biochemical, neurophysiological, and clinical methods. Such a multiaspect approach made it possible to follow the interrelationships between clinical, neurophysiological, and biochemical parameters during drug-induced changes in brain mediation and electrical stimulation of various brain areas.

The biochemical data for Parkinsonian patients show that in all patients studied the excretion rates for catecholamines and 5-HIAA are considerably lower than normal, a fact which is consistent with the large body of work linking Parkinsonism with dysfunction of the central adrenergic (dopaminergic) and serotonergic systems. The data on circadian excretion rhythms in different patients and in the same patients on different days are significant because they are essential for the discussion of neurophysiological and clinical parameters, and they suggest an explanation for the high day-to-day variability in clinical and neurophysiological parameters observed during background studies.

It may be assumed that during the period of increased DA and D excretion following L-dopa administration there is an increase in DA and D concentrations in the brain. This assumption is based on data that suggest that L-dopa can penetrate the blood–brain barrier and on findings by Bertler (1964) that the level of DA in the corpus striatum and hypothalamus reaches a maximum 15–25 min after L-dopa administration.

The finding that L-dopa administration tends to reduce the already depressed 5-HIAA excretion level in Parkinsonian patients suggests something about the pharmacodynamics of the drugs used by us. Reduced 5-HIAA excretion occurs probably because L-dopa suppresses serotonin metabolism by blocking the enzyme common to the synthesis of both catecholamines and serotonin. This assumption is supported by a number of studies showing a correlation between L-dopa administration and decrease in serotonin levels (Everett *et al.,* 1970; Goodwin, 1971).

In the light of the decreased level of serotonin in Parkinsonian patient, it would be interesting to consider the probable effect on the CNS of the serotonintropic drug, dezeril. If the assumption is correct that dezeril is a specific competing antagonist of serotonin which decreases brain serotonin levels ("Sandoz," Fanchaps *et al.,* 1960; Ansell *et al.,* 1969), it would be therapeutically inexpedient to use dezeril in the treatment of Parkinsonian patients whose serotonergic functions are already suppressed. However, clinical studies show that dezeril treatment has a positive clinical effect in Parkinsonian patients, relaxing muscle tone and accelerating movements at least during the first hour of examination. This effect may be due to the action of the competing antagonist which, in the absence of normal concentrations of the proper mediator, reacts with the reactive portion of the serotonergic receptor, reproducing the mediator's effect. This effect may also be explained by the action of the antagonists of the lizergine group (LSD, dezeril) which raise brain and blood serotonin levels within 1–1.5 hr after administration (Freedman, 1961; Kambarova, 1967). The resulting accumulation of serotonin in the organism is accompanied by increased serotonergic activity.

The neurophysiological studies should be considered from the standpoint of the change in the functional level of neuromediatory systems. The administration of L-dopa plus iprazid was most effective in the rehabilitation of the malfunctioning neurohormonal system: DA, serotonin, noradrenalin (pathogenic therapy). The administration of cholinolytics helped to restore the functional balance between adren-, cholin- and serotonergic mediation (symptomatic therapy). Dezeril treatment probably partly compensated for the deficit in serotonergic mediation systems. These three forms of treatment differed in their dynamics and their effects on movement speed, but they all produced a relaxation of muscle tone.

It would be interesting to know the mechanisms which account for the observed drug-induced changes in muscle tone and for the dissociation of muscle relaxation and deceleration of movement speed. While these mechanisms remain illusive, our assumption is that tremor speed and muscle tone are regulated by different mechanisms, and that some understanding of the mechanisms involved can be derived from analysis of electrophysiological data. In this respect, the LRSF data for different brain structures under the effects of different drugs are particularly interesting. It does not seem accidental that there is a correlation between LRSF changes in the globus pallidus and the VLT, and a practically linear decrease in muscle tone after the combined effect of L-dopa, iprazid, and dezeril. It also seems significant that there is a correlation between certain LRSF and muscle tone changes after drug administration. For example, after *m*-cholinolytic (metamyzil) administration there are minimal LRSF changes in all brain structures together with a short-lived unstable change in muscle tone, while after *N*-cholinolytic (pediphen) administration there are diverse variations of LRSF in each brain structure together with oscillating changes in muscle tone.

It seems quite probable that the level of stable functioning of brain structures is associated with principal readjustments in those regulation systems for motor automatism which determine the character of disease symptoms and the degree to which drugs can affect them. This assumption is of importance with respect to the pattern of reproducible SEP and IA responses occurring after neurotropic drug administration. Background studies showed that for each neuronal–glial population within a single structure and in different structures, there is a characteristic LRSF at which the SEP reproducible pattern in response to various kinds of activity may be observed. If this similarity in the patterns of the two SEP parameters reflects the mode of operation of the system maintaining motor automatism during disease, then, by correcting, to some extent, the pathological reactions by different means, it would be expected that if there were considerable changes in one parameter (LRSF), there would be substantial changes in the other one as well. Indeed, if the reproducibility phenomenon is taken as an index of a structure's participation in a given kind of activity, we have every reason to expect major changes in the reproducible patterns of the systems regulating motor automatism.

In this regard, Figure 11 is instructive. In background studies in response to the presented tests, there was a rather striking contrast between the "passivity" of the extrapyramidal structures (globus pallidus and caudate nucleus) and the "activity" of the VLT, where, according to the SEP data, most areas participate in either motor or mental activity. After the administration of L-dopa plus iprazid, and concurrent with the major clinical and LRSF changes, there was a reversal of the pattern of activity of the extrapyramidal structures and the VLT. In those studies the activity of the globus pallidus and caudate nucleus increased while that of the VLT decreased. From these data it may be concluded that the observed readjustments, to some degree, reflect changes in the mechanisms mediating the readjustments. Indirect evidence of the validity of this assumption is the fact that surgical destruction of the VLT is effective in producing clinical improvement in acute Parkinsonism.

The readjustments in IA patterns in different deep brain structures and in different areas of the same structures measured after neurotropic drug treatment in response to motor or mental tests have been discussed in detail elsewhere (Bechtereva, 1971; Bechtereva *et al.*, 1970).

In the present discussion we shall focus only on the data which support our thesis that the occurrence of reproducible responses correlates with the level of activity of neural populations, and that drugs modify the specialization of brain structures. Thus, L-dopa and, to a certain extent, dezeril tend to reduce the participation of the VLT and central thalamic nucleus in motor activity, and to involve the globus pallidus in the mediation of movement. These qualities of SEP patterns, and the changes after drug treatment in the SEP patterns of the extrapyramidal structures and the VLT, seem to partly confirm the thesis stated at the beginning of this chapter about the principles of pathogenic therapy.

It is not improbable that the above SEP pattern changes reflect the rehabilitation of mechanisms which inhibit reactions within certain physiological limits. In all probability the restored mechanisms are controlled by the striopallidar structures and the caudate nucleus (whose inhibitory effects are already known). Indeed, the administration of L-dopa plus iprazid is probably a form of pathogenic therapy, because together these drugs tend to compensate for a deficiency of DA, NA, and serotonin in the brain. Through·compensation it is possible not only to increase the range of function of the working neuronal–glial populations, but also to restore the activity of dysfunctional populations by normalizing a physiologically active substratum. With this concept in mind, it does not seem accidental that there should be a linear relationship between the restoration of function of those structures regulating motor automatism (the globus pallidus and caudate nucleus) where there is a severe dopamine and serotonin deficiency, and the suppression of activity in an anatomically and functionally related structure (the VLT) which is relatively poor in dopamin- and serotonergic mediation. It is quite probable that the background SEP pattern in the VLT in Parkinsonian patients partly reflects the existence of hyperreactions in the mediation of motor activity. After the administration of L-dopa plus iprazid these hyperreactions tend to be suppressed by the striopallidar system.

In Parkinsonian patients when drugs (cholinolytics and serotoninolytics) were administered which did not directly compensate for the chief biochemical dysfunction, their effect was associated with the cholin- and serotonergic receptor system, a diffuse network extending into many brain structures. The diffuse nature of the cholin- and serotonergic system suggests an explanation for the great number and variety of SEP pattern readjustments observed in all brain structures under study after the administration of cholin- and serotoninolytics. It should be noted that after the administration of metamyzil, pediphen, or dezeril, and SEP reproducible changes in the globus pallidus and the caudate nucleus were not followed by such a distinct "switching" of VLT activity as after L-dopa plus iprazid administration. Metamyzil, pediphen, or dezeril did not alter the general electrical activity of the VLT but merely modified the specialization of its neuronal–glial populations during mental and motor tests.

In Parkinsonian patients the pathology-compensating process induced by the administration of cholinolytics and dezeril probably involves brain stem and subcortical structures whose neurophysiological parameters cannot be studied in man for obvious reasons. Possibly the neuronal–glial populations of these structures undergo a partial transformation of specialization similar to that observed in the VLT. The character of the transformation would necessarily depend on the functional spectra of the populations and the types of biochemical mediators involved.

When discussing the effect of cholinolytics on Parkinsonian patients, it is not really possible to speak about the specific effect of the drugs on the pathologically altered systems controlling motor activity. The SEP patterns observed in pathological structures after cholinolytic administration differed significantly from those observed after the administration of L-dopa plus iprazid. Thus, it seems reasonable that symptomatic therapy (with cholinolytics) and pathogenic therapy (with L-dopa plus iprazid) produce the same positive clinical effect by entirely different mechanisms.

It should be noted that movements sometimes decelerate after L-dopa administration, accelerate after dezeril treatment, and reach maximal speed after the administration of L-dopa plus iprazid. The data from the biochemical studies show that dopamine levels increase while serotonin levels decrease; after dezeril treatment, DA levels remain low while serotonin concentration increases; and after L-dopa plus iprazid the concentrations of both mediators increase. Comparative analysis of these findings with those from clinical parameters reveals a relationship between serotonin concentration and movement speed. Assuming that movement speed is related more to tremor than to muscle tone, one could conclude that normal serotonergic function is necessary to abolish tremor in Parkinsonism. If this is the case, it seems logical that maximal therapeutic effect could be achieved in Parkinsonism through the administration of the serotonin precursors L-dopa and tryptophan. However, this mode of treatment has proved to be less than optimal; first, because there are competing interrelationships at the stage of decarboxylation (dopa → dopamine; 5-hydroxytryptophan → serotonin), and second, because sustained L-dopa treatment, particularly at high dosage levels, suppresses the intestinal absorption of phenylalanine (Granerus *et al.*, 1971). Since phenylalanine is a catecholamine precursor and a structural element of many proteins, long-term L-dopa treatment could lead to serious disorders in protein and neurotransmitter metabolism.

Thus, despite the progress made in Parkinsonian biochemistry and the contribution of clinical neurophysiology to the study of pathogenic mechanisms, the optimal therapy for Parkinsonism remains to be determined. The difficulty in finding a successful treatment is probably due to the fact that we do not yet know the full extent and complexity of the biochemical changes in the brain of a Parkinsonian patient and that the achievement of optimal compensation is extremely difficult, even for those biochemical dysfunctions which are already understood.

Parkinsonism is one of the diseases which provides an opportunity to demonstrate the use of complex methods of brain investigation in the study of pathological reactions in man. The comparative analysis of clinical, neurophysiological, and biochemical parameters in this kind of investigation can provide insight not only about CNS disease, but also about a wide range of methodological problems associated with the study of brain mechanisms involved in different kinds of activity.

In the history of biochemical research in CNS disease, the study of Parkinsonism is the exception rather than the rule. For the majority of diseases, the investigator more or less knows the clinical features, and he may also be aware of some bioelectrical correlates of pathological states, but he generally has little or no understanding of the central biochemical disorder. When so little is known about a disease, it is naturally very difficult to determine a suitable form of therapy. We have already noted that neuropharmacological investigation with drugs of specific lytic or mimetic neurotropic action is a useful method of studying CNS biochemical pathology. However, this method alone cannot provide a complete understanding of disease process, particularly in those diseases where CNS disturbances produce a complicated clinical picture.

Epilepsy is an example of a more typical CNS disease. It has an extremely complicated pathological structure, the limits of which still cannot be clearly defined. In fact, the term "epilepsy" may be thought of as a collective noun. In the epileptic condition there may be distinguished a rather diverse "specific" component, the paroxysmal state, as well as a similarly diverse, stable, and irreversible "unspecific" component—the changes, which usually take the form of mental disorders, occurring in the interseizure period. In many cases it is impossible to find any relationship between the two components, i.e., between the frequency of the seizures and the type or degree of the mental disorders. This and the fact that mental disorders sometimes precede the seizures and constitute the leading clinical symptoms, suggest that the paroxysmal component and the interseizure changes are equally important manifestations of the disease. With such a diversity of pathological symptoms, the search for adequate methods to study the pathogenic mechanisms becomes extremely difficult, and comparative methods are particularly complicated.

Apart from these problems, an understanding of epilepsy will require finding answers to a series of questions about the occurrence, spread, and termination of the paroxysmal state. During the last few decades biochemical changes during the epileptic seizure have been the focus of most biochemical studies of epilepsy and epileptiform states. Such studies have produced considerable data on the material substratum of the seizure or, in other words, on the biochemical basis of a generalized pathological excitation of the brain. In particular, it was found that during the seizure, when the processes of excitation dominates the brain, the metabolic processes are sharply increased. Oxygen consumption increases, and the rates of carbohydrate and phosphorous catabolism and protein metabolism accelerate. In addition, acetylcholine metabolism changes, and the distribution of ions in the brain is altered. During the interseizure period, these effects are not usually observed. Although not wanting to belittle the value of these studies, we should note that studies of this kind do not identify the biochemical processes which help to precipitate paroxysmal states or, no less important, the biochemical correlates of mental conditions. In fact, the search for biochemical changes occurring during the interseizure period may prove to be the most effective approach to finding a pathogenic therapy, for the interseizure changes may produce the irregularities which precipitate the seizure.

Thanks to the introduction of the intracerebral electrode into clinical practice, it has become possible to single out by electrical stimulation some of the symptoms of epilepsy and to study their electrophysiological and biochemical correlates. Methodical comparison of clinical, electrophysiological, and biochemical parameters following the administration of drugs which facilitate or suppress epileptogenesis will quite probably lead to the elucidation of some of the biochemical (mediatory) systems in epileptic patients.

We are quite aware that our findings do not yet allow us to answer some of the most important questions concerning epilepsy. We cannot determine what disturbances in mediation underlie the observed pathological symptoms, what effect changes in amine biochemistry have on the electrical activity of the brain, or which of the observed changes in excretory patterns correspond to a shift toward normalization.

However, the values of catecholamine and 5-HIAA excretion obtained during electrical tests following administration of L-dopa, corazol, and dezeril suggest that the increased excretion of DA during ES is usually associated with enhancement of epileptogenesis. Here it should be mentioned, however, that other excretory patterns are also correlated with a worsening of patient condition. Disease intensification was associated with (i) an increase in DA excretion and decrease in 5-HIAA excretion following EP of the right hippocampus and administration of corazol; (ii) an absence of any change in catecholamine excretion and an almost twofold increase in 5-HIAA excretion after dezeril administration. These seemingly contradictory data might be explained by the hypothesis that an epileptic seizure is not precipitated by an enhancement or reduction of one or another parameter, but by a movement from one functional state to another with the preservation of certain interrelationships (a functional balance) between the mediatory systems. This thesis was convincingly proposed by Verzeano (1972), who found that epileptic seizure may occur both following increase in synchronization in thalamic serotonergic structures after microinjections of 5-HT, and following desynchronization in thalamic cholinergic structures after microinjections of acetylcholine. On the basis of these findings he suggested that in the pathological state the balance between these two mediatory systems is disturbed, and the imbalance causes the development of the epileptic process. Our EEG and ESCoG data tend to confirm this theory.

Returning to our discussion of excretion patterns, there is another aspect of our data which should be considered. In those cases where we observed a decrease in 5-HIAA excretion with a simultaneous sharp increase in catecholamine excretion (after the administration of L-dopa and corazol and following EP of the right hippocampus), a decrease in serotonin concentrations probably played an important role in epileptogenesis and the development of mental disorders. It is quite possible that a 5-HT deficit could develop from a substantial release of D and synthesis of DA or from the administration of L-dopa if the author's belief is correct that the transformation of D to DA and of 5-HTP to 5-HT is accomplished by a decarboxylase which has broad substrate specifity and participates in both reactions.

Increase in 5-HIAA excretion after dezeril administration is quite probably the result of a mechanism in which dezeril, a competing antagonist of 5-HT, blocks the reactive portion of a receptor, and the released serotonin is inactivated by oxidative deamination. (Other means of inactivation are also possible.) Verification of these hypotheses requires some additional study of the final products of catecholamine and 5-HT inactivation.

We acknowledge objections that our suggestions are not justifiable solely on the basis of our data on excretion levels. And we are quite aware that the observed excretion patterns may be significantly affected by peripheral processes in those integrative structures (the hypothalamus and limbic systems) which are in one way or another affected by local electrical effects and neurotropic drugs. In considering the significance of our excretion findings, we were unable to find data relating biogenic amine levels in urine and the CNS. However, we did find a number of studies (Misyuk *et al.*, 1965; Giacalone and Kostowski, 1968; Kostowski and Giacalone, 1969; Kostowski *et al.*, 1968) on the changes in brain levels of 5-HIAA and 5-HT after stimulation of the midbrain and dorsal hippocampus, stimulation of the thalamus and the hypothalamus, and the administration of hexenal, ether, or N_2O anesthesia. These studies have provided some grounds for the comparisons and considerations presented here.

Our findings on the effect of electrical stimulation on the cerebral biochemical processes are worthy of consideration if the mechanisms of clinical and EEG effects are to be identified. Our data show that electrical effects produce gross and long-lasting changes in the functional condition of the CNS. The results of the therapeutic stimulations indicate that electrical stimulation may be used not only as a diagnostic tool but also as an effective therapeutic procedure. Stimulation's therapeutic effect is probably achieved by a pathogenic mode of action: stimulation creates favorable biochemical changes in the brain which, in turn, suppresses pathological signs. The effectiveness of electrical stimulation as a therapeutic measure depends on the ability to find and excite an area of the brain which is capable of suppressing pathological symptoms. If such a site is located, then electrical induction of changes in cerebral biochemical processes may be used as an effective way to exert a pathogenic influence on epilepsy.

The present study explores some of the biochemical and neurophysiological characteristics of two forms of CNS disease: Parkinsonism and epilepsy. The findings are rather promising with respect to the use of neuropharmacological tests and electrical stimulation to develop effective treatments for these pathological states.

4. REFERENCES

Ansell, G. B., Beeson, M. F., Bradley, P. B., 1969, The effects of stressful, stimuli and drugs of the concentrations and turnover rates of monoamine in rat brain, in: *The Present Status of Psychotropic Drugs*, pp. 299–301, Proc. CINP VI Intern. Congr. (Tarragone, 1968).

Barbeau, A., Murphy, C. F. and Sourkes, T. L., 1961, Excretion of dopamine in diseases of basal ganglia. *Science* **133**:1706.

Barbeau, A., Tétreault, L., Oliva, L., Morazain, L., and Gardin, L., 1966, Pharmacology of akinesia. Investigations on 3,4-dimethoxy-phenylethylamine, *Nature (London)* **209**:719.

Bechtereva, N. P., 1971, *The Neurophysiological Base of the Mental Activity in Man*, Leningrad.

Bechtereva, N. P., Grigorovitch, K. A., and Zontov, V. V., 1963, On the pathogenesis and the therapy of the Raynaud disease, *Zh. Nevropatol. i Psikhiatr.* **5**:641.

Bechtereva, N. P., Bondartchuk, A. N., and Zontov, V. V., 1965, *The Raynaud's Disease*, Leningrad.

Bechtereva, N. P., Bondartchuk, A. N., and Smirnov, V. M., Trochatchev A. I., 1967, *The Physiology and the Pathophysiology of the Deep Brain Structures in Man*, Leningrad–Moskva.

Bechtereva, N. P., Kambarova, D. K., and Matveev, Yu.K., 1970, The functional characteristic of the links of the cerebral control systems for mental and motor functions in man, *Fiziol. Zh. SSSR* **56**:1081.

Bertler, A., 1964, Dopamine in the central nervous system, in: *Biochemical and Neurophysio-*

logical Correlations of Centrally Acting Drugs (E. Trabucchi, R. Paoletti, and N. Canal. eds.), pp. 51–55, Pergamon Press, New York.

Carlsson, A., 1959, The occurrence, distribution and physiological role of catecholamines in the nervous system, Pharmacol. Rev. 11:490.

Carlsson, A., 1972, Biochemical and pharmacological aspects of parkinsonism, Acta Neurologica Scand. 48:11.

Connor, J. D., 1970, Caudate nucleus neurones: correlation of the effects of substantia nigra stimulation with iontophoretic dopamine, J. Physiol. 208(3):323.

Ehringer, H., and Hornykiewicz, O., 1960, Verteilung von Noradrenalin und Dopamin (3-Hydroxytyramin) im Gehirn des Menschen und ihr Verhalten bei Erkrankungen des extrapyramidalen Systems, Klin. Wochschr. 38:1236.

Everett, G. M., Borcherding, J. W., 1970, L-dopa: effect on concentrations of dopamine, norepinephrine, and serotonin in brains of mice, Science 168:849

Fanchaps, A., Daepfner, N., Weidmann, H., and Cerletti, A., 1960, Pharmakologische Charakterizierung von Deseril, einem Serotonin-Antagonisten, Schweiz. Med. Wochschr. 90:1040.

Feltz, P., 1970, Relation nigrostriatale: essai de différenciation des excitatins et inhibitions par micro-iontophorèse de dopamine, J. Physiol. Suppl. 62(1):151.

Freedman, D. X., 1961, Effect of LSD-25 on brain serotonin, J. Pharmacol. Exptl. Therap. 134:160.

Friedhoff, A. J., Hekimian, L., Alpert, M., and Tobach, E., 1963, DIhydroxyphenylalanine in extrapyramidial diseases, J. Am. Med. Assoc. 184:285.

Giacalone, E., and Kostowski, W., 1968, 5-hydroxytryptamine and 5-hydroxyindoleacetic acid in rat brain: effect of some psychotropic drugs and of electrical stimulation of various forebrain areas, Brit. J. Pharmacol. 34:662P.

Goodwin, F. K., Dunner, D. L., Cershon, E. S., 1971, Effect of L-dopa treatment on brain serotonin metabolism in depressed patients, Life Sci. 10:751.

Granerus, Ann-Katherine, Jagenburg, Rudolf, Stig, Rödjer and Alvar, Svanborg, 1971, Inhibition of L-phenylalanine absorption by L-dopa in patients with parkinsonism, Proc. Soc. Exptl. Biol. Med. 137,3:942.

Hornykiewicz, O., 1964, The role of dopamine (3-hydroxytyramine) in parkinsonism, in: Biochemical and Neurophysiological Correlations of Centrally Acting Drugs, (E. Trabucchi, R. Paoletti and N. Canal, eds.), pp. 57–68, Pergamon Press, New York.

Hornykiewicz, O., 1966, Dopamine (3-hydroxytyramine) and brain function, Pharmacol. Rev. 18:925.

Hull, C. D., Bernardi, G., and Buchwald, N. A., 1970, Intracellular responses of caudate neurons to brain stem stimulation, Brain Res. 22:163.

Iliukhina, V. A., 1972, The slow electrical processes in the human brain during mental and motor activity (with regard to the conditions of the central biochemical mediation), Avtoref. Kand. Diss., Leningrad.

Kambarova, D. K., 1967, The central mechanisms of the paroxysmal diseases of non-epileptic kind. Avtoref. Kand. Diss., Leningrad.

Kaminsky, L. S., 1959, Processing of the Clinical and Laboratory Data, Moskva.

Kaminsky, L. S., 1964, Statistical Processing of the Clinical and Laboratory Data, Moskva.

Kostowski, W., and Giacalone, E., 1969, Stimulation of various forebrain structures and brain 5HT, 5HIAA and behaviour in rats, in: The Present Status of Psychotropic Drugs, pp. 289–291 Proc. CINP. VI. Intern. Cong. (Tarragone, 1968).

Kostowski, W., Giacalone, E., Garattini, S. et al., 1968, Studies on behavioural and biochemical changes in rats after lesion of midbrain raphe, European J. Pharmacol. 4:371.

Matlina, E. Sh., and Menshikov, V. V., 1967, *The Clinical Biochemistry of the Cate-cholamines*, pp. 113–127, Moskva.

Misyuk, N. S., Prigun, P. P., Korenevskaia, A. A., and Misyuk, E. M., 1965, *The Data on the Serotonin Metabolism Under Inhibitory Condition of Brain*, Minsk.

Smirnov, V. M., 1967, In: *The Localization Problems in Psychoneurology*, Vol. X, pp. 22–48, (Tr. in-st im. Bechtereva), Leningrad.

Udenfriend, S., Titus, E., and Weissbach, H., 1955, The identification of 5-hydroxy-3-in-doleacetic acid in normal urine and a method for its assay, *J. Biol. Chem.* **216**:499.

Verzeano, M., 1972, Pacemakers, synchronization and epilepsy, in: *Synchronization of EEG Activity in Epilepsies* (H. Petsche and M. A. B. Brazier, eds.), pp. 155–188, Springer-Verlag, Wien, New York.

Chapter 6

Tremography as a Measure of Extrapyramidal Function in Study of the Dopamine Hypothesis

Murray Alpert

New York University
School of Medicine
New York, New York

1. ABNORMAL MOVEMENTS IN SCHIZOPHRENIA

Although an association between schizophrenia and abnormal movements has long been noted, recent behavioral research in schizophrenia has emphasized cognitive and emotional manifestations almost exclusively. Theoretical work has focused on "mental" phenomena [see, e.g., the behavioral topics considered in Cancro's reviews of schizophrenia (1971, 1972)], although clinicians recognize certain motor abnormalities as part of the schizophrenic syndrome (Fish, 1967). Movements such as posturing, mannerisms, waxy flexibility, etc., contribute to the establishment of the diagnosis, or to decisions as to the severity of illness.

In addition to the types of abnormal movements noted above, abnormal movements usually associated with extrapyramidal disorders, such as dyskinesia, dystonia, and choreoathetosis, etc., have been reported to occur at a greater than expected frequency in schizophrenics. This last assertion, which has been in the literature at least since Kraepelin (1918), is hard to establish unambiguously for a number of reasons: (i) Reports are usually based on impressions rather than survey data with adequate controls. (ii) For some workers diagnostic decisions may utilize, at least in part, the presence of the abnormal movements, so that diagnoses are not independent of the movement disorder. (iii) The wide prevalence of movement disorders subsequent to treatment with neuroleptic drugs now makes it very difficult to study the problem. (iv) Because neurological and psychiatric patients are frequently housed in the same hospitals, it is possible that hysterical patients or patients with echopraxia copy their neurologic wardmates.

Despite these problems it would be of great interest if it could be demonstrated that there is an increase in the frequency of abnormal movements in schizophrenia and that this increase could be attributed to shared pathophysiologic mechanisms. The relations between dopamine abnormalities and abnormal movements (Hornykiewicz, 1966; Lloyd and Hornykiewicz, Chapter 3, this volume) and the dopamine hypothesis in schizophrenia (Friedhoff and Van Winkle, 1964; Kety, 1970), taken together suggest a converging focus on the study of abnormal movements in schizophrenia.

Indirect evidence of a relationship between dopamine and schizophrenia, and between dopamine and abnormal movements continues to appear. For example, in a recent prospective longitudinal study, Yarden and Discipio (1971) showed that young schizophrenics who, on admission to hospital, have abnormal choreoathetotic movements are less well at outcome (about 3 yr) than a control group of schizophrenics free of abnormal movements. But here, again, the results cannot be interpreted as unambiguous evidence for a specific connection between the movement disorder and the schizophrenia, and may reflect the nonspecific effects of two distinct chronic disorders on outcome.

2. NEUROLEPTIC ACTION OF ANTISCHIZOPHRENIC DRUGS

Equally circumstantial but perhaps more convincing evidence for a relation between abnormal movements and schizophrenia may be found in the considerable body of literature concerning the extrapyramidal side effects that seem to characterize all drugs useful in the treatment of schizophrenia. The observation that antipsychotic drugs can produce abnormal movements, and the evidence that this side effect is linked with the tendency of these drugs to interfere with the action of dopamine in the central nervous system provides a large part of the support for the dopamine hypothesis of schizophrenia.

This "hypothesis" however, may need modification. Although therapeutically useful drugs share central antidopaminergic activity (among many other shared neuropharmacological actions), it has not been demonstrated that antidopaminergic agents are generally useful treatments in schizophrenia. For example, there are a number of phenothiazines with strong neuroleptic action which have little or no usefulness in schizophrenia (Cole et al., 1961; Davis, 1965). Also, dopamine precursor inhibitors, which should interfere with dopamine synthesis, have not proven to be therapeutically useful (Gershon et al., 1967), although these agents may interact with the antipsychotic action of neuroleptics (Carlsson et al., 1972, 1973).

Still, the "hypothesis" is robust since other lines of support come from evidence that interventions which tend to *increase* central dopaminergic activity can be accompanied by an increase in schizophreniclike behavior. These pharmacologic interventions have led to a number of animal model systems for the neuropharmacological study of some aspects of schizophrenia (Randrup and Mankvad, 1967). It is interesting that the animal models in general involve abnormal and stereotyped movement patterns. The movements studied differ from species to species, and it is not yet clear whether these abnormal movements are useful analogs for schizophrenic behaviors (Rubovits and Klawans, 1972).

3. RELATION BETWEEN NEUROLEPTIC AND THERAPEUTIC ACTIONS

Despite the consistency with which extrapyramidal side effects have been found among antischizophrenic drugs, the specificity of the relations between the therapeutic and side effects of neuroleptic drugs has been questioned because there is little correlation across drugs between frequency of extrapyramidal effects and therapeutic potency. Recently it has been shown that the different neuroleptic agents share both an antidopaminergic and an anticholinergic action, and the two actions vary independently (Miller and Hiley, 1974; Snyder et al., 1974). Since anticholinergic activity is important in the control of Parkinsonism (Duvoisin, 1967), intraclass variation in this action might explain the relative independence of the side effect and the therapeutic effect among neuroleptic agents.

We investigated the relation between extrapyramidal side effects (EPS) and therapeutic response in a relatively homogeneous group of ten female schizophrenics (Alpert et al., 1973). We were interested in whether individuals who are more vulnerable to EPS are more likely to show positive therapeutic response to that drug. We studied female schizophrenics between 18 and 45 yr of age because there are sex and age differences in relation to the severity of drug-induced EPS effects (Ayd, 1961). We correlated vulnerability to EPS from a fixed dose of chlorpromazine after one week of treatment with therapeutic response at the end of four weeks of treatment.

4. TREMOGRAPHY AS A MEASURE OF EXTRAPYRAMIDAL FUNCTION

Our measure of EPS was based on a quantitative analysis of each patient's digital tremor recorded bilaterally from each index finger (Alpert *et al.*, 1966). Tremor amplitude has certain advantages as an index of EPS because it is quantifiable, is sensitive to neuroleptics in clinical doses, and it is correlated within an individual with qualitative ratings of a range of signs and symptoms included in a standard clinical EPS rating scale. We also studied tremor spectrum because we had found that neuroleptic-induced tremor is characterized by low frequency irregular waveform as demonstrated in Figure 1 (Alpert and Diamond, 1967).

In earlier work we had found that individuals differed in their pattern of EPS, even to a fixed dose of the same neuroleptic. Some of the patients would show greater changes in one EPS sign, e.g., resistance to passive stretch or cogwheeling, while the EPS of other patients would be characterized by a different sign, e.g., drooling, or loss of associated movements, or tremor. However, in studying an individual patient repeatedly over time, as his EPS ratings waxed and waned, quantitative measures of digital tremor would wax and wane in a correlated manner (within individuals, correlations ranged from $r = 0.69$ to $r = 0.88$ in a number of experiments). This was true even if digital tremor was not an important part of the EPS syndrome for that patient, indeed, even if his digital tremor was not clinically apparent. Because of this we used tremography measures as a constant and quantitative marker for EPS.

5. STUDY OF NEUROLEPTIC AND THERAPEUTIC EFFECTS

In two pilot studies (Alpert *et al.*, 1973), one with chlorpromazine and one with trifluoperazine, we found statistically reliable correlations between the tendency of a patient to show an increase in tremor amplitude early in treatment and the magnitude of her therapeutic response to medication. Almost half the treatment variance could be predicted from the tremography. These pilot studies had small samples ($N = 10$ for each study) and had

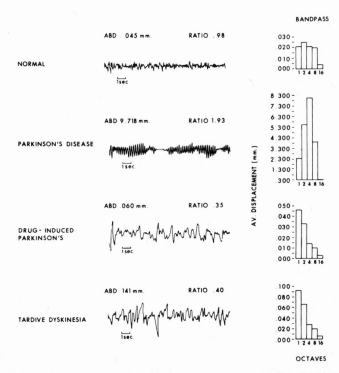

Figure 1. Comparison of some extrapyramidal tremor wave forms. ABD = Average Beam Displacement, a measure (in mm) of the average distance of the finger oscillations from the null point. The average displacement of the finger in each of five octave passbands (1–2 Hz, 2–4 Hz, 4–8 Hz, 8–16 Hz, and 16–32 Hz) is indicated in the bar graph to the right of each tracing. Time (1 sec) is indicated as a horizontal line.

methodological difficulties which limit the generalizability of interpretations. However, to-date the results suggest that EPS and therapeutic effects share common pharmacological mechanisms. Since the correlation is positive, the shared mechanism may simply be an artifact of drug dynamics such as absorption, penetration of the blood–brain barrier, or metabolism. However, the data are also consistent with (and may be seen as converging on) the dopamine hypothesis.

With our emphasis on abnormal movements we have continued in the classical tradition of considering the basal ganglia as restricted to motor functioning. In this volume, Krauthamer (Chapter 3) considers a wide range of other functions including sensory, association, memory, etc. These more subtle and complex mechanisms appear to have a greater potential as an explanation for the disturbances seen in schizophrenia. We should also note that the dopamine hypothesis of schizophrenia need not be restricted to basal ganglia dopamine mechanisms. Stevens (1973) has discussed the possible importance of limbic system dopamine in "An Anatomy of Schizophrenia." The action of neuroleptics on dopaminergic transmission in the limbic system could be expected to run in parallel with action in the basal ganglia, while providing a degree of freedom between the two areas in pharmacological actions.

6. EVIDENCE FROM PSYCHOTOXIC EFFECTS

This model would also be consistent with the vulnerability of schizophrenics to exacerbations of illness with MAO inhibitors (Himwich, 1971), with central stimulants which block catecholamine reuptake (Janowsky *et al.*, 1973), and with L-dopa (Yaryura-Tobias *et al.*, 1970, Angrist *et al.*, 1973). The dopamine hypothesis is *not* consistent with the vulnerability of Parkinsonian patients to the psychotoxic effects of these same treatments since these patients are hypodopaminergic. It is not clear whether dopamine depletion in Parkinson's disease is limited to cells of nigral origin or whether these cells also supply limbic structures (Hornykiewicz, 1966).

However, one must also consider the possibility that the psychotoxic picture seen in Parkinsonian patients is unrelated to schizophreniform disturbances. The frequent reports of a high incidence of psychotoxic reactions in these patients may reflect the fact that they tend to be an older, fragile group with a high incidence of non-drug-related mental changes, and also that they require relatively high doses of these compounds to control their movement disorders. By the same token, even among schizophrenics, there is question whether the psychotoxic effects of substances which increase dopaminergic activity reflect specific exacerbation of the schizophrenia or a nonspecific, toxic phenomenon. Taken individually, the many bits of information concerning the importance, for normal mental and motor functioning, of a well-modulated balance between central cholinergic and dopaminergic mechanisms (Friedhoff and Alpert, 1973) are not compelling, but the range of experiments in which relations can be demonstrated suggest that there may be fire somewhere in all of the smoke.

In Chapter 5, Volume 2, John Davis considers what is known of the significance and mechanism of action of amphetamine-induced psychoses. We have had the opportunity to study the effects of large doses of amphetamines on cardiovascular function, on digital tremor, and on psychiatric status in conjunction with the experiments of Angrist *et al.*, (1971;

1973) in which amphetamine-induced psychoses were studied under experimental conditions.

7. STUDY OF AMPHETAMINE MODEL PSYCHOSIS

A typical experiment is shown in Figure 2 in which racemic amphetamine in a total dose of 745 mg was administered to a volunteer over 64 hr. In the figure, time is depicted on the abscissa. At the bottom of the figure, the dosing schedule (doses ranged from 0 to 40 mg, and were administered hourly depending on the stability of vital signs) is presented. Above this pulse rate and then mean arterial blood pressure [diastolic plus one-third (systolic–diastolic)] are depicted. The horizontal dashed line indicates this subjects' average levels over five experiments. The amplitude of tremor for each hand and a histogram reflecting the spectral analysis of the tremor waveform are next above. At the top, the psychiatrically significant behavioral changes are shown, the filled symbols representing more severe, psychoticlike signs.

The study (Alpert *et al.*, 1972) involved three volunteers, each of whom participated in an induction with *dl-*, *l-*, and *d-*, amphetamine. One volunteer participated in two additional experiments, one involving pretreatment with reserpine and one with L-dopa. Experiments were continued until a clear psychotic end point was reached or until changes in vital signs precluded further study.

In earlier experimental amphetamine inductions (Griffith *et al.*, 1970), the remarkable similarity across subjects (*S*) in the sequence of symptoms preceding the psychosis and the type of psychosis elicited had been noted. However, in the crossover design one can see repeating individual variations on the common theme of the paranoid psychosis. This effect can be seen in Figures 3, 4, and 5 where the psychotoxic patterns in pairs of amphetamine inductions with the same individual are plotted together. The effect is even more striking when one examines the modality and content of hallucinations. *S* #1 in five different inductions had olfactory hallucinations and repeating similar delusions, while *S* #2 never had olfactory hallucinations and always showed a repeating pattern of mood changes.

The course toward psychosis is not monotonic and as can be seen in Figures 3, 4, and 5, the breakthrough of psychotic material may be followed by some restitution even though amphetamines are continued. In outline, the course of the syndrome was as follows: Early in the experiment there usually was some lability of mood, usually with early euphoria and later-ap-

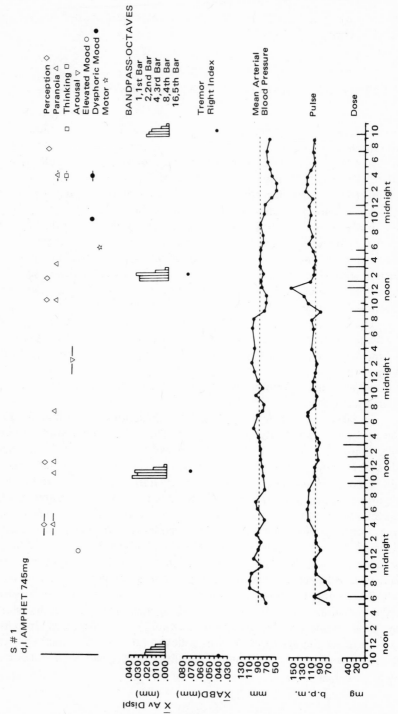

Figure 2. Time course of the response of S #1 to racemic amphetamine. See text for description of the figure.

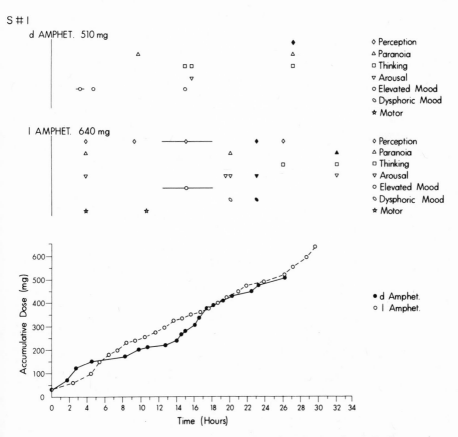

Figure 3. Cumulative *d*- or *l*-amphetamine dose and psychotoxic signs for *S* #1. See text for description.

pearing dysphoria. The effect on mood appeared earlier, and was marked with *l*-amphetamine. During the course of the experiments attention-deployment progressed through a stage of extreme distractability to a point of fixed obsessive brooding. Thinking changes ranged from vague ideas of reference to fixed delusions. There was usually some blunting of affect. Increasing illogicality could be seen progressing to concern with mutually exclusive or irrelevant ideas. Frequently, superimposed features included auditory hallucinations, frank persecutory delusions, transient telepathic ideas, and panic states. At advanced stages the subject was often too paranoid to reveal his preoccupations. These changes were not accompanied by confusion or disorientation, although at terminal points in the experiment clouding of consciousness and confusion can occur.

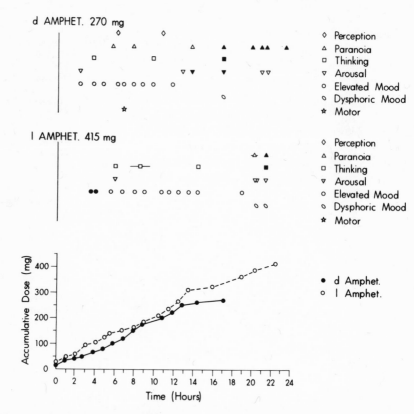

Figure 4. Cumulative *d*- or *l*-amphetamine dose and psychotoxic signs for *S* #2. See text for description.

In Table I the average cardiovascular effects of the experiments are summarized. *d*-Amphetamine tended to have a greater effect on mean pulse rate than *l*-amphetamine, but this was not always present. The effects on mean levels and variability of pulse and blood pressure differs from subject to subject and do not correlate with the psychotoxic effects seen in the experiments.

In Table II is presented the mean tremor displacement averaged for the two hands. The amplitudes are followed by the hour and total dosage. *S* #1 showed increase in tremor amplitude in the first three experiments, each of which culminated in the development of psychotic symptoms. *S* #2 showed a slight decrease in tremor amplitude for all three experiments. These experiments also culminated in psychotic manifestations which were of somewhat greater floridness than those of *S* #1 (compare Figures 2 and 3). *S* #3 showed increase in tremor in response to the *d*- and *l*-isomers (dosage in the *dl* experiment was proceeding very slowly at the time the measurements were taken). This increase in tremor was accompanied by a mild psychotoxic effect (see Figure 5). In the reserpine experiment the psychotoxic effects (see Figure 6) as well as the cardiovascular and tremor effects (see Tables I and II) of amphetamine were all diminished. In the *l*-dopa experiment tremor was reduced initially, and never showed this subject's usual increase. The experiment could be continued only to 265 mg at 24 hr because at that point a tachycardia developed and cardiovascular changes persisted for 4 hr. However, up to this point the *S* showed fewer psychotoxic effects of amphetamine than in other experiments (cf. Figure 6 with Figures 2 and 3).

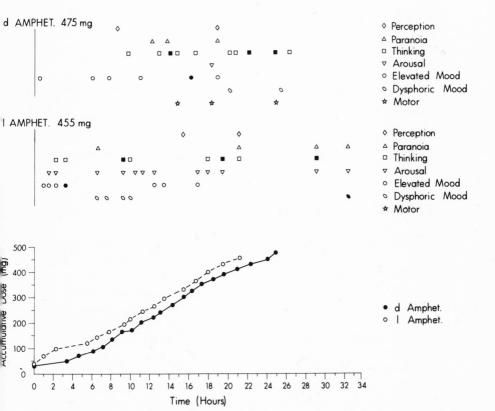

Figure 5. Cumulative *d*- or *l*-amphetamine dose and psychotoxic signs for *S* #3. See text for description.

Table I. Cardiovascular Effects of Amphetamine Isomers for the Volunteers

Subjects	dl	l	d	dl and Reserpine	DL and L-dopa
S #1					
Dose (mg)	745	640	510	950 & 14.5	265 & 8.5
Time (hr)	64	30	26	53	24
Pulse X	108	98	105[a]	100	97
S.D.	14.3	8.7	12.1	11.4	11.1
M.A.B.P. ×	87	96	107	88	85
S.D.	12.0	5.5	10.8	10.9	7.9
S #2					
Dose (mg)	465	415	270		
Time (hr)	22	23	17		
Pulse X	74	72	81[b]		
S.D.	12.6	15.2	10.2		
M.A.B.P. ×	116	115	115		
S.D.	6.1	6.6	7.2		
S #3					
Dose (mg)	400	455	475		
Time (hr)	25	21	25		
Pulse X	73	79	80		
S.D.	7.3	5.9	8.1		
M.A.B.P. ×	110	110	109		
S.D.	8.2	10.1	7.7		

[a] l vs. d $t = 2.53$ $p < 0.02$ df = 51.
[b] l vs. d $t = 2.03$ $p < 0.05$ df = 37.

8. CARDIOVASCULAR EFFECTS OF AMPHETAMINE ISOMERS

Within an experiment there was no indication that moment to moment changes in cardiovascular function were correlated with psychotoxic effects. This was also true of cross-isomer comparisons within a subject and cross-subject comparisons. In two subjects the d-isomer reliably provoked more cardiovascular arousal than the l-isomer. This finding would be consistent with the hypothesis of a greater stereospecific effect involving mechanisms under noradrenergic control (Snyder, 1972). Pretreatment with both reserpine and L-dopa appears to have reliably reduced cardiovascular arousal. These results are of interest because of the several suggestions implicating a relationship, even a causal one, between hyperarousal and schizophrenia (Epstein and Coleman, 1970). In our experiments hyperarousal appeared more regularly with the d-isomer of amphetamine, although the d- and l-isomers appeared to have equal psychotoxic effects.

These experiments permitted us to observe the relation between the

Table II. Effects of Amphetamine Isomers on Amplitude of Tremor for the Three Volunteers

Subjects	dl	l	d	dl and Reserpine	DL and L-dopa
S #1					
Dose (mg)	745	640	510	950 & 14.5	265 & 8.5
Time (hr)	64	30	26	53	24
X̄ RH&LH (hr) (mg)	0.0452 (−7)	—	0.0531 (−2)	0.0437 (−1)	0.0314 (−0.50)
X̄ RH&LH (hr) (mg)	0.0710 (+17) (185)	0.0358 (+4) (60)	0.0487 (+5) (150)	0.0955 (+5) (105)	0.0223 (+3) (60)
X̄ RH&LH (hr) (mg)	0.1049 (+44) (555)	0.0779 (+22) (475)	0.1043 (+22) (430)	0.0572 (+24) (375)	0.0465 (+23) (245)
X̄ RH&LH (hr) (mg)	0.0644 (+64) (745)	0.0951 (+28) (555)	0.0788 (+30)	0.0842 (+42) (760)	
X̄ RH&LH (hr)				0.0506 (+72)	
S #2					
Dose (mg)	465	415	270		
Time (hr)	22	23	17		
X̄ RH&LH (hr)	0:0653 (033)	0.0879 (−31)	0.0766 (−8)		
X̄ RH&LH (hr) (mg)	0.0735 (+14)	0.0703 (+16) (325)	0.0597 (+16) (260)		
X̄ RH&LH (hr) (mg)	0.0524 (+20) (420)	0.0631 (+23) (415)	0.0490 (+22) (270)		
X̄ RH&LH (hr)	0.0584 (+37)				
S #3					
Dose (mg)	400	455	475		
Time (hr)	25	21	25		
X̄ RH&LH (hr)	0.0462 (−6)	0.0955 (−13)	0.0650 (−72)		
X̄ RH&LH (hr) (mg)	0.0637 (+18) (345)	0.0920 (+4) (100)	0.0487 (+5) (70)		
X̄ RH&LH (hr) (mg)	0.0484 (+24) (385)	0.1774 (+22) (455)	0.1768 (+23) (430)		

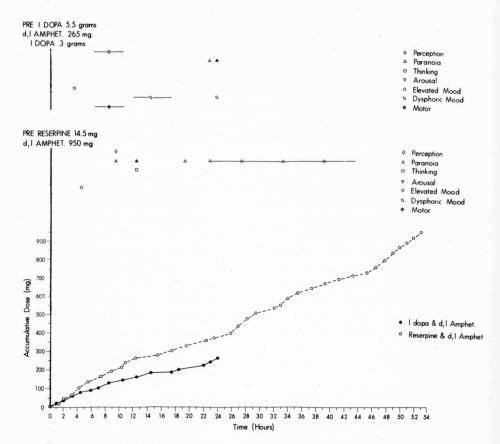

Figure 6. Cumulative dose of racemic amphetamine and psychotoxic signs in experiments involving pretreatment with L-dopa or reserpine for *S* #1

development of the "amphetamine model psychosis" and changes in tremor. Some of these results are presented in Table II which has been discussed above. In our experience tremor amplitude tends to increase with amphetamines, perhaps more with the *d-* than with the *l*-isomer. The increase in amplitude appears to reflect increase in higher frequency components (see Figure 7).

The waveform typically seen with amphetamines is presented in Figure 8, along with representations of tracings seen in anxiety, alcoholism, and under conditions in which anticholinergics produce an increase in tremor. In the experiments with amphetamine isomers we found that two volunteers showed increases in tremor to both the *l, d,* and racemic preparations of amphetamine while one volunteer's tremor-amplitude decreased for the three preparations. In these nine experiments all subjects developed their idiosyncratic version of the "amphetamine model psychosis."

Thus, both changes in autonomic arousal and in tremor-amplitude could be dissociated from the psychotoxic effects of amphetamines. One subject participated in two additional experiments, one involving pretreatment with reserpine and one involving pretreatment with L-dopa. In both experiments the autonomic changes, the tremor changes, and the psychotoxic effects were attenuated. However, in the second experiment (L-dopa) a breakaway tachycardia developed, and the experiment had to be terminated after only 265 mg of racemic amphetamine. In other experiments this subject had shown greater psychotoxic effects at this dose (compare Figure 6 with Figures 2 and 3). While not conclusive, the experiment may be interpreted as suggesting that the L-dopa pretreatment did not potentiate amphetamines' psychological effects.

As John Davis has indicated (Chapter 5, Volume II), the results of the experiments with the "amphetamine model psychoses" both support and complicate the dopamine hypothesis. Certainly no simple increase in activity of a transmitter would seem consistent with the range of data we have discussed. Although *ad hoc* (*post hoc*) explanations could be invoked to explain the various exceptions to the dopamine hypothesis, such ra-

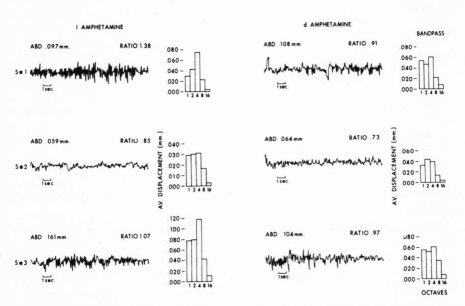

Figure 7. Comparison of effects of *d*- or *l*-amphetamines on tremor in three volunteers. The right hand is shown in each case. The tremors were recorded at approximately the same point in the course of the induction in each case. The dose and time are as given in Table II.

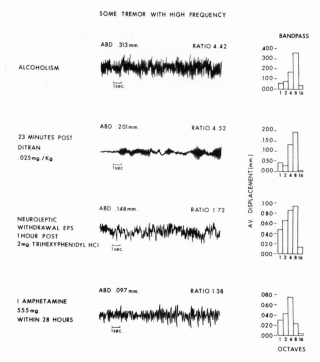

SOME TREMOR WITH HIGH FREQUENCY

Figure 8. Comparison of tremor with higher frequency components.

tionalizations can be engaged in only at a price. We must be aware of the reduced utility of an hypothesis which is not subject to disconfirmation.

9. THE USEFULNESS OF TREMOGRAPHY

The use of tremography has contributed to our study of the relations between abnormal movements and schizophrenia. However, we do not yet have a clear understanding of the parameters of tremography and can anticipate that it will become more useful as a dependent measure as understanding of its' mechanisms increases. Although tremor amplitude or, perhaps, the amplitude of the *low frequency components* of *resting* tremor, appears most related to the action of dopamine as a central neurotransmitter, the relevant independent measure does not seem to be the *rate* of dopamine turnover but, rather, the rate of turnover in relation to turnover of other transmitters. Brimblecombe and Pinder (1972), in an excellent and extensive review of work in tremor mechanisms, mainly in animals, have presented compelling evidence that the balance of activity of dopamine and acetylcholine and also of dopamine and serotonin are associated with alterations in tremor.

To date, the study of schizophrenia is heavily dependent on the use of human subjects so that noninvasive procedures for the estimation of biological parameters are required. The correlation between abnormal movements, tremor, and dopamine, although less than perfect, appears sufficiently strong to make them useful dependent measures. One should recognize that "schizophrenic behavior" as seen in human subjects is almost certainly imperfectly correlated with any discrete measure of brain function. The advantages of an objective and quantitative measure suggest a role for tremography in schizophrenia research.

10. SUMMARY

The main support for the dopamine hypothesis derives from a number of sources: pharmacologic effects of antischizophrenic drugs; pharmacological manipulations that make schizophrenics worse, including MAO inhibitors, anticholinergics, L-dopa, and methylphenidate; and experiments with amphetamines insofar as this can be considered a model psychosis in nonschizophrenics. Although the burden of this evidence is considerable, we have cited a number of experiments in which alterations in psychotic level appears to be dissociable from changes in dopamine. In addition, the time course of alterations in dopamine does not coincide with the time course of the psychosis. Changes in dopamine appear to lead the changes in psychosis by hours or even days. While this may be taken as evidence that the changes in dopamine are not a consequence of the psychotic state, some explanation of the factors involved in the time lag would make the hypothesis more precise and more testable. However, it seems fair to state that the relations between abnormal movements and schizophrenia appear to be greater than chance, although less than causal.

ACKNOWLEDGMENTS

This work was supported, in part, by U.S. Public Health Service grants #MH08618 and MH08638, and by a grant from the Bitker Foundation. I appreciate the assistance of Florence Diamond and Edward M. Laski. We acknowledge with appreciation Dr. Angrist's generosity in making the volunteers available for our study.

11. REFERENCES

Alpert, M., and Diamond, F., 1967, Regularity of tremor in extrapyramidal disease, in: *Progress in Neuro-Genetics,* Vol. I, pp. 040–405, Excerpta Med Intern. Congr. Series #175.

Alpert, M., Lomask, M., and Friedhoff, A. J., 1966, Instrumentation for the recording and predictive analysis of physiological tremor, in: *Instrumentation Methods for Predictive Medicine* (T. B. Weber and J. Poyer, eds.), Instrument Society of America, Los Angeles.

Alpert, M., Angrist, B., Diamond, F., and Gershon, S., 1972, Neurohumoral mechanisms mediating the autonomic, CNS, and psychotoxic effects of amphetamines in humans, Presented at the 27th Annual Meeting of the Society of Biological Psychiatry, Texas.

Alpert, M., Diamond, F., Kesselman, M., and Mas, F., 1973, Association between therapeutic and extrapyramidal effects in pharmacotherapy of schizophrenia, Presented at the 28th Annual Meeting of the Society of Biological Psychiatry, Montreal.

Angrist, B., Shopsin, B., and Gershon, S., 1971, Comparative psychotomimetic effects of stereoisomers of amphetamine, *Nature* **234**:152.

Angrist, B., Sathananthan, G., and Gershon, S., 1973, Behavioral effects of L-dopa in schizophrenic patients, *Psychopharmacologia* **31**:1.

Ayd, F., 1961, A survey of drug-induced extrapyramidal reactions, *J. Am. Med. Assoc.* **175**:1054

Brimblecombe, R. W., and Pinder, R. M., 1972, *Tremors and Tremorgenic Agents,* Scientechnica, Bristol.

Cancro, R., (ed.), 1971, 1972, *Annual Review of the Schizophrenic Syndrome* Vols. 1 and 2, Brunner-Mazel, New York.

Carlsson, A., Persson, T., Roos, B. E., and Walinder, 1972, Potentiation of phenothiazines by α-methyltyrosine in treatment of chronic schizophrenia, *J. Neural Transmission* **33**:83–90.

Carlsson, A., Persson, T., Roos, B. E., Walinder, and Skott, A., 1973, Further studies on the mechanisms of antipsychotic action, *J. Neural Transmission* **34**:125.

Cole, J. O., and Clyde, D. J., 1961, Extrapyramidal side effects and clinical response to the phenothiazines, *Rev. Can. Biol.* **20**:565–574.

Davis, J. M., 1965, The efficacy of the tranquilizing and antidepressant drugs, *Arch. Gen. Psychiat.* **13**:552.

Davis, J. M., and Janowsky, D., 1973, Amphetamine and methylphenidate psychoses, in: *Frontiers in Catecholamine Research* (E. Usdin and S. H. Snyder, eds.), Pergamon Press, New York.

Duvoisin, R. C., 1967, Cholinergic–anticholinergic antagonism in parkinsonism, *Arch. Neurol.* **17**:124.

Ellinwood, E. H., Jr., 1967, Amphetamine psychosis: I, Description of the individuals and process, *J. Nervous Mental Disease* **144**:273.

Ellinwood, E. H., Jr., 1968, Amphetamine psychosis: II, Theoretical implications, *J. Neuropsychiat.* **4**:45.

Epstein, S., and Coleman, M., 1970, *Psychosomat. Med.* **32**:113.

Fish, F., 1967, *Clinical Psychopathology,* John Wright and Sons, Bristol.

Friedhoff, A., and Alpert, M., 1973, A dopaminergic-cholinergic mechanism in the production of psychotic symptoms, *Biol. Psychiat.* **6**:165.

Friedhoff, A. J., and Van Winkle, E., 1964, Biological *O*-methylation and schizophrenia, *Psychiat. Res. Rep. Am. Psychiat. Assoc.* **19**:149.

Gershon, S., Hekimian, J. J., Floyd, A., Jr., and Hollister, L. E., 1967, Methyl-*p*-tyrosine (AMT) in schizophrenia, *Psychopharmacologia* **11**:189.

Griffith, J. D., Cavanaugh, J. H., and Oates, J. A., 1970, Psychosis induced by the administration of d-amphetamine to human volunteers, in: *Psychotomimetic Drugs* (D. H. Efron, ed.), Raven Press, New York.

Himwich, H. E., 1971, *Biochemistry, Schizophrenia, and Affective Illnesses* Williams and Wilkins, Baltimore.

Hornykiewicz, O., 1966, Dopamine (3-hydroxytyramine) and brain function, *Pharmacol. Rev.* 18:925.

Janowsky, D. S., El-Yousef, M. K., Davis, *et al.,* 1973, Provocation of schizophrenic symptoms by intravenous administration of methylphenidate, *Arch. Gen. Psychiat.* 28:185.

Kety, S., 1966, Current biochemical research in schizophrenia, in: *Psychopathology of Schizophrenia* (P. H. Hoch and J. Zubin, eds.), Grune and Stratton, New York.

Kety, S., 1970, The hypothetical relationships between amines and mental illness: a cortical snythesis, in: *Amines and Schizophrenia* (H. E. Himwich, S. Kety, and J. R. Smythies, eds.), pp. 271–277, Pergamon Press, New York.

Kraeplin, E., 1918, *Dementia Praecox* E. and S. Livingstone, London.

Miller, R. J., and Hiley, C. R., 1974, Anti-muscaric properties of neuroleptics and drug-induced parkinsonism, *Nature* 248:596.

Randrup, A., and Munkvad, S., 1966, Role of catecholamines in the amphetamine excitatory response, *Nature* 211:540.

Randrup, A., and Munkvad, S., 1967, Stereotyped activities produced by amphetamine in several animal species and man, *Psychopharmacologia* 11:300.

Rubovits, R., and Klawans, H. L., 1972, Implications of amphetamine-induced stereotyped behavior as a model for tardive dyskinesia, *Arch. Gen. Psychiat.* 27:502–507.

Smythies, J. R., and Ansun, F., 1970, The biochemistry of psychosis, *Scot. Med. J.* 15:34–40.

Snyder, S. H., 1972, Catecholamines in the brain as indicators of amphetamine psychosis, *Arch. Gen. Psychiat.* 27:169–179.

Snyder, S., Greenberg, D., and Yamarura, H. J., 1974, Antischizophrenic drugs and brain cholinergic receptors, *Arch. Gen. Psychiat.* 31:58–61.

Stevens, J. R., 1973, An anatomy of schizophrenia, *Arch. Gen. Psychiat.* 29:177.

Ungerstedt, U., 1971, Stereotaxic mapping of the monoamine pathways in the rat brain, *Acta Physiol. Scand. Suppl.* 367:1.

Yardin, P. E., and Discipio, W. J., 1971, Abnormal movements and prognosis in schizophrenia, *Am. J. Psychiat.* 128:317–323.

Yaryura-Tobias, J. A., Diamond, B., and Merlis, S., 1970, The action of L-dopa on schizophrenic patients, *Current Therap. Res.* 12:528–531.

Chapter 7

Mammalian Biosynthesis of Potential Psychotogens Derived from Dopamine

Arnold J. Friedhoff and Jack W. Schweitzer

Millhauser Laboratories of the Department of Psychiatry
New York University Medical Center
New York, New York

1. INTRODUCTION

Normal mental functions can be disrupted by many kinds of drugs. Hallucinogens are of special interest because of their ability to impair higher centers without producing substantial effect on other functions of the central nervous system. While the mechanism of action of hallucinogens has not been clarified, the striking structural resemblance between certain of these agents and several central nervous system transmitters has not gone unnoticed (Osmond and Smythies, 1952; Snyder and Merril, 1965). Mescaline, for example, bears a strong structural similarity to dopamine, and, among indoles, *N,N*-dimethyltryptamine and bufotenin resemble serotonin (Figure 1). The hallucinogenic properties of these biogenic amine congeners are well documented for mescaline (Kapadia and Fayez, 1970) and for the indoles (Fujimori and Alpers, 1970).

2. BEHAVIORAL AND BIOCHEMICAL EFFECTS OF 3,4-DIMETHOXYPHENETHYLAMINE

3,4-Dimethoxyphenethylamine (DMPEA), the di-*O*-methylated derivative of dopamine (see Figure 1), appears not to induce hallucinations on oral

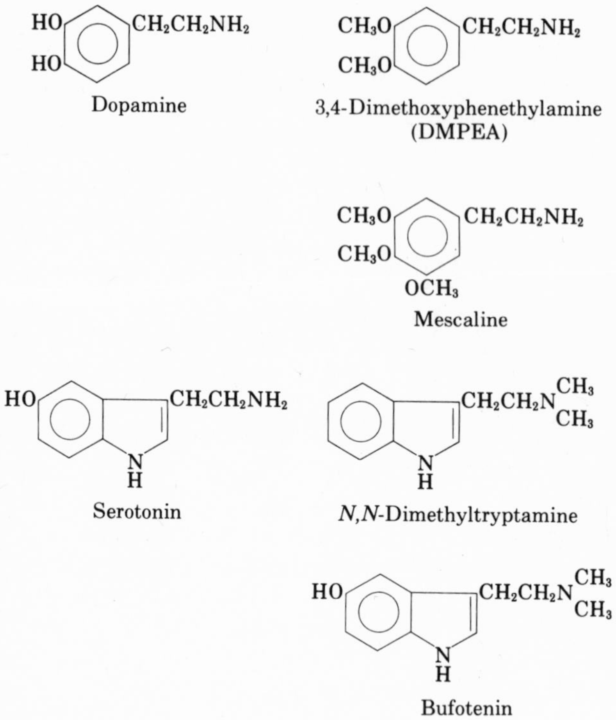

Figure 1. Biogenic amines and structurally related hallucinogens.

administration (Hollister and Friedhoff, 1966; Shulgin et al., 1969; Chara-lampous and Tansey, 1967), but has some psychotropic effects when injected iv to subjects pretreated with nialamide, a monoamine oxidase inhibitor (Charalampous, 1971). DMPEA does, however, induce strong behavioral and physiological reactions when tested in lower animals. Ernst (1965) found that DMPEA can induce a hypokinetic syndrome with mydriasis, salivation and, with large doses, piloerection and a catatonic state in cats. The 3,5- and 2,3-dimethoxy isomers induced salivation only, as did 3-hydroxy-4-methoxyphenethylamine. DMPEA mimics the activation effects seen with mescaline when postsynaptic cortical potentials are measured in the cat (Vacca et al., 1968). Bindler et al., (1968) found that both negative and positive postsynaptic cortical potentials are increased with DMPEA. Takeo and Himwich (1965) reported that both DMPEA and mescaline induce arousal at the medullary level in rabbits, in contrast to adrenaline-induced arousal which takes place at the midbrain level. An increase in evoked responses following DMPEA administration was also demonstrated in the rat (Dear and Malcolm, 1967). In shock-induced avoidance studies in rats, Levis and Caldwell (1971) were unable to separate the effects on altered behavior produced by mescaline and DMPEA. Bridger and Mandel (1967) have also noted the similarity of behavioral effects induced by mescaline and DMPEA.

Biochemically, DMPEA can exert effects on dopamine pathways. It has been shown to reverse the inhibition of prolactin release produced by dopamine (Smythe and Lazarus, 1973). Barbeau *et al.* (1966) found that, in monkeys, DMPEA increased the excretion of dopamine and a metabolite, dihydroxyphenylacetic acid, but not of other catecholamines. In rats it caused an increase in dopamine concentration in the central gray masses of the brain. The fact that DMPEA fails to elicit psychotomimetic effects in man unless preceded by a monoamine oxidase inhibitor is very likely related to its rapid metabolism. When 500 mg doses of DMPEA were administered to eight psychotic subjects, a mean of 0.4% (range: 0.1–0.7%) was excreted unchanged. In contrast, when a mean of 443 mg mescaline was administered to each of the same subjects, 23.1% was excreted as mescaline (Friedhoff and Hollister, 1966). In light of these observations it seems premature to eliminate DMPEA as a potential hallucinogen. It might produce significant effects if its degradation were retarded or if its biosynthesis occurred at selective central nervous system sites.

3. THE METHYLATION HYPOTHESIS

Perhaps as a reaction to the overelaboration of limited data in the past, it is currently fashionable to accept only the narrowest interpretation of any finding. However, broader hypotheses can be very useful in the heuristic sense, if they are based on established observations and are consistent with most, if not all, of the known data. It should be expected that most such hypotheses will ultimately be replaced or drastically revised as new data are accumulated. The transmethylation hypothesis is one such. It suggests that psychotics may be capable of synthesizing one or more psychotogens by excessive or abnormal methylation, using as substrates structurally related biogenic amines or their normal metabolites (Osmond and Smythies, 1952). Support for this early hypothesis has emerged from several areas. A chronology of some of the evidence might be as follows:

1. Cantoni (1952) identified S-adenosylmethionine as an active methyl donor in biological methylation reactions. This substance is formed enzymatically from methionine and ATP.

2. Armstrong *et al.* (1957) identified urinary 3-methoxy-4-hydroxymandelic acid as a metabolite of adrenaline.

3. Axelrod (1957) demonstrated *in vitro* that catecholamines form mono-*O*-methylated metabolites.

4. Pollin *et al.* (1961) produced exacerbations of schizophrenic symptoms upon feeding methionine to iproniazid-treated patients.

5. Axelrod (1961) detected an enzyme in rabbit lung capable of converting tryptamine to *N*,*N*-dimethyltryptamine, and serotonin to bufotenin.

6. Friedhoff and Van Winkle (1962) detected DMPEA in the urine of schizophrenics but not in the urine of normal subjects. Subsequently, they showed the possible origin of urinary DMPEA by means of *in vivo* and *in vitro* studies with labeled dopamine (Friedhoff and Van Winkle, 1963).

7. Daly *et al.* (1965) converted several catecholamine metabolites to trioxy metabolites, thereby demonstrating a confluence between catecholamine and mescaline metabolism in mammalian tissue.

8. Various investigators have implicated dopamine overproduction in the etiology of schizophrenia (see for example, Friedhoff and Van Winkle, 1964).

9. Recently it has been demonstrated that mescaline can be formed in mammalian tissues from an appropriate precursor. (Friedhoff *et al.*, 1972*a*, *b*, *c*).

Discussions of the validity of many of these observations can be found in reviews by Weil-Malherbe and Szara (1971), Wyatt *et al.* (1971), and Friedhoff and Alpert (1973). Some aspects of biological *O*-methylation in reference to the formation of psychotogens will now be reviewed.

4. ASPECTS OF BIOLOGICAL *O*-METHYLATION

4.1. Catechol-*O*-methyltransferase

Biological mono-*O*-methylation in animal tissue was first observed by Axelrod (1957). In subsequent studies it was demonstrated (see, e.g., Axelrod, 1965) that the soluble enzyme catechol-*O*-methyltransferase (COMT) utilizes the methyl donor *S*-adenosylmethionine (SAM) and Mg^{++}. Alberici *et al.*, (1965) found that as much as 50% of brain COMT can be retained by the particulate nerve ending fraction. It is now commonly accepted that COMT participates in the rapid deactivation of catecholamine neurotransmitters at the synapse.

COMT has broad substrate specificity, but rates of *O*-methylation vary with different catechols. Drugs that contain the catechol moiety or that can be enzymatically hydroxylated to catechols, can be subsequently *O*-

methylated, *in vivo* or *in vitro* to mono-*O*-methylated catechols (guaiacols). Thus, apomorphine (McKenzie and White, 1973), diphenylhydantoin (Chang *et al.*, 1972), and even chlorpromazine (Daly and Manian, 1969) are excreted, in part, as guaiacols. The enzyme can even methylate ascorbic acid, a nonbenzenoid 5-membered heterocyclic compound. It was shown by Blaschke and Hertting (1971) to be mono-*O*-methylated both *in vivo* and *in vitro*.

Either of the two hydroxyl groups of catechols can be methyated. The extent of *meta-* to *para-O*-methylation of 1-substituted 3,4-dihydroxy-aromatics depends on the electronic nature and size of functional groups (Creveling *et al.*, 1972). Despite an earlier observation that stereospecificity was not apparent, these authors have shown that enantiomorphs do yield different *meta/para* (*m/p*) ratios. The most extreme example is that of D- and L-dopa which yield *m/p* ratios of 3.4 and 19.8, respectively.

Axelrod and Vesell (1970), Assicot and Bohuon (1971), and Frere and Verly (1971), have reported the presence of at least two distinct forms (isoenzymes) or COMT in various mammalian tissues. The possibility exists that differences seen in specificity, *m/p* ratio formation, and localization may be divided between the isoenzymes, in the same way that some of the mystery surrounding the nonspecificity of monoamine oxidase has been dispelled since the discovery that this enzyme is actually a composite of at least two related oxidases (Youdim *et al.*, 1969).

Changes in COMT activity have been reported in affective disorders, schizophrenia, and Down's syndrome (Gustavson *et al.*, 1973). Cohn *et al.* (1970) found that women with primary affective disorders were deficient in blood cell COMT. Matthysse and Baldessarini (1972) demonstrated a significant rise in COMT activity of red blood cells of schizophrenics. Thus some evidence exists for alterations in *O*-methylation activity in psychotics.

4.2. *O*-Methylating Enzymes Capable of Forming Hallucinogens

In addition to our studies on the formation of di-*O*-methyl metabolites of dopamine, referred to earlier, there have been occasional reports on the excretion of other di-*O*-methylated substances in man. Price (1969) has provided evidence that conjugated di-methoxybenzoic acid (Figure 2) is a metabolite of isovanillic acid in man. Ubiquinone or coenzyme Q (Folkers, 1967), one of the cofactors in the electron transport system found in all life forms, possesses an *ortho*-dimethoxy structure (Figure 2).

On the basis of findings like these we undertook a reexamination of the *O*-methylating properties of the soluble supernatant of liver, using a variety of guaiacols as substrates. With most substrates we were able to

DMPEA
Dimethoxybenzoic acid
DMPAA
Ubiquinone 10
(Coenzyme Q_{10})

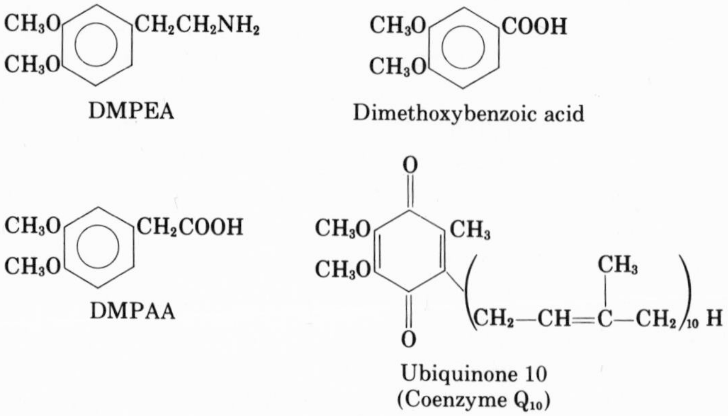

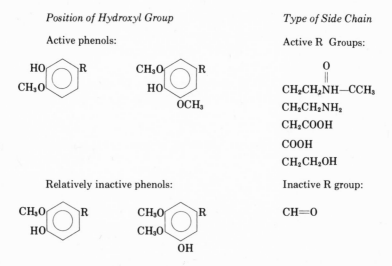

Figure 2. Di-*O*-methylated compounds isolated from human urine.

demonstrate that further *O*-methylation had indeed taken place (Friedhoff *et al.*, 1972*a*). Subsequent work has shown that the formation of di-*O*-methylated compounds works best when substrates contain a *p*-methoxy group and a *m*-hydroxy group, as shown in Figure 3. Thus, the major mono-*O*-methylated catecholamine metabolites are not preferred substrates for this enzyme. The simplest substance capable of further methylation is guaiacol and, therefore, the enzyme, if it is distinct from COMT, could be called guaiacol-*O*-methyltransferase (GOMT), in conformity with the common nomenclature used for other methyltransferases.

Position of Hydroxyl Group
Type of Side Chain
Active phenols:
Active R Groups:
$CH_2CH_2NH—CCH_3$
$CH_2CH_2NH_2$
CH_2COOH
COOH
CH_2CH_2OH
Relatively inactive phenols:
Inactive R group:
CH=O

Figure 3. Substrates for guaiacol-*O*-methyltransferase.

The optimum pH for this reaction is about 9, whereas COMT activity is best at pH 8. The other known O-methylating enzymes, hydroxyindole-O-methyltransferase, phenol-O-methyltransferase, and iodophenol-O-methyltransferase, cannot be considered as being responsible for the activity we ascribe to GOMT since these enzymes are not Mg^{++} dependent. Other criteria that eliminate from consideration the possible participation of these methyltransferases have been discussed by Friedhoff et al. (1972c).

The relative activity of various isoguaiacols is shown in Table I. N-Acetyl-3-hydroxy-4-methoxyphenethylamine (iso-NAMT), an in vitro metabolite of dopamine, upon further O-methylation, forms N-acetyl-3-4-dimethoxyphenethylamine (NADMPEA), an active in vivo metabolite of DMPEA (Friedhoff and Schweitzer, 1968; Schweitzer and Friedhoff, 1966). The O-methylation of iso-NAMT, as shown in Table II, demonstrates the requirement for enzyme and substrate. In these experiments, ^{14}C-methyl-S-adenosylmethionine is used as methyl donor. In this way the product is radioactive, and its identity can be ascertained by its ability to undergo the same reactions as authentic, unlabeled NADMPEA.

In order to firmly establish the location of the ^{14}C-methyl group, labeled products from two separate incubations with iso-NAMT were subjected to microsomal O-demethylation. Synthetically prepared 3-^{14}C-methyl-NADMPEA and 4-^{14}C-methyl-NADMPEA were tested in the same way. The products, upon enzymatic mono-O-demethylation, should be a mixture of N-acetyl-3-methoxy-4-hydroxyphenethylamine (n-NAMT) and iso-NAMT, since the microsomal enzyme is not specific, but only one of the demethylated products should retain the label. As shown in Table III, enzymatically formed NADMPEA behaved, as expected, like synthetic 3-^{14}C-NADMPEA. The metabolic formation of NADMPEA from iso-NAMT and to a lesser extent by n-NAMT has been confirmed by Hartley and Smith (1973) using a bovine pineal extract.

We next examined the methylation of phenolic trioxy precursors of mescaline and its metabolites. In contrast to dioxy substrates, favored

Table I. O-Methylation of Various Isoguaiacols by Guaiacol-O-Methyltransferase[a]

Substrate	Relative activity	Product
iso-Homovanillic acid	100	DMPAA
iso-N-Acetylmethoxytyramine	45	NADMPEA
iso-Vanillyl alcohol	23	Dimethoxybenzyl alcohol
iso-Methoxytyramine	5	DMPEA
iso-Vanillin	1	Veratraldehyde

[a] From Friedhoff et al., 1972c.

Table II.   Conversion of iso-NAMT to NADMPEA by Rat Liver Supernatant

Experiment	Sample	Incubation system[a]	iso-NAMT concentration	Product dpm/hr per mg protein
1	1	Complete—boiled	1.5×10^{-3} M	9
	2	Complete	1.5×10^{-3} M	10,980
	3	Complete	1.5×10^{-3} M	11,000
2	1	Complete—no substrate	0	4
	2	Complete	4.8×10^{-4}	8,650
	3	Complete	4.8×10^{-4}	6,880

[a] Incubation conditions: 50 mg protein from $100,000 \times g$ for 1 hr supernatant from rat liver, iso-NAMT in amount shown, 96 mμmole ^{14}C-SAM (52.5 μCi/μmole), 100 μmole MgCl$_2$ and 1 mmole tris-HCl, pH 9.0, and water to make a final volume of 10 ml. Incubations were carried out for 15 min. From Friedhoff et al., 1972a.

precursors for O-methylation are those in which the hydroxy group is located at the *para* position (see Figure 3). The activity towards these substrates is roughly ten times greater than toward isoguaiacols. In addition, while iso-NAMT is about nine times more active (see Table I) than the corresponding free amine (iso-methoxytyramine), N-acetyl-4-desmethylmescaline (NA4DMM) is only about twice as active as 4-desmethylmescaline (4DMM, or 3,5-dimethoxy-4-hydroxyphenethylamine), as shown in Table IV (Friedhoff et al., 1972b).

Table III.   Location of Position of Label of ^{14}C-NADMPEA Formed Enzymatically from iso-NAMT and ^{14}C-S-Adenosylmethionine by Means of Microsomal O-Demethylation[a]

Compound subjected to O-demethylation[c]	Products retaining ^{14}C after microsomal demethylation			
	Found		Expected	
	% iso-NAMT	% n-NAMT	% iso-NAMT	% n-NAMT
Product 1[b]	4	96	0	100
Product 2[b]	3	97	0	100
3-^{14}C-NADMPEA	5	95	0	100
4-^{14}C-NADMPEA	90	10	100	0

[a] Unpublished data. See text for rationale.
[b] ^{14}C-labeled material obtained from two separate incubations of iso-NAMT, ^{14}C-S-adenosylmethionine and GOMT, as described in Table II.
[c] Each incubation contained microsomes from 0.5 g rat liver, 100 μmole phosphate buffer pH 7.4, 25 μmole MgCl$_2$ and 4.8 mg NADPH in a final volume of 1.0 ml. Incubations were carried out for 1 hr. After extraction with CHCl$_3$, the compounds were separated by silica gel thin-layer chromatography in the system benzene-heptane-diethylamine, 10 : 5 : 1.

Table IV. Enzymatic Formation of Mescaline and N-Acetylmescaline in Rat Liver
Homogenate[a]

Conditions[b]	Substrate concentration	Mescaline from 4DMM dpm/mg per hr	N-Ac-mescaline from NA4DMM dpm/mg per hr
Complete	5×10^{-4} M	35,800	63,200
No substrate	0	325	280
No Mg^{++}, 10^{-3} EDTA added	5×10^{-4}	1,650	920
Boiled protein	10^{-3}	200	185

[a] From Friedhoff et al., 1972b.
[b] The complete system contained 2 mg protein from $100,000 \times g$ for 1 hr dialyzed rat liver homogenate, 200 μmole tris-HCl buffer, pH 9.0, 10 μmole MgCl$_2$, 4 nmole ^{14}C-S-adenosylmethionine, (52.3 mCi/mmole) and the concentration of substrate given above in a final volume of 1 ml. Incubations were carried out for 15 min.

The radioactive product in incubations with 4DMM was identified as mescaline by chromatography in four solvent systems, by cocrystallization with authentic mescaline hydrochloride, and by subsequent successive derivatization and cocrystallization. This sequence included acetylation to form N-acetylmescaline and bromination of this derivative to form N-acetyl-2,6-dibromomescaline. After each step the molar specific activity remained constant. Another portion of the metabolic product was mixed with unlabeled mescaline and subjected to oxidation with alkaline permanganate. The expected product, identified as 3,4,5-trimethoxybenzoic acid, retained the label without loss of molar specific activity. The identification of metabolically formed N-acetylmescaline, from NA4DMM, was confirmed by similar techniques.

Rat liver GOMT activity responds to stress. In one study, rats were subjected to warm water swim stress for 1 or 2 hr per day for 5 days. Livers and brains from these rats and control animals were tested, using NA4DMM as substrate. A 20% rise, significant at the 0.01 level, was obtained in liver but no change was seen in brain (Schweitzer et al., 1973). Neither 5-day adaptation to a 4°C environment nor intermittent foot-shock yielded a significant elevation in GOMT.

Studies pursuant to GOMT isolation and to the measurement of levels in blood fractions of psychotic patients are in progress in our laboratories.

In studying the formation of mescaline and other trioxy compounds, we have been prompted by the observations of two independent groups of investigators. Catecholamine metabolites have been shown to be capable of forming trioxy metabolites (Daly et al., 1965). The microsomal hydroxylation of 3-methoxy-4-hydroxyphenethanol, metanephrine, and N-methyl-metanephrine yielded 3-methoxy-4,5-dihydroxyphenethanol, 3-methoxy-4,5-dihydroxy-N-methylphenethanolamine, and 3-methoxy-4,5-dihydroxy-N,N-dimethylphenethanolamine, respectively. While these investigators were unable to demonstrate the formation of 3-methoxy-4,5-dihydroxyphenethylamine (4,5-di-desmethylmescaline, 4,5DMM) from methoxytyramine, Benington and Morin (1968) have argued that the slow release of tritium from 5-^{3}H-3-methoxytyramine under typical microsomal hydroxylation conditions provides evidence that 4,5DMM was the product.

We have carried out O-methylation studies, using rat liver supernate, with 4,5DMM as substrate. Both 3,4-dimethoxy-5-hydroxyphenethylamine and 3,5-dimethoxy-4-hydroxyphenethylamine (4DMM) are formed. These unpublished results are in agreement with studies of Masri *et al.* (1964) in which both 3,4-dimethoxy-5-hydroxybenzoic acid and 3,5-dimethoxy-4-hydroxybenzoic acid are formed upon enzymatic mono-O-methylation of 3-methoxy-4,5-dihydroxybenzoic acid. In contrast, Daly *et al.* (1962) were unable to form 4DMM using unlabeled 4,5DMM (and unlabeled SAM) as substrate. In that study equimolar amounts of 4,5-DMM and SAM were incubated. It has been shown that S-adenosylhomocysteine, the product that is formed when S-adenosylmethionine releases the methyl group, is a powerful COMT inhibitor (Deguchi and Barchas, 1971). It is therefore not surprising that under the conditions of Daly *et al.* (1962) the less favored product (4DMM) might be formed in an undetectable amount.

5. CONCLUSIONS

Pertinent studies have been discussed that bear on the methylation hypothesis, or as suggested by Faurbye (1968), the mescaline hypothesis, of schizophrenia. We have provided evidence from more recent studies from our laboratories that enzymes exist in mammalian tissue, including man, for the production of mescaline and related compounds, such as DMPEA. Also it has been found (Daly *et al.*, 1965; Benington and Morin, 1968) that catecholamine metabolites can be further ring-hydroxylated to form trioxy derivatives that could serve as precursors in the formation of mescaline.

The identification and characterization of mammalian enzymes that can catalyze the formation of methylated hallucinogenic derivatives of biogenic amines (rabbit lung N-methyltransferase and GOMT) raises an alternative to the transmethylation hypothesis, namely, that certain endogenous hallucinogens may serve a normal function. If mescaline is formed physiologically from dopamine under any circumstances (this remains to be demonstrated, even though the appropriate enzymes appear to be present), then exogenously administered mescaline may have hallucinogenic activity because it disrupts the normal function served by its endogenous counterpart. We would appear to be a long way from establishing such a mechanism, but in many ways this view is more consistent with the mechanism by which a related compound, the endogenous catecholamine precursor, L-dopa, can induce psychotic reactions. Alternatively, the problem in psychosis may result from an overproduction of dopamine or serotonin, the precursors of the psychotogens. The evidence pointing to hyperdopaminergia as a factor in psychosis is discussed extensively elsewhere in this volume.

Considerable pharmacological evidence points to the possibility that the interaction of several transmitters may also play a role in the development of psychotic symptoms, rather than the aberrant activity of a single system. The effect of anticholinergic hallucinogens like ditran, an experimental anti-Parkinson drug, cannot be readily reconciled with the methylation hypothesis, or with the notion that dopaminergic function alone is disturbed. For this reason we (Friedhoff and Alpert, 1973) have arrived at a wider view: "... an increase in dopaminergic activity or a decrease in cholinergic activity produces psychotic symptoms and relieves Parkinsonian symptoms. Conversely, a decrease in dopaminergic activity or an increase in cholinergic activity relieves psychotic symptoms, but produces Parkinsonian symptoms."

It is possible that the various outward manifestations of schizophrenia relate to the dominant biogenic amine in a particular individual. Perhaps in some individuals excessive dopamine, in relation to acetylcholine, might lead to excessive methylation and thereby produce hallucinations in that individual.

The above models, despite inconsistencies, make possible a degree of predictiveness with regard to the action of psychotropic drugs and also have implications for the regulation of normal mental function. We should therefore ask: What is the normal function that is being disrupted when a symptom is produced? It seems logical that if a system when disturbed induces hallucinations, the same system must have been involved in the regulation of some normal function (dreaming?) of which an hallucinogen is but an extreme manifestation. Viewed from this perspective, development of a model of psychopathology may also make possible the elucidation of aspects of normal regulatory function.

6. REFERENCES

Alberici, M., Rodriquez de Lores Arnaiz, G., and De Robertis, E., 1965, Catechol-*O*-methyltransferase in nerve endings of rat brain, *Life Sci.* **4**:1951.

Armstrong, M. D., McMillan, A., and Shaw, K. N. F., 1957, 3-methoxy-4-hydroxy-D-mandelic Acid, a urinary metabolite of norepinephrine, *Biochim. Biophys. Acta* **25**:422.

Assicot, M., and Bohuon, C., 1971, Presence of two distinct catechol-O-methyltransferase activities in red blood cells, *Biochimie* **53**:871.

Axelrod, J., 1957, O-Methylation of epinephrine and other catechols *in vitro* and *in vivo, Science* **126**:400.

Axelrod, J., 1961, Enzymatic formation of psychotomimetic metabolites from normally occurring compounds, *Science* **134**:343.

Axelrod, J., 1965, The formation and metabolism of physiologically active compounds by N- and O-methyltransferases, in: *Transmethylation and Methionine Biosynthesis* (S. K. Shapiro, and F. Schlenk, eds.), p. 71, University of Chicago Press, Chicago.

Axelrod, J., and Vesell, E. S., 1970, Heterogeneity of N- and O-methyltransferases, *Mol. Pharmacol.* **6**:78.

Barbeau, A., Singh, P., and Joubert, M., 1966, Effect of 3,4-dimethoxyphenylethylamine injections on catecholamine metabolism in rats and monkeys, *Life Sci.* **5**:757.

Benington, F., and Morin, R. D., 1968, Enzymatic 5-hydroxylation of 3-methoxytyramine, *Experientia* **24**:33.

Bindler, E., Sanghvi, I., and Gershon, S., 1968, Pharmacological and behavioral characteristics of 3,4-dimethoxyphenylethylamine and its N-acetyl derivative, *Arch. Intern. Pharmacodyn.* **176**:1.

Blaschke, E., and Hertting, G., 1971, Enzymic methylation of L-ascorbic acid by catechol-O-methyltransferase, *Biochem. Pharmacol.* **20**:1363.

Bridger, W. H., and Mandel, I. J., 1967, The effects of dimethoxyphenylethylamine and mescaline on classical conditioning in rats as measured by the potentiated startle response, *Life Sci.* **6**:775.

Cantoni, G. L., 1952, The nature of the active methyl donor formed enzymatically from L-methionine and adenosinetriphosphate, *J. Am. Chem. Soc.* **74**:2942

Charalampous, K. D., 1971, Comparison of metabolism of mescaline and 3,4-dimethoxyphenylethylamine in humans, *Behav. Neuropsychiat.* **2**:26.

Charalampous, K. D., and Tansey, L. W., 1967, Metabolic fate of β-(3,4-dimethoxyphenyl)-ethylamine in man, *J. Pharmacol. Exptl. Therap.* **155**:318.

Chang, T., Okerholm, R. A., and Glazko, A. J., 1972, A 3-O-methylated catechol metabolite of diphenylhydantoin (dilantin) in rat urine, *Res. Commun Chem. Path. Pharmacol.* **4**:13.

Cohn, C. K., Dunner, D. L., and Axelrod, J., 1970, Reduced catechol-O-methyltransferase activity in red blood cells of women with primary affective disorder, *Science* **170**:1323.

Creveling, C. R., Morris, N., Shimizu, H., Ong, H. H., and Daly, J. W., 1972, Catechol-O-methyltransferase IV. Factors affecting *m*- and *p*-methylation of substituted catechols, *Mol. Pharmacol.* **8**:398.

Daly, J. W., and Manian, A. A., 1969, The action of catechol-O-methyltransferase on 7,8-dihydroxychlorpromazine-formation of 7-hydroxy-8-methoxychlorpromazine and 8-hydroxy-7-methoxy chlorpromazine, *Biochem. Pharmacol.* **18**:1235.

Daly, J., Axelrod, J., and Witkop, B., 1962, Methylation and demethylation in relation to the *in vitro* metabolism of mescaline, *Ann. N.Y. Acad. Sci.* **96**:37.

Daly, J., Inscoe, J. K., and Axelrod, J., 1965, The formation of O-methylated catechols by microsomal hydroxylation of phenol and subsequent enzymatic catechol O-methylation. Substrate specificity, *J. Med. Chem.* **8**:153.

Dear, E. M. A., and Malcolm, J. L., 1967, A study of the effect of 3,4-dimethoxyphenylethylamine on cortical evoked potentials in the rat, *Intern. J. Neuropharmacol.* **6**:529.

Deguchi, T., and Barchas, J., 1971, Inhibition of transmethylations of biogenic amines by S-adenosylhomocysteine, *J. Biol. Chem.* **246**:3175.

Ernst, A. M., 1965, Relation between the structure of certain methoxyphenethylamine derivatives and the occurrence of a hypokinetic rigid syndrome, *Psychopharmacologia* 7:383.

Faurbye, A., 1968, The role of amines in the etiology of schizophrenia, *Comprehensive Psychiat.* 9:155.

Folkers, K., 1967, Research on coenzyme Q, in: *Phenolic Compounds and Metabolic Regulation* (B. J. Finkle, and V. C. Runeckles, eds.), p. 94, Appleton-Century-Crofts, New York.

Frere, J. M., and Verly, W. G., 1971, Catechol-*O*-methyltransferase. The *para*- and *meta*-*O*-methylations of noradrenaline, *Biochim. Biophys. Acta* 235:73.

Friedhoff, A. J., and Alpert, M., 1973, A dopaminergic-cholinergic mechanism in production of psychotic symptoms, *Biol. Psychiat.* 6:165.

Friedhoff, A. J., and Hollister, L. E., 1966, Comparison of the metabolism of 3,4-dimethoxyphenylethylamine and mescaline in humans, *Biochem. Pharmacol.* 15:269.

Friedhoff, A. J., and Schweitzer, J. W., 1968, An effect of *N*-acetyl-dimethoxyphenethylamine, *Diseases Nervous System* 29:455.

Friedhoff, A. J., and Van Winkle, E., 1962, Isolation and characterization of a compound from the urine of schizophrenics, *Nature* 194:897.

Friedhoff, A. J., and Van Winkle, E., 1963, Conversion of dopamine to 3,4-dimethoxyphenylacetic acid in schizophrenic patients, *Nature* 199:1271.

Friedhoff, A. J., and Van Winkle, E., 1964, Biological *O*-methylation and schizophrenia, *Psychiat. Res. Rep. Am. Psychiat. Assoc.* 19:149.

Friedhoff, A. J., Schweitzer, J. W., and Miller, J. C., (1972a). The enzymatic formation of 3,4-di-*O*-methylated dopamine metabolites by mammalian tissues, *Res. Commun Chem. Path. Pharmacol.* 3:293.

Friedhoff, A. J., Schweitzer, J. W., and Miller, J., 1972b, Biosynthesis of mescaline and *N*-acetylmescaline by mammalian liver, *Nature* 237:454.

Friedhoff, A. J., Schweitzer, J. W., Miller, J. C., and Van Winkle, E., 1972c, Guaiacol-*O*-methyltransferase: A mammalian enzyme capable of forming di-*O*-methylcatecholamine derivatives, *Experientia* 28:517.

Fujimori, M., and Alpers, H. S., 1970, Psychotomimetic compounds in man and animals, in: *Biochemistry, Schizophrenias, and Affective Illnesses,* (H. E. Himwich, ed.), p. 361, Williams and Wilkins Co., Baltimore.

Gustavson, K. H., Wetterberg, L., Backstrom, M., and Ross, S. B., 1973, Catechol-*O*-methyltransferase activity in erythrocytes in Down's syndrome, *Clin. Genet.* 4:279.

Hartley, R., and Smith, J. A., 1973, Formation *in vitro* of *N*-acetyl-3,4-dimethoxyphenethylamine by pineal hydroxyindole-*O*-methyltransferase, *Biochem. Pharmacol.* 22:2425.

Hollister, L. E., and Friedhoff, A. J., 1966, Effects of 3,4-dimethoxyphenylethylamine in man, *Nature* 210:1377.

Kapadia, G. J., and Fayez, M. B. E., 1970, Peyote constituents: chemistry, biogenesis and biological effects, *J. Pharm. Sci.* 59:1699.

Levis, D. J., and Caldwell, D. F., 1971, The effects of a low dose of mescaline and 3,4-dimethoxyphenylethylamine under two levels of adversive stimulation, *Biol. Psychiat.* 3:251.

Mandell, A. J., and Morgan, M., 1970, Human brain enzyme makes indole hallucinogens, *Proc. Am. Psychol. Assoc.* p. 228.

Masri, M. S., Robbins, D. J., Emerson, O. H., and De Eds, F., 1964, Selective para- or meta-*O*-methylation with catechol-*O*-methyltransferase from rat liver, *Nature* 202:878.

Matthysse, S., and Baldessarini, R. J., 1972, *S*-Adenosylmethionine and catechol-*O*-methyltransferase in schizophrenia, *Am. J. Psychiat.* 128:1310.

McKenzie, G. M., and White, H. L., 1973, Evidence for the methylation of apomorphine by catechol-*O*-methyltransferase *in vivo* and *in vitro*, *Biochem. Pharmacol.* 22:2329.

Osmond, H., and Smythies, J., 1952, Schizophrenia: a new approach, *J. Mental Sci.* **98**:309.

Pollin, W., Cardon, P. V., and Kety, S. S., 1961, Effects of amino acid feeding in schizophrenic patients treated with iproniazid, *Science* **133**:104.

Price, J., 1969, The metabolites of isovanillic acid in man, with special reference to the formation of 3,4-dimethoxybenzoic acid, *Clin. Chim. Acta* **25**:31.

Schweitzer, J. W., and Friedhoff, A. J., 1966, The metabolism of α-C^{14}-3,4-dimethoxyphenethylamine, *Biochem. Pharmacol.* **15**:2097.

Schweitzer, J. W., Stone, E. A., and Friedhoff, A. J., 1973, Increased *in vitro* O-methylation in swim-stressed rats, Presented at the 4th meeting of the International Society for Neurochemistry, Tokyo.

Shulgin, A. T., Sargent, T., and Naranjo, C., 1969, Structure–activity relationships of one-ring psychotomimetics, *Nature* **221**:537.

Smythe, G. A., and Lazarus, L., 1973, Blockade of the dopamine-inhibitory control of prolactin secretion in rats by 3,4-dimethoxyphenylethylamine (3,4-di-O-methyldopamine), *Endocrinology* **93**:147.

Snyder, S. H., and Merril, C. R., 1965, A relationship between the hallucinogenic activity of drugs and their electronic configuration, *Proc. Natl. Acad. Sci. (U.S.)* **54**:258.

Takeo, Y., and Himwich, H. E., 1965, Mescaline, 3,4-dimethoxyphenylethylamine, and adrenaline: sites of electroencephalographic arousal, *Science* **150**:1309.

Vacca, L., Fujimori, M., Davis, S. H., and Marrazzi, A. S., 1968, Cerebral synaptic transmission and behavioral effects of dimethoxyphenylethylamine: a potential psychotogen, *Science* **160**:95.

Van Praag, H. M., 1967, The possible significance of cerebral dopamine for neurology and psychiatry, *Psychiat. Neurol. Neurochir.* **70**:361.

Weil-Malherbe, H., and Szara, S. I., 1971, *The Biochemistry of Functional and Experimental Psychoses,* Charles C. Thomas, Springfield.

Wyatt, R. J., Termini, B. A., and Davis, J., 1971, Biochemical and sleep studies of schizophrenia: a reveiw of the literature—1960–1970. Part I. Biochemical studies, *Schizophrenia Bull.* **4**:10.

Youdim, M. B. H., Collins, C. G. S., and Sandler, M., 1969, Multiple forms of rat brain monoamine oxidase, *Nature* **223**:626.

Chapter 8

Regulation of Brain Dopamine Turnover Rate: Pharmacological Implications

E. Costa and M. Trabucchi

Laboratory of Preclinical Pharmacology
National Institute of Mental Health
Saint Elizabeths Hospital
Washington, D.C.

1. INTRODUCTION

The ability of brain dopaminergic neurons to maintain the concentration of their transmitter at steady state in the face of continuous changes of their activity patterns depends critically upon the way in which metabolic enzymes, storage mechanisms, and regulatory dopamine receptors are organized in dopaminergic synapses (Costa, 1973; Costa and Meek, 1974, Glowinski 1973; Carlsson *et al.*, 1972*a*). There is incomplete information concerning this organization, and there are only scant details concerning their molecular arrangements and interactions. Thus, the current understanding makes the study of dopaminergic function a most ambitious undertaking. Indeed, the problem would appear to be insuperable unless conceptual models can be made available to deal with the gaps in our knowledge.

The study of the dynamics of the dopaminergic system while it is functioning is facilitated by the pattern of distribution of dopaminergic axons in brain (Ungerstedt, 1971). In the rat brain the cell bodies of these neurons are located in the pars compacta of the substantia nigra (A_9, A_{10}) or within the nucleus arcuatus hypothalami, the nucleus dorsalis medialis hypothalami, and the nucleus periventricularis. These cell bodies generate three main dopaminergic pathways: nigrostriatal system, mesolimbic system and

the tubero-infundibular system. The nigrostriatal system fans out in the'
globus pallidus and enters the nucleus caudatus putamen. From here the
axons running lateroventrally from the capsula interna extend to the nucleus
amygdaloideus centralis. The mesolimbic system enters the nucleus accumbens and the nucleus interstitialis striae terminalis while another branch
enters the tuberculum olfactorium and probably the frontal and other parts
of the telencephalon. The terminals of the tubero-infundibular system dis-
tribute to various hypothalamic nuclei, to the median eminence, and form
an ascending pathway which has not yet been clearly described. It is still de-
bated where the cell bodies for the dopaminergic terminals of cerebral
cortex are located. Some authors have suggested that the cortex may
contain dopaminergic interneurons: this suggestion is supported by uptake
(Descarries and Lapierre, 1973) and by lesion studies (Thierry and Glowinski, 1973).

    In this review we shall discuss separately the theoretical and technical
difficulties one faces when the dopaminergic neurons are studied *in vivo* to
detect how drugs and environment affect their function.

2. PROBLEMS IN INTERPRETING THE COMPARTMENTATION
AND THE FUNCTIONAL IMPLICATIONS OF TURNOVER
RATE MEASUREMENT OF NEURONAL DOPAMINE

    Recently several approaches have been followed to measure dopamine
(DA) turnover rate in brain structures. Claims have been made that one
method yields more reliable information than others (Glowinski, 1973;
Costa, 1973). However, it is safe to say that all the methods used up to now
have their intrinsic difficulties. Before discussing the significance in psychopharmacology of *in vivo* measurements of DA turnover rate, let us
review the present state of the art. Each of the three neuronal systems that
releases DA can be considered as comprising sets of interacting subsystems.
These subsystems function at various levels of organization. When the
turnover of DA is studied in homogenates of whole brain, the problems of
interpretation are enhanced because this sample includes two types of
neuronal pathways that contain DA. In one of them, norepinephrine (NE) is
the transmitter and DA serves as a precursor of NE, in another, DA is the
transmitter. Obviously the measurement of DA turnover rate in structures
where DA is the precursor of NE has a different meaning from that of
structures where the DA is the transmitter. This problem is bypassed by
microdissection techniques. Recently, several discrete dopaminergic units
have been studied by taking the measurements in specific tel-diencephalic
nuclei (Koslow *et al.*, 1974). From the data reported in Table I some

guidelines can be proposed to estimate the presence of dopaminergic and/or noradrenergic pathways in discrete brain nuclei.

From these data, it appears that N. preopticus medialis, N. anterior hypothalami, and cortex pyriformis are probably exclusively innervated by noradrenergic axons. This conclusion implies that the amount of DA which serves as a precursor of NE can be estimated to be less than 1% of that of the transmitter. Higher proportions of DA may indicate that in a nucleus innervated by NE terminals there is a contamination by dopaminergic cells or fibers. If this inference is correct, then cerebellum, superior cervical ganglia, and locus coeruleus contain a contamination by dopaminergic fibers or cells. N. caudatus putamen and nucleus accumbens appear to be almost exclusively innervated by dopaminergic axons, whereas the N. septi lateralis et medialis and the nucleus amygdaloideus centralis are equally innervated by dopaminergic and noradrenergic terminals. If the amount of DA that functions in noradrenergic nerves as a precursor of NE is only 5–7% of the NE contained in these nerves (Koslow et al., 1974), the error in the measurement of the DA turnover rate in brain nuclei containing about equal amounts of NE and DA appears to be rather insignificant.

To understand neuronal interaction at synaptic level, ideally the dynamics of a single neuronal entity should be investigated; however, such studies are not feasible because the accuracy of our methods for microdissection would be inappropriate. Although the resolution of mass

Table I. Concentrations of Norepinephrine and Dopamine in Discrete Brain Nuclei or Other Neural Tissues

Nucleus or brain area	Catecholamines (pmole/mg protein) mean ± SEM[a]		
	NE	DA	DA/NE
N. Caudatus-putamen[b]	14 ± 1.7	570 ± 18	40.7
N. Accumbens[b]	33 ± 5.2	610 ± 46	18.4
N. Septi Lateralis et medialis[b]	73 ± 12	85 ± 23	1.1
N. Preopticus medialis[b]	210 ± 11	13 ± 4.1	0.061
N. Anterior hypothalami[b]	210 ± 34	12 ± 1.4	0.057
Cortex pyriformis[b]	93 ± 21	6.8 ± 0.75	0.073
N. Amygdaloideus centralis[b]	95 ± 21	238 ± 13	2.5
Locus coeruleus[c]	200 ± 16	32 ± 2.5	0.16
Cerebellum[c]	11 ± 2.64	1.3 ± 0.4	0.11
Superior cervical sympathetic ganglion[c]	714 ± 61	128 ± 16	0.17

[a] Each analysis included 0.6 to 0.8 mg of fresh tissue containing about 60 to 80 μg protein.
[b] Koslow et al., 1974.
[c] Koslow et al., 1972.

fragmentography, the most sensitive method available to assay the concentration of NE and DA, may reach the level of a single brain neuron (Koslow *et al.*, 1972), its sensitivity will be insufficient to assay the DA turnover rate in single neurons. In fact, the incorporation of ^{18}O into DA after 10 min of ^{18}O inhalation averages 1.2% to 3% of the transmitter pool, and the mass fragmentography cannot measure 1% of the catecholamine present in a single neuron (LeFevre and Koslow, unpublished observations). Hence, studies of the dynamics of the various subsystems included in the dopaminergic pathways of rat brain can be focused on the collection of the nerve terminals reaching a given brain nucleus but not on single cells. By studying the dynamics of DA in various brain nuclei, we can appreciate whether drugs selectively affect the dopaminergic input to a given brain nucleus. Not only can we evaluate differences of drug effects on nigrostriatal, mesolimbic, and tubero-infundibular dopaminergic systems but also among the various telencephalic nuclei that are innervated by each of the three dopaminergic neuronal systems. Such selectivity may derive from a drug action on other neuronal systems regulating presynaptically the function of a given set of dopaminergic terminals, but also regulating interneurons involved in the regulation of a given nucleus.

2.1. Mathematical Formulation of the Subsystems

In general, any subsystem participating in a complex dynamic regulation is defined by a set of variable attributes. A very simple model is reported here.

Input $\longrightarrow$ SUBSYSTEM

$\longrightarrow$ Output (Y)

(U) $\longrightarrow$ (A)

Unobserved variables

Let a subset of these attributes be an input U and an output Y, we attach to the input–output pair a parameter $x(t_o)$ such as Y is uniquely determined by U and $x(t_o)$. Therefore, the vectors U and Y are to be understood as a set of time variable functions defined in some interval (t_o,t). In practice, to measure the dynamic state of the subsystem we introduce a special label at t_o without changing the steady state. We then use this label to trace the way in which the input is elaborated by the subsystem and we study the output Y

as a function of time by measuring the intrinsic incorporation of the label in the chemical entity that exhibits the vectorial changes described by Y. So far three types of labels have been used to study the dynamic state of dopaminergic subsystems: (i) the intravenous injection of the labeled amino acid, tyrosine (Sedvall *et al.*, 1968; Neff *et al.*, 1969, 1971) which is the substrate of the rate-limiting step for DA biosynthesis (Udenfriend, 1966); (ii) the inhalation of the stable isotope ^{18}O (Sedvall *et al.*, 1973a); and (iii) the intraventricular injection of the labeled DA (Iversen and Glowinski, 1966) or the intracerebral injection of labeled tyrosine (Javoy *et al.*, 1974). The intraventricularly injected DA is taken up into the metabolic compartments of the neuronal DA by specific processes located in the membrane of dopaminergic neurons. The decay of the radioactive DA injected intraventricularly is the least useful of the three methods because of the limited degree of specificity of the DA uptake in the dopaminergic nerves and the change of the steady state of brain DA that is involved. Therefore, some of the DA administered intraventricularly enters noradrenergic neurons where it is metabolized into NE; the decay of this radioactivity is faster than that of DA entering dopaminergic neurons because this pool of DA is only 5–7% that of NE. In addition, the fate of DA which enters other monoaminergic neurons creates further complications because it remains metabolically inert. The labeling with tritiated tyrosine injected intracerebrally and the measurement of the accumulation of ^{3}H H_2O has been proposed to estimate tyrosine hydroxylation (Udenfriend, 1966), the rate-limiting process for DA synthesis. This method may be of value to study mechanisms of drug action on dopaminergic neurons but not to estimate DA synthesis; however, the precision of the localization of the injection becomes highly relevant for this estimation, because the distribution of DA along the longitudinal axis of N. caudatus putamen varies (Koslow *et al.*, 1974). When the labeling procedures involve the intravenous injection of ^{3}H tyrosine or the inhalation of $^{18}O_2$ without changing the steady state of tyrosine or O_2, the label traces the dynamic of catecholamine synthesis. Both conversion of ^{3}H tyrosine into DA and ^{18}O incorporation into DA describe the kinetics of the system at the step that is rate-limiting for the operation. With ^{3}H tyrosine or ^{18}O the label is included simultaneously in various brain subsystems (for instance, in all tel-diencephalic nuclei receiving dopaminergic innervation) and by using a recently developed microdissection technique (Koslow *et al.*, 1974) (see Table I), the turnover rate of DA in the cell bodies and nerve endings of the various brain nuclei can be analyzed simultaneously.

A procedure frequently used to gain information on details of a dopaminergic subsystem is that of administering drugs that perturb the subsystem in a known and predictable way. The operation of various subsystems in the brains of normal and drug-treated animals is then compared. However, if the perturbation determines a change of the steady state, the comparison must be performed while the normal and the perturbed systems are at steady state. Data collected while the steady state is changing cannot be interpreted using principles of steady state kinetics (Costa, 1973). Specific equations can be derived to measure the turnover rate using the basic equation that describes the steady state operation of a kinetic compartment open at both ends. The assumption made is that input and output are balanced, SAU and SAY are the specific activities of input U and output Y, which are measured, and k_y is the first-order rate constant describing the output of SAY.

$$\frac{dy}{dt} = k_y (SAU - SAY)$$

2.2. Analytical Problems

When the label is either ^{18}O or ^{3}H tyrosine and the output measured is the change with time of either the mass or the specific radioactivity of DA, one should try to measure either the change of specific activity or the incorporation of ^{18}O into 3,4-dihydroxyphenylalanine (dopa). This measurement is difficult because dopa is unstable. Moreover, if the measurement is performed in brain areas that contain abundant NE and DA neurons, the changes in the dopa cannot be readily interpreted in terms of DA or NE turnover since dopa is the precursor for both amines. The study of the change with time of the specific activity of tyrosine in brain parts cannot be readily taken as the expression of the change with time of the specific activity of the catecholamine precursor because tyrosine is involved in other metabolic activities in addition to the biosynthesis of catecholamines. The pool size of tyrosine involved in the synthesis of catecholamines in rat heart was estimated by kinetic analysis and found to correspond to 12% of the total tyrosine pool in heart (Costa et al., 1972). Moreover, it was calculated that the first-order rate constant of this pool is 10 hr^{-1}. The rate constant of the remaining pools of heart tyrosine was estimated to be 0.67 hr^{-1} (Costa et al., 1972). In rat heart ventricles, the fast turning over pool of tyrosine relates to the pool of DA; by making the assumption that the DA present in heart ventricles is only the precursor of NE, the turnover rate of synthesis of this transmitter was measured. In the light of the present knowledge (see Table I), we may advance some doubts on the validity of the assumption that heart DA, which reaches a concentration of about 10% that of NE, functions exclusively as a NE precursor. Because of these complications, one cannot extrapolate that the tyrosine compartmentation in brain resembles that of heart. Therefore, the compartmentation of striatal tyrosine was investigated (Doteuchi *et al.,* 1974). The strategy followed was that of comparing the specific activity of tyrosine and dopa at various times after a pulse injection of radioactive tyrosine. The results obtained in these studies are summarized in Table II and show that within the time limit of about 20 min the specific activity of striatal dopa is comparable to that of striatal tyrosine (TY). This rapid equilibration between the specific activity of striatal dopa and tyrosine may relate to the differences between the sizes of these two pools that of dopa being only 0.38% that of tyrosine.

These data suggest that by plotting on semilogarithmic paper the decay of striatal DA specific activity versus time expressed as a function of the turnover time of tyrosine SA, it is possible to calculate the turnover rate of striatal DA with some accuracy (Doteuchi *et al.,* 1974). The measurement of dopa concentrations in striatum involves two types of problems. One relates to the sensitivity of the assay procedure, and the other relates to the postmortem stability of this amino acid. The former requires that striata from five to six rats be pooled to perform the assay, the latter has been solved utilizing a microwave radiation focused to the skull of rats for 2 sec (Guidotti *et al.,* 1974).

The data of Table III indicate that tissue concentrations of dopa after microwave radiation are identical to the dopa concentrations that are measured in tissues obtained with the freeze-blowing technique which allows for the collection of frozen brain samples in 0.5 sec (Lust *et al.,* 1973). Since freeze-blowing does not allow for brain dissection, it cannot be used to measure the dynamic state of DA in discrete brain structures. Previous reports had indicated that in rats killed with a microwave application, the dopa concentrations of striatum were below 0.14 μmole/g per striatum

Table II. Steady State and Specific Activities of Striatal Tyrosine and Dopa[a] at Various Times after L-(3,5³H) Tyrosine

Minutes after Labeling	Tyrosine		Dopa	
	nmole/g	dpm/nmole	nmole/g	dpm/nmole
3	72	5420	0.29	4990
6	80	5140	0.29	4850
9	73	4670	0.31	3910
12	77	4400	0.29	4100
15	82	3480	0.34	3600
18	81	2990	0.33	2790

[a] Each value was obtained by pooling the striate of eight rats. Each rat received 0.4 mCi/ kg iv L-(3,5³H) tyrosine (30 Ci/mmole) at zero time.

Table III.   Dopa Concentrations in Brain of Rats Killed by Various Procedures

Killing procedure	Minutes between death and homogenization	Dopa pmole/mg protein ± SEM
Microwave[a]	1	2.6 ± 0.20
Microwave	5	2.6 ± 0.21
Decapitation	1	1.6 ± 0.10[c]
Decapitation	5	1.6 ± 0.13[c]
Freeze-blowing[b]	—	2.7 ± 0.26

[a] A beam of microwaves produced by a magnetron that operates with a nominal input of 2.0 kw at 2.45 GHz was focused by a metal wave guide to the skull of a rat. A 2-sec irradiation inactivates the enzymes in the rat brain (Guidotti et al., 1974).
[b] According to Lust et al. (1973) it extracts and freezes the brain in 0.5 sec.
[c] $p < 0.01$ Versus values of rats killed by freeze-blowing.

(Carlsson et al., 1972a). The commercial microwave radiator used by Carlsson et al. (1972b) produces a homogeneous microwave field in about 20.000 cm³. We have modified this microwave radiation to deliver concentrated energy in a few cubic centimeters, thus causing instantaneous inactivation of brain enzymes. Since the rate of the expected temperature rise which inactivates brain enzymes is directly proportional to the product of the power (energy delivery rate) by time, a precise control of the radiation time assures the appropriate calibration of the instrument. To estimate the action of neuroleptics on the turnover rate of DA in striatum and N. accumbens of rats, we have injected pulses of L-(3′,5′-³H) tyrosine and have killed the rats with 2 sec of microwave radiation and have measured the specific activity of tyrosine and DA in striatum and N. accumbens (see Table V).

2.3. Compartmentation of Striatal DA

Javoy and Glowinski (1971) have reported that in dopaminergic nerve terminals of rat striatum there are two distinct storage forms of DA. A functional pool of transmitter that includes about 26% of the total striatal DA and a main storage pool that includes the remaining striatal DA. They calculated that the functional pool has a fractional rate constant (k_{DA}) of 4.6 hr⁻¹, while the k_{DA} of the main storage pool is 0.34 hr⁻¹. Doteuchi et al. (1974) have calculated how the specific activity of DA should change if the two pools with the characteristics described by Javoy and Glowinski were operative in regulating the change with time of the specific activity of striatal DA stores in rats receiving a pulse intravenous injection of radiactive tyrosine. By working with a model similar to that proposed by Javoy and Glowinski (1971), we have calculated the changes of tyrosine and DA specific activity and compared these theoretical data with those obtained by direct experimentation. As shown in Figure 1, the proposed model is at variance with the experimental data. We believe that this substantiates the conclusion that the store of striatal DA may not be compartmentalized in the way proposed by Javoy and Glowinski (1971). To probe the concept of a DA compartmentation even further, we have assumed that the size of the functional pool of DA may be only 5% of the total store. We have found that even this size would be a little too large to comply with the experi-

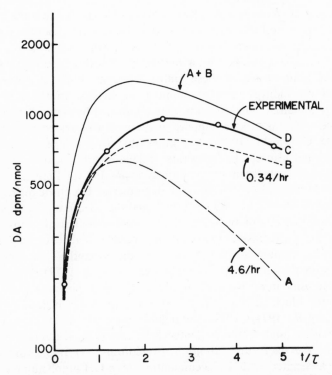

Figure 1. Calculated values of S_{NDA}, assuming compartmentation of striatal dopamine (DA) proposed by Javoy and Glowinski (1971). One compartment is proposed to have a k_{DA} of 4.6 hr^{-1}, and the other a k_{DA} of 0.34 hr^{-1}; the first functional compartment is 26% of the total dopamine in striatum, and the other includes 74% of the total dopamine. Data are plotted as S_{NDA} (t/τ), where $\tau = 1/k_{Tyr}$. Curve A = S_{NDA} in the "functional" compartment (k_{DA} = 4.6 hr^{-1}, including 26% of striatal dopamine); B = S_{NDA} of the "main storage" compartment (k_{DA} = 0.34 hr^{-1}, including 74% of striatal dopamine); C = experimental S_{NDA}; D = A + B, where data are plotted as $S_{NDA}(t/\tau)$ with $\tau = 1/k_{Tyr}$. (From Doteuchi *et al.*, 1974, with permission.)

mental data point of the change with time of DA specific activity in striatum of rats receiving a tracer pulse of radioactive tyrosine.

A number of alternatives can be adduced to explain the biphasic decay of striatal DA after intraperitoneal injections of α-methyltyrosine (Costa 1973; Doteuchi *et al.*, 1974), which was the main experimental evidence that led Javoy and Glowinski (1971) to formulate their model of striatal DA compartmentation. In addition, we have also shown that the injection of α-methyltyrosine does not block instantaneously the synthesis of DA (Doteuchi *et al.*, 1974). This and the accumulation in striatum of *p*-OH-norephedrine formed from α-methyltyrosine (Doteuchi *et al.*, 1974) can account for the distortion from the linearity in the decay of striatal DA of rats injected with α-methyltyrosine.

A report by Weissman and Koe (1965) had suggested that the action of (+) amphetamine on the motor activity of rats directly depends on the synthesis rate of brain catecholamines. They showed that when the synthesis of catecholamines was blocked by a pretreatment with α-methyltyrosine, although the brain stores of these amines was only partially depleted, the activity of the indirect sympathomimetic to increase motor activity was completely impaired. These results were confirmed by a number of investigators and were taken as a support to the two pool systems proposed by Javoy and Glowinski (1971). We know that (+) amphetamine releases striatal DA but also blocks firing rate of dopaminergic neurons of the pars compacta of the substantia nigra (Bunney *et al.*, 1973a). Perhaps, when the firing rate of a neuron is blocked, the dynamics of DA through the various compartments of striatum are perturbed, and the release of DA depends exclusively from its rate of synthesis which is impaired after high doses of (+) amphetamine (Kuczenski, 1974). It is possible that (+) amphetamine increases the amount of DA present in the synaptic cleft which then interacts with presynaptic DA receptors (Kehr *et al.*, 1972). Moreover, α-methyl-*p*-tyrosine in rat is metabolized into *p*-OH-amphetamine and *p*-OH-norephedrine which accumulates in various brain nuclei including striatum (Doteuchi *et al.*, 1974). These compounds exert a complex action on the storage, release, and synthesis (Doteuchi *et al.*, 1974; Kuczenski, 1974) of DA which deserves further attention. In addition, (+) amphetamine injections are associated with an accumulation of *p*-OH-amphetamine and *p*-OH-norephedrine in brain (Groppetti and Costa, 1969). Preliminary work by Dr. Doteuchi (personal communication) appears to indicate that a pretreatment with *p*-OH-norephedrine given intraventricularly reduces the effects on motor activity elicited by successive injections of (+) amphetamine. In the light of these results, the experiments showing that a pretreatment with α-methyltyrosine reduces the stimulation of motor activity elicited by (+) amphetamine are now open to a number of alternative interpretations.

A plausible alternative is that p-OH-amphetamine and p-OH-norephedrine accumulate in striatum and modify the regulation of synthesis and/or the release of DA. From several lines of evidence has emerged the concept that catecholaminergic nerves possess regulatory presynaptic receptors (Langer, 1973). In dopaminergic nerves the DA presynaptic receptors participate in a negative feedback control mechanism through which the DA present in the synaptic cleft may inhibit its own release and reduce its own synthesis (Kehr et al., 1972).

2.4. Problems in Measuring Turnover Rate of Striatal DA from the Accumulation of Dopa after Inhibition of Dopa Decarboxylase

The discovery that supramolecular mechanisms controlled by presynaptic receptor sites regulate synthesis and release of DA has created a number of stimulating new avenues of research (Andén et al., 1972; 1973). These include a new methodology to measure the turnover rate of striatal DA from the accumulation of striatal dopa after inhibition of dopa decarboxylation (Carlsson et al., 1972b; Kehr et al., 1972). In addition, new interpretations are now possible to explain the relationship between changes of DA turnover rate and unit activity of dopaminergic neurons. When nigrostriatal axons are severed or lesioned electrothermically, there is a rapid increase in the striatal DA and dopa content (Andén et al., 1972) and an increase of the conversion of tyrosine into dopa (Andén et al., 1973; Roth et al., 1973; Walters and Roth, 1974). An increase of striatal DA turnover and of dopa concentrations can also be obtained by injecting γ-hydroxybutyrolactone (GBL) (Roth and Surh, 1970; Gessa et al., 1966) which causes a reduction in the extraneuronal release of DA and in the firing rate of DA units located in the pars compacta of the substantia nigra (Roth et al., 1973). Thus, the increased rate of dopa formation after specific lesions of the nigrostriatal system or after injection of γ-hydroxybutyric acid can be measured after a blockade of dopa decarboxylase with 3-hydroxybenzylhydrazine (NSD 1015). This measurement of dopa accumulation in striatum of lesioned or normal rats receiving NSD 1015 has been taken as a method to estimate dopamine biosynthesis (Kehr et al., 1972; Carlsson et al., 1972b). This technique assumes that dopa, within broad limits of concentrations, does not operate as a feedback regulator by product inhibition of DA synthesis as previously suggested (Costa, 1972). This assumption is contrary to in vitro studies of tyrosine hydroxylase (Udenfriend et al., 1965) and to recent in vivo documentation (Javoy et al., 1974). Calculations of the data published (Carlsson et al., 1972a) suggest that the molar accumulation of dopa only partially accounts for the turnover rate of striatal DA as evaluated by other methods (Costa and Meek, 1974). Although the measurement of dopa concentrations does not estimate absolute synthesis rates, it may be of value for comparative drug studies.

2.5. The Use of ^{18}O to Measure the Turnover Rate of DA in Terminals and Cell Bodies of Dopaminergic Axons

This laboratory has developed quantitative mass fragmentographic methods for the determination and structural identification of very small amounts of catecholamines and their metabolites (Koslow et al., 1972). These methods had been developed to make possible the use of ^{18}O to label DA stores in discrete brain nuclei and to measure the turnover rate of the transmitter at synaptic level by changes of the relative abundance of ^{18}O in DA molecules (Cattabeni et al., 1972; LeFevre et al., 1975).

Sedvall et al. (1973a) have shown that when rats inhale ^{18}O$_2$ for 3 hr, this stable isotope is incorporated in the brain homovanillic acid (HVA) pool. The rate of ^{18}O incorporation in this metabolite of DA is increased when the rats receive chlorpromazine. These ^{18}O studies confirm earlier reports that the turnover rate of brain DA increased following injections of this neuroleptic. Long-term exposure to ^{18}O$_2$ appears to be devoid of toxicity (Samuel, 1973, in Sedvall et al., 1973b). The labeling of brain dopamine with ^{18}O was successively published by Sedvall et al. (1973a) who reported that exposure of the rats to an atmosphere containing ^{18}O$_2$ for approximately 3 hr labels 50% of the brain DA. Of course, the rate of this incorporation relates to the rate of change ^{18}O in the inhaled gas (LeFevre et al., 1975).

In our laboratory, we (LeFevre et al., 1975) have obtained evidence that a significant incorporation of ^{18}O can be obtained in discrete brain nuclei containing either dopaminergic axon terminals (N. accumbens, N. amygdaloideus centralis, and N. caudatus putamen) or dopaminergic cell bodies (pars compacta of substantia nigra area A$_8$, A$_9$, A$_{10}$) of rats breathing for 30 min in an atmosphere in which the ^{16}O$_2$ is replaced by 30% ^{18}O$_2$. The instrumentation is designed in such a way that the rate of this replacement depends on the utilization rate of ^{16}O$_2$. These preliminary data obtained by LeFevre et al. (1975) show that the ratio between m/e 428 and 430, the base peaks of the mass spectrum of the perfluoropropionate derivative of DA and of its isotopically deviant form, differ in various brain nuclei. It appears to increase faster in the pars compacta and A$_{10}$ nucleus of substantia nigra that contain dopaminergic cell bodies than in N. accumbens, tuberculus olphactorium, or in those brain nuclei which contain DA axon terminals emanating from these cells.

2.6. Interpretation of DA Turnover Rate Measurements in Terms of Dopaminergic Neuronal Function

In Table IV, we list the action of various drugs on striatal dopaminergic unit activity, turnover of striatal DA measured *in vivo,* and the concentration of dihydroxyphenylacetic acid (Dopac), DA, and $3',5'$-cyclic adenosine monophosphate (cAMP) in rat striatum. This table is compiled using various data in the literature and shows that the changes of unit activity in DA neurons correlates directly with the changes of the concentrations of Dopac or dopa but not with the turnover rate measurements of striatal DA. However, these data also show that the increase of unit activity does not correlate with the increase of striatal cAMP elicited by (+) amphetamine and by the direct DA receptor stimulant apomorphine (Andén *et al.,* 1967). Hence, the concentration of striatal cAMP appears to be a reliable index of the activation of dopaminergic receptor function. It is therefore clear that none of the measurements listed in Table IV can reliably define the action of a drug on the dopaminergic neurons, or the change of their activity due to environmental stimuli. Only a number of simultaneous measurements can define the profile of the changes caused by various experimental conditions on dopaminergic function.

3. MOLECULAR MECHANISMS FOR THE REGULATION OF DOPAMINERGIC NEURONS

3.1. Regulation of Striatal Tyrosine Hydroxylase

When neuroleptic drugs of various chemical classes are injected into rats, they increase the turnover rate of striatal DA measured *in vivo* (Carlsson and Lindqvist, 1963; Corrodi *et al.,* 1967; Neff and Costa, 1967; Gey and Pletscher, 1968), and enhance the rate of unit activity of dopaminergic cells in the pars compacta of substantia nigra that innervate the striatum (Aghajanian and Bunney, 1973). It is currently believed that these actions are linked to a blockade of postsynaptic DA receptors (Carlsson and Lindqvist, 1963). Reserpine and some neuroleptics which are chemically related to butyrophenones, diphenylbutylamines, and dibenzthiopines, increase the affinity of striatal tyrosine hydroxylase (TH) for pteridine cofactors when these neuroleptics are injected into rats (Zivkovic *et al.,* 1974). This change is specific for TH of dopaminergic brain nuclei but fails to occur when the drugs are added *in vitro* to striatal homogenates. The decrease of the apparent k_m of striatal TH for the pteridine cofactor which is elicited by injections of methiothepin, haloperidol, and reserpine

Table IV. Action of Various Drugs on Different Parameters Defining the Function of Nigrostriatal Dopaminergic Neurons[a]

Treatment	Unit activity of substantia nigra neurons	DA Turnover rate in vivo	Dopamine concentrations	Dopa concentrations	Dopac concentrations	cAMP concentrations
S.N. Stimulation[b]	↑	—	—	—	↑	↑
S.N. Lesion[b]	↓	—	↑	↑	↓	No change
Amphetamine	↓	↑	No change	↑	↓	↑
Haloperidol	↑	↑	No change	↑	↑	No change
Morphine	↓	↑	No change	—	↑	No change
Apomorphine	↓	No change	No change	↓	—	↑
γ-Hydroxybutyrate	↓	↑	↑	↑	↓	No change

[a] This table was compiled from data published by Costa et al. (1972); Roth et al. (1973); Costa et al. (1973).

[b] For the details in the procedure followed to cause the substantia nigra (S.N.) stimulation and lesions see Roth et al. (1973). The data on cAMP concentrations are taken from Carenzi et al. (1975).

can be readily antagonized by injections of apomorphine which directly stimulates the postsynaptic dopaminergic receptors (Andén et al., 1967). These doses of apomorphine when given alone fail to change the kinetic properties of striatal TH but apomorphine readily normalizes the affinity of TH for pteridine cofactors when it is increased by various neuroleptics. Since the increase of striatal TH affinity for the cofactor is not associated with an apparent increase of V_{max} any inference concerning its physiological significance with regard to the control of TH activity in vivo should be made with great caution. In fact, the validity of any physiological inference made from these data strictly depends on the concentrations of pteridine cofactor present in the dopaminergic nerve terminals of rat brain. However, since the increase of striatal and accumbens TH affinity for the pteridine cofactor elicited by various doses of neuroleptics parallels the increase of the turnover rate of striatal and accumbens DA measured in vivo (Table V), it is probable that the concentration of pterdine cofactor present in dopaminergic terminals of rat brain is below the apparent k_m for the cofactor measured in vitro using a crude enzyme preparation in the presence of a detergent to prevent adsorption of TH onto membranes.

The in vitro inhibition of TH by DA is enhanced when the affinity of TH for the pteridine cofactor is increased by the neuroleptics (Zivkovic et al. 1974). These findings suggest that neuroleptics increase the activity of TH when the cofactor is present in concentrations below enzyme saturation, but they do not weaken the TH inhibition by DA which in vivo appears to

Table V. Activity of Various Neuroleptics on Tyrosine Hydroxylase and Turnover Rate of DA in Striatum and N. Accumbens

Drug	Striatum[a]		N. Accumbens[a]	
	TH	DA turnover	TH	DA turnover
Methiotepin	0.43	0.43	0.60	0.60
Pimozide	0.64	—	6.0	—
Haloperidol	1.6	2.1	7.8	4.2
Chlorpromazine	8.6	5.6	15	5.6
Clozapine	79	11	38	7.6
Thioridazine	54	—	27	—
Promethazine	>86	—	>86	—

[a] The doses (μmole/kg iv) listed under TH are those that when injected iv significantly increased TH activity measured 30 min after the drug. Tyrosine hydroxylase activity was measured as described by Zivkovic et al. (1974). The doses listed under DA turnover (μmole/kg ip) are those that increase the conversion of L-(3',5'-³H) tyrosine into ³H DA. The drugs were injected 10 min before the label and the rats were killed 10 min after the label.

be operative in the feedback control of TH by product inhibition (Zivkovic
et al., 1974).

The binding of soluble TH to synaptic intracellular membranes is currently viewed as a cause of an allosteric activation of this enzyme
(Kuczenski and Mandell, 1972; Kuczenski, 1973). It has been speculated
that such a change may have a regulatory value for the enzyme *in vivo*. The
experiments with neuroleptics reported in Table V indicate that the
increased affinity of TH for the pteridine cofactor may be the molecular
basis for the increased turnover of striatal and N. accumbens DA elicited by
various neuroleptics. Other studies (Roth *et al.*, 1974) indicate that striatal
TH is allosterically activated by the removal of Ca^{++} which is produced by
the addition of EGTA 10^{-6}M. When Ca^{++} is removed the k_i for DA
increases from 1.07×10^{-4}M to 7.39×10^{-2} M. Perhaps, during cessation of
impulse flow, when the Ca^{++} influx and the transmitter release are blocked,
the lack of available intracellular Ca^{++} results in the allosteric change of
TH. This increases the k_i for DA and reduces the efficiency of feedback
control by product inhibition. In fact, Roth *et al.* (1974) have shown that
the injection of γ-hyroxybutyrate causes an increase of the k_i for DA from
0.11 mM to 60 mM. These findings support the view that cessation of unit
activity in DA neurons causes an increased accumulation of dopa and DA
because the TH is now relieved from the feedback control by product inhibition. It becomes then of consequence to evaluate the increase of TH activity
as it relates to the increase of the turnover rate of brain DA elicited by
drugs. The leading points for such a discussion are shown in Table VI.

From this table it appears that in striatum a strict correlation between
the increase of DA turnover rate and that of the affinity of TH for the
pteridine cofactor exists only for a number of neuroleptics, but it does not
extend to the indirect sympathomimetic, (+) amphetamine, and to the two
analgesics (viminol R_2 and morphine) which, as shown in Table VI, also
increase the turnover rate of striatal DA. The question then arises: Which
molecular mechanisms differentiate the increase of DA turnover elicited by
analgesics and by indirect sympathomimetics? Shall we assume that their
action on dopaminergic tracts is similar? In order to gain further information of the similarity and differences in the mechanisms whereby various
drugs affect DA turnover rates in striatum and N. accumbens, we studied
how receptor mechanisms at DA central synapses were changed by various
drugs.

3.2. Regulation of Striatal Adenylcyclase

The discovery that striatum contains an adenylate cyclase which is selectively stimulated by DA (Kebabian *et al.*, 1972) has opened new avenues

Table VI. Increase of Striatal TH Activity Elicited by Doses of Various Drugs that Increase DA Turnover *in Vivo*

Drug	TH[a] Activity	DA Turnover
Viminol R$_2$	No change	↑
Morphine	No change	↑
Amphetamine	No change	↑
Haloperidol	↑	↑
Methiotepin	↑	↑
Chlorpromazine	↑	↑
Clozapine	↑	↑

[a] TH activity was measured with concentrations of pteridine cofactor (DMPH$_4$, 0.3 mM) which is below k_m (about 0.9 mM); thus an increase of TH activity indicates an increased affinity of TH for the cofactor.

for the understanding of drug actions on synaptic mechanisms. It was reported (Costa *et al.*, 1973) that (+) amphetamine in doses that increase motor activity enhance striatal cAMP concentrations in striatum and increase the turnover rate of striatal DA. It was also shown that injections of dopa also selectively increase the concentrations of cAMP in striatum (Garelis and Neff, 1974). That the increase of striatal cAMP is associated with a stimulation of DA postsynaptic receptors was shown by using apomorphine and dopa which cause an increase of striatal cAMP (Table VII). We then tested morphine in doses that increase the turnover rate of

Table VII. Striatal Concentrations of cAMP after Drugs that Act on Striatal Dopaminergic Synapses

Drug	cAMP[c] nmole/mg protein
Saline[a]	5.2 ± 0.6
Morphine (26)[d]	5.9 ± 0.8
Amphetamine (6.4)[d]	9.2 ± 0.5[c] (+76%)
Apomorphine (3.2)[d]	8.7 ± 0.7[c] (+67%)
Haloperidol (1.3)[d]	4.6 ± 0.3
Saline[b]	2.4 ± 0.4
L-Dopa (507)	4.5 ± 0.2[c] (+73%)

[a] The data reported are from Costa *et al.* (1973) and Carenzi *et al.* (1975).
[b] The data reported are from Garelis and Neff (1974).
[c] $p < 0.01$ Versus values of respective controls.
[d] The number in parentheses is the dose in μmole/kg, ip.

striatal DA and found that it does not increase the concentrations of striatal cAMP (Costa et al., 1973). The neuroleptics that in vitro lower the DA stimulation of adenylcyclase but fail to modify the basal adenylcyclase activity (Clement-Cormier et al., 1974) also fail to alter the striatal concentrations of cAMP when injected in doses that increase the turnover rate of striatal DA in vivo. These experiments therefore not only differentiate biochemically the action of (+) amphetamine from that of morphine and haloperidol but add some insight in the interpretation of the various parameters that can be measured to characterize drug effects on dopaminergic synapses (Carenzi et al., 1975). As shown in Table IV, the recording of unit activity does not give any indication that the action of amphetamine and haloperidol differ with regard to receptor activation. Actually, from these data one might infer that haloperidol but not (+) amphetamine stimulates DA receptors. The striatal cAMP can increase when the unit activity recording is practically abolished [(+) amphetamine or apomorphine]; conversely, the units can be extremely active (morphine and neuroleptics) but the cAMP levels in striatum are normal. Of special significance is the measurement of dopa and Dopac concentrations; these are increased when the unit activity is decreased (Table IV). However, these measurements by themselves fail to differentiate between a drug that activates the postsynaptic receptor [(+) amphetamine] and a drug that blocks the function of dopaminergic terminals (γ-OH-butyrate) (Roth et al., 1973).

The present understanding of the function of dopaminergic synapses indicates that the recording of unit activity of dopaminergic neurons in the pars compacta of substantia nigra is insufficient to define the action of drugs on dopaminergic synapses. In contrast, the biochemical parameters listed in Table IV unveil differences in the mechanism of drug action which fail to be clarified by electrophysiological measurements. The turnover rate measurement of striatal DA coupled with the assay of striatal TH, striatal cAMP, and dopa can define without apparent discrepancies the action of drugs on dopaminergic neurons.

3.3. Specificity of Drug Action in Mesolimbic and Nigrostriatal Dopaminergic Systems

Anticholinergic drugs have been administered to overcome the extrapyramidal effects elicited by neuroleptics. The antipsychotic action of neuroleptics remains unimpaired when they are associated with anticholinergics, suggesting that the blockade of cholinergic synapses antagonizes the extrapyramidal effects but not the antipsychotic effects of phenothiazines and butyrophenone neuroleptics.

The possibility that these two actions can be dissociated is supported by studies with clozapine, an effective antipsychotic devoid of cataleptic action and incapable of antagonizing stereotype behavior elicited by apomorphine (Stille and Hippius, 1971; Stille *et al.*, 1971). This drug accelerates the turnover rate of DA in striatum but the doses required for this effect are higher than those required to inhibit the arousal reaction. The effects of clozapine on the turnover rate of DA in the limbic system and in striatum of rabbits was compared; all doses of clozapine tested induced a greater percentage of HVA increase in the limbic system than in corpus striatum (Andén and Stock, 1973). On the other hand, all doses of haloperidol tested increased equally well the content of HVA in limbic structures or striatum. Similar selectivity of action for dopaminergic terminals in limbic system versus those of striatum was reported when haloperidol and anticholinergic drugs were associated (Andén, 1972). In addition, we know that clozapine is a potent blocker of central muscarinic receptors (Miller and Hiley, 1974).

In Table V we have compared the DA turnover rate and TH activity in striatum and N. accumbens of rats receiving various neuroleptics. Clozapine and thioridazine are the only two neuroleptics which can increase the TH activity in N. accumbens when given in doses that are unable to change the TH activity in striatum. Moreover, clozapine shows similar differential activity on the turnover rate of DA in striatum and N. accumbens. These data are of interest because: (i) they reveal a great parallelism between the increase of TH activity and that of DA turnover rate; (ii) they indicate that a differential effect on TH activity in N. accumbens and striatum may be an index to separate antipsychotic activities from extrapyramidal side effects in new classes of neuroleptics; (iii) they stress the possibility that the N. accumbens and, perhaps, the nucleus amygdaloideus centralis can be viewed as possible sites for the action of antipsychotic drugs. That these nuclei posseses a different type of dopaminergic receptor appears rather improbable (Horn *et al.*, 1974). Perhaps, the regulatory interneuronal loops are different in the N. accumbens and striatum, the latter involving a cholinergic link. It is possible that protection from side effects caused by neuroleptics is due to a selectivity in drug action deriving from the coupling of two pharmacological actions into one molecule. From a therapeutic standpoint the association of the two actions in a single molecule is far more advantageous than the administration of an anticholinergic with a neuroleptic. Titration of the two effects with the administration of two drugs is hampered by the different half-life and affinity constant of the two drugs. Moreover, the DA uptake is inhibited by anticholinergic drugs (Coyle and Snyder, 1969). To test whether the selectivity of the action on TH by various neuroleptics is modified by the cholinergic mechanisms present in striatum and N. accumbens, we have associated haloperidol and benztropine and we have measured the TH activity in striatum and N. accumbens. We have found that benztropine reduces the increase in the affinity of TH for the cofactor elicited by haloperidol (Zivkovic, personal communication); this action is dose-related and appears selective for striatum.

4. INTERACTION OF THE NIGROSTRIATAL DOPAMINERGIC SYSTEM WITH OTHER NEURONAL SYSTEMS

Available studies of the cholinergic mechanisms in the striatum of rats indicate that this nucleus contains a very high concentration of acetylcholine (ACh), acetylcholinesterase, and choline acetylase (Yamamura *et al.*, 1974). By histochemical methods it was shown that cholinesterase activity resides in small striatal neurons (Lynch *et al.*, 1972). The activity of enzymes related to cholinergic function and the striatal ACh content are not changed when the main anatomically established striatal afferent systems are severed (Butcher and Butcher, 1974). This finding suggests that most of the cholinergic activity detected in striatum may be localized in interneurons. Moreover, it has been reported that these interneurons contain axons which are extremely fine in diameter and which show a tendency to bifurcation (Kemp and Powell, 1971). Other cytochemical evidence suggests that GABA terminals innervating the substantia nigra originate in striatum and reach the substantia nigra via globus pallidus and nucleus interpeduncularis (Fonnum *et al.*, 1974; McGeer *et al.*, 1973). Thus the following model appears probable:

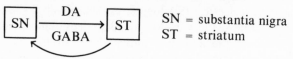

SN = substantia nigra
ST = striatum

In striatum the link between cholinergic, dopaminergic, and GABA neurons can be expressed by the following model:

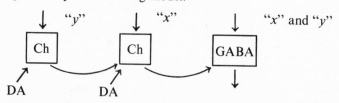

where cholinergic neurons are connected in parallel with each other and exert a facilitatory influence on each other, and they inhibit GABA feedback through a muscarinic synapse. DA nerve terminals of striatum inhibit cholinergic interneurons. These and GABA neurons may be activated by other transmitters (in our scheme represented as "y" or "x"). Assuming that a decrease of activity in cholinergic striatal interneurons is associated with a decrease of ACh turnover rate, it can be predicted that (i) stimulation of DA receptors reduces the turnover rate of striatal ACh; (ii) blockade of DA receptors increases the turnover of ACh (Stadler et al., 1973); (iii) blockade of cholinergic receptors should not change ACh turnover rate, but blockade of these receptors when DA receptors are blocked should bring to normal the accelerated turnover rate. If we take the TH activity in striatum as an index of the functional activation of GABA neurons then TH activity should decrease when GABA neurons are activated and TH should increase when the activity of GABA neurons is reduced.

We are currently testing this model. The data reported in Table VIII show that, as predicted, haloperidol which inhibits DA receptors increases the turnover rate of striatal ACh. In contrast, dopa and apomorphine which stimulate DA receptors inhibit the turnover rate of striatal ACh. The increase of the striatal ACh turnover rate elicited by the DA receptor blocker was blocked by the muscarinic receptor blocker, benztropin, which failed to influence the turnover of ACh when given alone.

The data of Table VIII appear to suggest that the effects of dopaminergic receptor blockers and stimulants are unique for the striatum and cannot be obtained in cortex. It is therefore tempting to speculate that the antagonism of the extrapyramidal affects of neuroleptics by anticholinergics is due to interferences with the regulatory interneuronal chain DA → ACh → GABA, which is operative in striatum but not in N. accumbens.

Table VIII. Turnover Rate of ACh in Striatum and Occipital Cortex after Various Drugs Acting on Striatal Dopaminergic Synapses

Drug	μmole/kg ip	Turnover rate of ACh[a] (μmole/g per hr)	
		Striatum	Occipital cortex
Saline	—	0.82	0.20
Apomorphine	10	0.24	0.21
Dopa	500	0.43	0.21
Haloperidol	8	1.8	0.22
Clozapine	12	0.79	0.21
Benztropine	12	0.91	0.18
Benztropine + haloperidol	8	0.82	—

[a] The turnover rate of ACh in various brain parts was estimated from the change with time of the specific activity of choline and acetylcholine measured in the brain parts of rats killed by microwave exposure, between 2 and 6 min of a constant rate infusion of Me-^{14}C phosphorylcholine (S.A. 49 μCi/μmole; 30 μCi/min/kg iv).

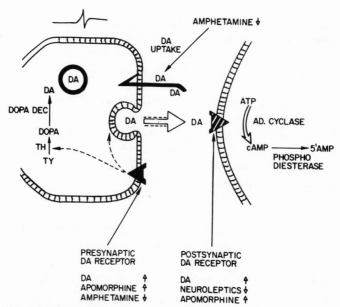

Figure 2. Site of action of various drugs on post- and presynaptic parts of a brain DA synapses. The description is purely speculative and is an attempt to reconcile possible discrepancies in the light of the present understanding of DA function.

5. CONCLUSIONS

The hypothetical model of Figure 2 can be proposed to interpret how various drugs modify the function of striatal dopaminergic synapses. The various drugs listed are seen as acting either at the postsynaptic or at the presynaptic parts of DA nerve terminals. We believe that in these two sites there are two structurally different DA receptors which also differ with regard to the affinity constant for DA. We assume that the affinity for DA is greater for the postsynaptic than for the presynaptic receptors.

The quantal of DA released by nerve impulses might be related to the difference in these two affinities. That is, DA can be released until the DA concentration in the cleft reaches the level for stimulation of the DA presynaptic receptor. When this receptor is stimulated, the release of DA by nerve impulses is blocked as long as the receptor is occupied by DA. Amphetamine releases DA and blocks its reuptake. Initially, the turnover rate of striatal DA is increased, but after about 1-hr (+) amphetamine injections, the release and turnover of DA decrease because the DA-sensitive presynaptic receptor is continuously occupied by DA. The firing rate of the units in substantia nigra is reduced by (+) amphetamine almost immediately because the stimulation of DA receptors enhances the inhibitory effects of GABA terminals in substantia nigra. It would be of interest to test whether picrotoxin applied iontophoretically stimulates the units depressed by iv (+) amphetamine.

Apomorphine and morphine have an affinity for the DA receptor: apomorphine has maximal affinity for the postsynaptic DA receptor (Andén et al., 1967). Thus, it increases striatal cAMP concentrations in a dose-related fashion and in high doses blocks DA turnover rate (Carenzi et al., 1974). Moreover, it stops unit activity in substantia nigra by a mechanism similar to that of (+) amphetamine. Morphine fails to change cAMP concentrations although it accelerates the turnover rate of striatal DA. The unit activity of substantia nigra neurons is decreased by (+) amphetamine and apomorphine (Bunney et al., 1973a) but is activated by morphine (Bunney, personal communication) and by neuroleptics (Bunney et al., 1973b). One could propose that morphine and haloperidol have a similar mode of action. However, morphine action on the firing rate of dopaminergic neurons of substantia nigra is not reversed by (+) amphetamine which promptly reverses the increase unit activity of DA neurons elicited by neuroleptics. We propose that this important difference between neuroleptics and analgesics can be explained only if morphine acts on the input of dopaminergic neurons and perhaps interferes with the regulation of these neurons by the inhibitory effects of GABA (McGeer et al., 1973). This possibility is in agreement with electrophysiological experiments which show that morphine blocks the inhibition caused by iontrophoretically applied GABA on spinal neurons (Dostrovsky and Pomerans, 1973). This possibility is in keeping with pharmacological experiments which have indicated a difference in the catalepsy induced by chlorpromazine and morphine (Kuschinsky and Hornykiewicz, 1972; Wand et al., 1973). In high doses morphine may inhibit extraneuronal release of DA by nerve impulses (Kuschinsky and Hornykiewicz, 1972).

The following possibilities can be predicted from the model of the cholinergic and dopaminergic neuronal intersections in striatum that is emerging: (i) the effects on DA turnover elicited by morphine should not be blocked by benztropine; (ii) the effect on unit activity of apomorphine and amphetamine should be blocked by picrotoxin; (iii) the electrical stimulation of the substantia nigra should elicit an increase of cAMP in striatum and promote an increase of TH. Some of these experiments are now in progress. Before closing, we would like to make it clear that this model may apply to average doses of the drugs discussed and that specificity of action may be lost when the doses are enhanced.

6. REFERENCES

Aghajanian, G. K., and Bunney, B. S., 1973, Central dopaminergic neurones: neurophysiological identification and responses to drugs, in: *Frontiers in Catecholamine Research* (E. Usdin and S. Snyder, eds.), pp. 643–648, Pergamon Press, New York.

Andén, N. E., and Stock, G., 1973, Effect of clozapine on the turnover of dopamine in the treatment with neuroleptic and anti-acetylcholine drugs, *J. Pharm. Pharmacol.* 24:905.

Andén, N. E., and Stock, G., 1973, Effect of closapine on the turnover of dopamine in the corpus striatum and in the limbic system, *J. Pharm. Pharmacol.* 25:346.

Andén, N. E., Bedard, P., Fuxe, K., and Ungerstedt, U., 1972, Early and selective increase of brain dopamine levels after axotomy, *Experientia* 28:300.

Andén, N. E., Magnusson, T., and Stock, G., 1973, Effect of drugs influencing monoamine mechanisms on the increase in brain dopamine produced by Axotomy or treatment with γ-hydroxybutyric acid, *Naunyn-Schmiedebergs. Arch. Exptl. Pathol. Pharmakol.* 278:363.

Andén, N. E., Rubenson, A., Fuxe, K., and Hökfelt, T., 1967, Evidence for dopamine receptor stimulation by apomorphine, *J. Pharm. Pharmacol.* 19:627.

Bunney, B. S., Aghajanian, G. K., and Roth, R. H., 1973a, Comparison of effects of L-Dopa, amphetamine and apomorphine on firing rate of rat dopaminergic neurons, *Nature (New Biol.)* 245:123.

Bunney, B. S., Walters, J. R., Roth, R. H. and Aghajanian, G. K., 1973b, Dopaminergic neurons: effect of antipsychotic drugs and amphetamine on single cell activity, *J. Pharmacol. Exptl. Therap.* 185:560.

Butcher, S. G., and Butcher, L. L., 1974, Origin and modulation of acetylcholine activity in the neostriatum, *Brain Res.* 71:167.

Carenzi, A., Guidotti, A., Revuelta, A., and Costa, E., 1975, The action of morphine and viminol on the dopaminergic neurons of rat striatum. *J. Pharmacol. Exptl. Therap.* (accepted for publication).

Carlsson, A., and Lindqvist, M., 1963, Effect of chlorpromazine or haloperidol on the formation of 3-methoxytyramine and normetanephrine in mouse brain, *Acta Pharmacol. Toxicol.* 20:140.

Carlsson, A., Kehr, W., Lindqvist, M., Magnusson, T., and Atack, C. V., 1972a, Regulation of monoamine metabolism in the central nervous system, *Pharmacol. Rev.* 24:371.

Carlsson, A., Davis, J. N., Kehr, W., Lindqvist, M., and Atack, C. V., 1972b, Simultaneous measurements of tyrosine hydroxylase and triptophan hydroxylase activities in brain *in vivo* using an inhibitor of the aromatic amino acid decarboxylase, *Naunyn-Schmiedebergs Arch. Exptl. Pathol. Pharmakol.* 275:153.

Cattabeni, F., Koslow, S. H., and Costa, E., 1972, Gas chromatography–mass fragmentography in a new approach to the estimation of amines and amine turnover, in: *Advances in Biochemical Psychopharmacology Vol. 6* (E. Costa, L. Iversen, and Paoletti, R., eds.), Raven Press, New York.

Clement-Cormier, Y. C., Kebabian, J. W., Petzold, F. L. and Greengard, P., 1974, Dopamine-sensitive adenylate cyclase in mammalian brain: a possible site of action of antipsychotic drugs, *Proc. Natl. Acad. Sci. (U.S.)* 71:1113.

Corrodi, H., Fuxe, K., and Hökfelt 1967, The effect of psychoactive drugs on the central monoamine neurons, *European J. Pharmacol* 11:363.

Costa, E., 1972, Appraisal of current methods to estimate the turnover rate of serotonin and catecholamines on human brain, in: *Advances in Biochemical Psychopharmacology, Vol. 4,* (E. Costa and M. S. Ebadi, eds.), Raven Press, New York.

Costa, E., 1973, The fundamental role of immediate precursors to estimate turnover rate of catecholamines by isotopic labeling, in: *Pharmacology and the Future of Man, Vol. 4* (F. E. Bloom and G. H. Acheson, eds.), pp. 215–226, S. Karger Publishing Co., Basel.

Costa, E., and Meek, J. L., 1974, Regulation of biosynthesis of catecholamines and serotonin in CNS, *Ann. Rev. Pharmacol.* **14:**491.

Costa, E., Green, A. R., Koslow, S. H., LeFevre, H. F., Revuelta, A. V., and Wang, C., 1972, Dopamine and norepinephrine in noradrenergic axons: A study in vivo of their precursor product relationship by mass fragmentography and radiochemistry, *Pharmacol. Rev.* **24:**167.

Costa, E., Carenzi, A., Guidotti, A., and Revuelta, A., 1973, Narcotic analgesics and the regulation of neuronal catecholamine stores, in: *Frontiers in Catecholamine Research* (E. Usdin and S. Snyder, ed.), pp. 1003–1010, Pergamon Press, New York.

Costa, E., Guidotti, A., and Zivkovic, B., 1974, Short- and long-term regulation of tyrosine hydroxylase, in: *Adv. Biochem. Psychopharmacol.* **12:**161.

Coyle, J. T., and Snyder, S. H., 1969, Antiparkinsonian drugs: inhibition of dopamine uptake in the corpus striatum as a possible mechanism of action, *Science* **166:**899.

Descarries, L., and Lapierre, Y., 1973, Noradrenergic axon terminals in the cerebral cortex of rat. Radioautographic visualization after topical application of DL-[³H] norepinephrine, *Brain Res.* **51:**141.

Dostrovsky, J., and Pomerans, B., 1973, Morphine blockade of amino acid putative transmitters on cat spinal cord sensory interneurons. *Nature* (*New Biol.*) **246:**222.

Doteuchi, M., Wang, C., and Costa, E., 1974, Compartmentation of dopamine in rat striatum, *Mol. Pharmacol.* **10:**225.

Fonnum, F., Grofova, I., Riuvik, E., Storm-Mathisen, J., and Walbey, F., 1974, Origin and distribution of glutamate decarboxylase in substantia nigra of the cat, *Brain Res.* **71:**77.

Garelis, E., and Neff, N. H., 1974, Cyclic adenosine monophosphate: collective increase in caudate nucleus after administration of L-dopa, *Science* **183:**532.

Gessa, G. L., Vargiu, L., Crabai, F., Boero, G. C., Caboni, G., and Camba, R., 1966, Selective increase of brain dopamine induced by γ-hydroxybutyrate, *Life Sci.* **5:**1921.

Gey, K. F., and Pletscher, A., 1968, Acceleration of turnover of ¹⁴C-catecholamines in rat brain by chlorpromazine, *Experientia* **24:**335.

Glowinski, J., 1973, The "functional pool" in central catecholaminergic neurons, in: *Pharmacology and the Future of Man* (F. E. Bloom and G. H. Achesson, eds.), pp. 204–214, Pergamon Press, New York.

Groppetti, A., and Costa, E., 1969, Tissue concentrations of *p*-hydroxynorephedrine in rats injected with *d*-amphetamine, effect of pretreatment with desipramine, *Life Sci.* **8:**653.

Guidotti, A., Cheney, D. L., Trabucchi, M., Doteuchi, M., Wang, C., and Hawkins, P. A., 1974, Focussed microwave radiation: a technique to minimize postmortem changes of cyclic nucleotides, dopa, and choline and to preserve brain morphology, *Neuropharmacology* **13:**1115.

Horn, A. S., Cuello, A. C., and Miller, R. J., 1974, Dopamine in the mesolimbic system of the rat brain: endogenous levels and the effects of drugs on the uptake mechanism and stimulation of adenylate cyclase activity, *J. Neurochem.* **22:**265.

Iversen, L. L., and Glowinski, J., 1966, Rate of turnover of catecholamines in various brain regions, *J. Neurochem.* **13:**671.

Javoy, F., and Glowinski, J., 1971, Dynamic characteristics of the "functional compartment" of dopamine in dopaminergic terminals of the rat striatum, *J. Neurochem.* **18:**1305.

Javoy, F., Agid, D., Bouvet, L., and Glowinski, J., 1974, *In vivo* estimation of tyrosine hydroxylation in the dopaminergic terminals of the rat neostriatum, *J. Pharm. Pharmacol.* **26:**179.

Kebabian, J. W., Petzold, G. L., and Greengard, P., 1972, Dopamine-sensitive adenylate cyclase on caudate nucleus of rat brain and its similarity to the "dopamine receptor," *Proc. Natl. Acad. Sci. (U.S.)* **69:**2149.

Kehr, W., Carlsson, A., Lindqvist, M., Magunsson, T., and Atack, C., 1972, Evidence for a receptor mediated feedback control of striatal tyrosine hydroxylase activity, *J. Pharm. Pharmacol.* **24:**744.

Kemp, J. M., and Powell, T. P. S., 1971, The structure of the caudate nucleus of the cat: light and electron microscopy, *Phil. Trans. Roy. Soc. Lond. Ser. B.* **262:**383.

Koslow, S. H., Cattabeni, F., and Costa, E., 1972, Norepinephrine and dopamine: assay by mass fragmentography in the picomole range, *Science* **176:**177.

Koslow, S. H., Racagni, G., and Costa, E., 1974, Mass fragmentographic measurement of NE, DA, 5HT, and ACh in seven discrete nuclei of the rat tele-diencephalon, *Neuropharmacology* **13:**1123.

Kuczenski, R. T., 1973, Striatal tyrosine hydroxylase with high and low affinity for tyrosine: implications for the multiple-pool concept of catecholamines, *Life Sci.* **13:**247.

Kuczenski, R., 1975, Effect of catecholamine releasing agents on synaptosomal DA biosynthesis: multiple pools of DA or multiple forms of tyrosine hydroxylase, *Neuropharmacology* **14:**1.

Kuczenski, R. T., and Mandell, A. J., 1972, Regulating properties of soluble and particulate rat brain tyrosine hydroxylase, *J. Biol. Chem.* **247:**3114.

Kuschinsky, K., and Hornykiewicz, O., 1972, Morphine catalepsy in the rat: relation to striatal dopamine metabolism, *European J. Pharmacol.* **19:**119.

Langer, S. Q., 1973, The regulation of transmitter release elicited by nerve stimulation through a presynaptic feed-back mechanism, in: *Frontiers in Catecholamine Research* (E. Usdin and S. Synder, eds.), pp. 543–549, Pergamon Press, New York.

LeFevre, H. F., Costa, E., Koslow, S. H., 1975, *Fed. Proc.* **34:**778.

Lynch, G. S., Lucas, P. A., and Deadwyler, S. A., 1972, The demonstration of acetylcholinesterase containing neurones within the caudate nucleus of the rat, *Brain Res.* **45:**617.

Lust, W. D., Passouneau, J. V., and Veech, R. L., 1973, Cyclic adenosine monophosphate, metabolites, and phosphorylase in neural tissue. A comparison of methods of fixation, *Science* **181:**280.

McGeer, E. G., Fibiger, H. C., McGeer, P. L., and Brooke, S., 1973, Temporal changes in amine synthesizing enzymes of rat extrapyramidal structures after hemitransection or 6-hydroxydopamine administration, *Brain Res.* **52:**289.

Miller, R. J., and Hiley, C. R., 1974, Antimuscarinic properties of neuroleptics and drug-induced parkinsonism, *Nature* **248:**596.

Neff, N. H., and Costa, E., 1967, Effect of tricyclic antidepressant and chlorpromazine on brain catecholamine systems, in: *Proceedings of the Internation Symposium on Antidepressant Drugs* (S. Garattini and M. N. C. Burkes, eds.), pp. 28–34, Excerpta Med. Foundation, New York.

Neff, N. H., Lin, R. C., Ngai, S. H., and Costa, E., 1969, Turnover rate measurements of brain serotonin in anesthesized rats, *Adv. Biochem. Psychopharmacol.* **1:**92.

Neff, N. H., Spano, P. F., Groppetti, A., Wang, C. T., and Costa, E., 1971, A simple procedure for calculating the synthesis rate of norepinephrine, dopamine and serotonin in rat brain, *J. Pharmacol. Exptl. Therap.* **176:**701.

Roth, R. H., and Surh, Y., 1970, Mechanism of the γ-hydroxybutyrate-induced increase in brain dopamine and its relationship to sleep, *Biochem. Pharmacol.* **19:**3001.

Roth, R. H., Walters, J. R., and Aghajanian, G. K. (1973) Effect of impulse flow in the release and synthesis of dopamine in the rat striatum, in: *Frontiers in Catecholamine Research* (E. Usdin and S. Synder, eds.), pp. 567–574, Pergamon Press, New York.

Roth, R. H., Walters, J. R., and Morgenroth, V. H., 1974, Effects of alterations in impulse flow on transmitter metabolism in central dopaminergic neurons, *Adv. Biochem. Psychopharmacol.* **12**:369.

Sedvall, G. C., Weise, V. K., and Kopin, I. J., 1968, The rate of norepinephrine synthesis measured in vivo during short intervals; influence of adrenergic nerve impulse activity, *J. Pharmacol. Exptl. Therap.* **159**:274.

Sedvall, G., Mayevsky, A., Fri, C. G., Sjöquist, B., and Samuel, D., 1973*a*, The use of stable oxygen isotopes for labeling of homovanillic acid in rat brain in vivo, *Adv. Biochem. Psychopharmacol.* **7**:57.

Sedvall, G., Mayevsky, A., Samuel, D., and Fric, G. (1973*b*) Oxygen-18 in measurement of dopamine turnover in rat brain, in: *Frontiers in Catecholamine Research* (E. Usdin and S. Snyder, eds.), pp. 1071–1075, Pergamon Press, New York.

Stadler, H., Lloyd, K. G., Gadea-Ciria, M., and Bartholini, G., 1973, Enhanced striatal acetylcholine release by chlorpromazine and its reversal by apormorphine, *Brain Res.* **55**:476.

Stille, G., and Hippius, H., 1971, Kritische Stellungsnahme zum Begriff der Neuroleptika, *Pharmakopsychiatry Neuropsychopharmakol.* **4**:182.

Stille, G., Lavener, H., and Eichenberger, E., 1971, The pharmacology of 8-chloro-11-(4-methyl-1-piperazinyl) 5-H-Dibenzo [b, e,] [1, 4] diazepine (clozapine), *Farmaco (Sci.)* **26**:603.

Thierry, A. M., and Glowinski, J., 1973, Existence of dopaminergic nerve terminals in the rat cortex, in: *Frontiers in Catecholamine Research* (E. Usdin and S. Snyder, eds.), pp. 649–651, Pergamon Press, New York.

Udenfriend, S., 1966, Tyrosine hydroxylase, *Pharmacol. Rev.* **18**:43.

Udenfriend, S., Zaltzan-Nirenberg, P., and Nagatsu, T., 1965, Inhibitors of purified beef adrenal tyrosine hydroxylase, *Biochem. Pharmacol.* **14**:837.

Ungerstedt, U., 1971, Stereotoxic mapping of the monoamine pathways in the rat brain, *Acta Physiol. Scand. Suppl.* **367**:1.

Walters, J. R., and Roth, R. M., 1974, Dopaminergic neurones: drug induced antagonism of the increase of tyrosine hydroxylase activity produced by cessation of impulse flow, *J. Pharmacol. Exptl. Therap.* (in press).

Wand, P., Kuschinsky, K., and Sontag, K.-H., 1973, Morphine-induced muscular rigidity in rats, *European J. Pharmacol.* **24**:189.

Weissman, A., and Koe, B. K., 1965, Behavioral effect of L-α-methyl-tyrosine, an inhibitor of tyrosine hydroxylase, *Life Sci.* **4**:1037.

Yamamura, H. I., Kuhar, M. J., Greenberg, D., and Snyder, S. H., 1974, Muscarinic cholinergic receptor binding: regional distribution in monkey brain, *Brain Res.* **66**:541.

Zivkovic, B., Guidotti, A., and Costa, E., 1974, Effect of neuroleptics on striatal tyrosine hydroxylase: changes in the affinity for the pteridine cofactor, *Mol. Pharmacol.* **10**:727.

Index